D0057018

CASE STUDIES
IN MEDICAL ETHICS

Robert M. Veatch is widely known as a writer and lecturer on medical ethics. After undergraduate and graduate preparation in pharmacology, he turned to the study of ethics, in which he received his Ph.D. degree from Harvard University. Since 1970 he has been at the Institute of Society, Ethics and the Life Sciences in Hastings-on-Hudson, New York, where he is currently Senior Associate.

LIBRARY

CASE STUDIES
IN MEDICAL ETHICS

Robert M. Veatch

HARVARD UNIVERSITY PRESS
Cambridge, Massachusetts
and London, England   1977

LIBRARY

MAR 1 3 1978

UNIVERSITY OF THE PACIFIC

341808

for
Carl

Copyright © 1977 by Robert M. Veatch
All rights reserved
Printed in the United States of America

Library of Congress Cataloging in Publication Data

Veatch, Robert M.
    Case studies in medical ethics.

    Bibliography: p.
    Includes index.
    1. Medical ethics—Case studies.   I. Title.
R724.V4   174'.2'0926   76-50932
ISBN 0-674-09931-1

The biological revolution has given great new powers to medicine. It is possible to keep a creature's cells alive virtually indefinitely with artificial respirator, artificial cardiac pacemaker, artificial tissues, and intravenous feeding of artificial food, which give rise to what some would call an artificial human being. Electrodes can now be implanted in the human brain to evoke movements, repress aggressive impulses, and relieve heretofore intractable pain. Human life has been created in a laboratory, and soon such life may be carried through to "birth." Medical ethical problems that once were no more than entertaining speculations about the future are now a reality.

There was a day when the issues of medical ethics seemed plain: how big to make a physician's sign, whether to prescribe over the telephone, whether to split fees with persons referring patients. These are still important questions, which help to define the role of the physician. Today, however, the biological revolution has forced us to deal with another set of problems with a new sense of urgency. Although the exotic ethical issues get the headlines, the less dramatic problems are still the most important: when to withhold the truth from a patient, when to break a confidence, why the patient's consent is important, how the dying patient can be treated humanely. Yet now that the typical physician treating the typical patient has at least a fifty-fifty chance of benefiting him, the stakes are much higher. Because a moral mistake can be literally a life-or-death disaster, medical ethics can no longer be regarded as dessert in the smorgasbord of medical education. Physicians must no longer be educated as technical geniuses and moral imbeciles. More important, medical ethics can no longer be left to the medical professional. Medical ethics is not restricted to physician ethics. The case studies collected here are designed to urge the student—both future physician and future patient—to struggle with the social and ethical impact of decisions made in the medical context. Although some of the cases are ethically exotic, they also deal with the more ordinary, and therefore more important, problems of everyday medicine.

This collection of case studies originated with the founding of the Institute of Society, Ethics and the Life Sciences. In 1970 the institute began a Program in Medical Ethics at Columbia University's College of Physicians and Surgeons as part of a larger emphasis on systemic development of the teaching of medical ethics. It soon became apparent that carefully developed case studies were one of the major needs of a teaching program. While the need was great in medical schools, it was even greater in other schools where medical ethics courses were developing— in departments of biology, sociology, philosophy, and religion; in professional schools of law, theology, education, and social work; and in other health-science schools, including nursing, occupational therapy, dentistry, and the new paramedical programs. Some of the cases grew out of the program at Columbia. Many more have come from the participants in the research groups at the institute and from a larger number of colleagues who shared with me their experiences as clinicians, teachers, and patients. Some are from the court records of cases marking crucial historical precedent.

With few exceptions, all of the cases are rooted in real experiences. Except for the cases based on public records, such as court documents, the details, including names and places, have been changed to ensure anonymity and clarity. A few cases dealing with problems that will face medicine in the future, such as cloning and national health insurance, are fictional. Since all the cases are numbered in sequence for this book, some cases are numbered differently from earlier appearances elsewhere. The present numbers are completely independent of numbers previously associated with those cases.

Some of the cases have appeared in the series Case Studies in Bioethics, which is a regular feature of the *Hastings Center Report,* the institute's journal. New cases will appear there in future issues. At this point in history it is certain that new problems will emerge in the field tomorrow, raising new moral issues in medical ethics. While I have generally tried to pinpoint the crucial issues raised by a case, commentaries by others representing different and opposing views are also included. Some cases and commentaries are quite brief, others more extended. At times questions are presented for discussion. At other times several cases in sequence are followed by a single commentary discussing the crucial differences among them. The object is to provide sufficient information on each case to pursue adequately the relevant points of ethical controversy and at the same time to avoid redundancy.

The fellows and staff of the institute have been partners in this project. They have learned to expect me to insist that they either reduce to writing their own case stories or criticize and verify cases obtained from other sources. Daniel Callahan and Willard Gaylin, the Director and the President of the institute respectively, have done more than encourage me in the six-year task of collecting the cases. They first envisaged such a volume and then saw to it that the project became an integral part of the medical ethics teaching program for which I have administrative responsibility. They freed time for me not only to collect the cases but also to meet with students at about fifty colleges, universities, and medical schools where these cases were tested. They encouraged teaching programs in which I was involved not only at Columbia but also at Dartmouth College, Vassar College, the State University of New York at Purchase, and Manhattanville College, as well as at countless seminars and lectures where a wide variety of students, from high schoolers to practicing physicians, wrestled with the cases. Certainly without their support this volume would never have been written. Marc Lappé, Peter Steinfels, Susan Peck, Joel Meister, Sharmon Sollitto, Tabitha Powledge, Patricia Pierce, Martha Bush, and Marilynn Nelson have each spent hours on various phases of the project, and to them appreciation is gratefully acknowledged.

I must acknowledge the help received in constructing and presenting the more theoretical ethical issues from Ralph Potter, Arthur Dyck, Harvey Cox, Roderick Firth, and John Rawls of Harvard University; Paul Ramsey of Princeton University; and Robert Neville, formerly on the institute staff and now at the State University of New York at Purchase. Others who have helped supply or develop cases include Daniel Burke, Eric Cassell, Victor Sidel, George Dyck, Frank Freemon, and Albert R. Jonsen. Those who have suffered most for this volume are certainly the members of my family: Laurie, Paul, and Carl. To them goes my special appreciation. For the future patients and practitioners of the art and science of medicine the challenge now begins.

CONTENTS

CASE STUDIES
IN MEDICAL ETHICS

Five Questions
of Ethics

Medical ethics as a field presents a fundamental problem. As a branch of applied ethics, medical ethics becomes interesting and relevant only when it abandons the ephemeral realm of theory and abstract speculation and gets down to practical questions raised by real, everyday problems of health and illness. Much of medical ethics, especially within the profession itself, is indeed oriented to the practical questions of what should be done in a particular case. Medicine, even more than business and law, is case oriented. Yet if those who must resolve the ever-increasing ethical dilemmas in medicine—including patients, family members, physicians, nurses, hospital administrators, and public policy-makers—treat every case as something entirely fresh, entirely novel, they will have lost perhaps the best way of reaching solutions: to understand the general principles of ethics and face each new situation from a systematic ethical stance.

This is a volume of case studies in medical ethics. It begins by recognizing the fact that one cannot do any ethics, especially medical ethics, in the abstract. It is real-life, flesh-and-blood cases which raise the fundamental questions. But a general framework is also needed from which to resolve the dilemmas of life. The cases in this volume are therefore organized in a systematic way. The chapters and issues within the chapter are arranged in an order to work systematically through the questions of ethics. Since the main purpose of the book is to provide a collection of case studies from which may be built a more comprehensive scheme for one's own medical ethics, the first few pages are addressed to the more theoretical issues. The object is to construct a framework of the basic questions in ethics which must be answered in any complete and systematic medical ethics.

Five fundamental questions must be answered in order to take a complete and systematic ethical position. Each question has several plausible answers, which have been developed over two thousand years of Western thought. For normal day-to-day decisions made in a medical context, it is not necessary to deal with each question. In fact, to do so would paralyze the decision-maker, whether lay person or professional. Most medical decisions are quite ordinary—such as choosing aspirin or endurance for a headache, bandage or air exposure for a wound, and practical or registered nurse for a chronically ill patient—and do not always demand full ethical analysis. Other decisions, as in the case of emergency intervention, are not ordinary at all, but the moral choices are so obvious that, in the moment of crisis, the value alternatives pale in comparison with the immediate needs for rapid action. Still, in both the ordinary and emergency situations it is only possible to act without being immobilized by the ethical and other value problems because some general rules or guidelines have emerged from previous experience and reflection. If the ethical dilemma is serious enough, it will be necessary to deal, at least implicitly, with all five of the fundamental questions.

What Makes Right Acts Right?

At the most general level, which ethicists call the level of metaethics, the first question is, What makes right acts right? What are the meaning and justification of ethical statements?

The meaning of the terms *right* and *wrong* must be understood at least to the point where the subtle and pervasive presence of ethical and other value judgments in medicine can be recognized. The problem is first to distinguish between evaluative statements and statements presenting nonevaluative facts. Evaluative language is much more common in medicine and biology than is often realized. It is logically impossible to decide on a course of action—to choose one medical approach over another—without appealing at least implicitly to some set of values. Thus every medical decision, no matter how trivial, requires evaluation. The key is learning to spot evaluative language when it occurs. Such words include *should, ought, prefer, desire, must,* and related verbs. They also include characterizations such as *preferable, desirable, responsible, good,* and *bad,* as well as *right* and *wrong.*

It is also necessary to distinguish between moral and nonmoral evaluation. This can be much harder, since often the difference cannot be discerned from the language itself. To say that abortion prior to twenty-four weeks is right may be to say that it is moral or only that it is legal. To say that morphine is desirable may mean that it is morally called for or only that it is pleasant and possibly immoral. Chapter 1 presents a series of cases where both moral and nonmoral evaluations are made in what appear to be quite ordinary medical situations. The main task is to discern the value dimensions and to separate them from the physiological, psychological, and other facts.

A closely related problem which depends on the question of what makes right acts right is the question, Who ought to decide? This is the focus of chapter 2. If rightness is a matter of personal taste, it seems reasonable that the decision-maker might be different than if rightness is a matter of scientific knowledge or of divine approval. Having learned to recognize the difference between the factual and evaluative dimensions of a case in medical ethics, one will constantly encounter the problem of who ought to decide, of where the locus of decision-making ought to rest. The technological advances in biology and medicine have so mystified us that we often assume that the proper decision-maker is the one who knows the medical facts the best. This may be true if there is no significant disagreement over values, but such is not often the case. Chapter 2 presents cases with a wide range of decision-makers, from patients, families, physicians, hospital administrators, and professional committees to lawyers, clergymen, politicians, legislators, and the general public.

The choice between these decision-makers depends at least in part on what it is that ethical terms mean, or more generally what it is that makes right acts right. Several answers to this question have been offered. One reflects the cynicism of a person who recognizes that different societies seem to reach different conclusions about whether a given act is right or wrong. From this perspective, to say that an act is morally right means nothing more than that it is in accord with the values of the speaker's society or simply that it is approved by the speaker's society. Some societies practice and approve of infanticide, while other societies consider abortion as well as infanticide the most heinous of moral offenses. This position, called social relativism, explains rightness or wrongness on the basis of whether the act fits with social customs, mores, and folkways.

One problem with this view is that it seems to make sense to say that some act is wrong even though it is approved by the society of the speaker. A second answer to the question of what makes right acts right attempts to correct this problem. According to this position, to say that an act is right means that it is approved by the speaker himself. This position, called personal relativism, reduces ethical meaning to personal preference. It too creates problems, however, for behavior thought to be immoral by some is approved by others. Birth control, euthanasia, and research on children for the benefit of others are medical examples. But such differences in judgment may have another explanation than that ethical terms refer to the speaker's own preferences. Those disagreeing might simply not be working with the same facts. The approver of an experiment on a child might believe that there is a reasonable chance for the experiment to save the child's own life, while the critic might see it as simply for the purpose of benefiting others. The supporter of euthanasia in a particular case might believe that the dying person is in great pain, while the opponent might believe that the person is producing reflex muscle twitches and feels no pain at all. This kind of factual disagreement was an issue in the interpretation of muscle movement in response to external stimulation in the widely publicized case of Karen Quinlan, in which the parents wanted to stop extraordinary treatment on an irreversibly comatose young woman. To claim that two people are in moral disagreement simply because the same act is seen as right by one person or society and wrong by another requires proof that both see the facts in the same way. Differences of circumstance or belief about the facts could easily account for many moral differences.

The social or personal relativist's understanding of ethical terms seems to conflict with the very notion of calling an act right or wrong. Certainly social and personal relativism minimize ethical dispute. In this case the only purpose of ethical debate is to exchange personal or social preferences or to clarify the different beliefs about the facts. The two positions are thus potentially conservative. An ethical challenge to immoral behavior is weak and rather pointless if right and wrong mean nothing more than expressions of taste, for there is little reason to change one's behavior only to make it conform to another's personal or societal tastes.

In contrast with social and personal relativism, there is another more universal group of answers to the question of what makes right acts right. These positions, collectively called universalism or sometimes absolutism, hold that, in principle, acts which are called morally right or wrong are right or wrong independent of social or personal biases. Certainly some choices merely involve personal taste: flavors of icecream or hair lengths vary from time to time, place to place, and person to person. But these are matters of preference, not morality. No one considers the choice of vanilla morally right and chocolate morally wrong. But other evaluations appeal beyond the standards of social and personal taste to a more universal frame of reference. When these are concerned with acts or character traits—as opposed to, say, paintings or music—they are thought of as moral evaluations. When a universal standard is assumed to exist, it makes more sense to dispute whether an act is right or wrong.

The nature of the universal standard is disputed even among absolutists or universalists. For the theologically oriented, it may be a divine standard. According to this view, to call it right electrically to stimulate the brain of a patient suffering from intractable pain is to say that God would approve of the act. This position is often called theological absolutism.

Still another view among universalists takes empirical observation as the model. The standard in this case is nature or external reality. The problem of knowing whether an act is right or wrong is then the problem of knowing what is in nature. Empirical absolutism, as the view is sometimes called, sees the problem of knowing right and wrong as analogous to knowing scientific facts. As in the empirical sciences, ethics requires that people observe and record their perceptions, only in ethics they observe and record their perceptions of right and wrong, of moral requiredness. As in the empirical sciences, they also make use of devices to avoid the errors of the naive observer. And as in the empirical sciences, they can never know for sure that their senses are not deceiving them. Some observers may differ from others in their account of what they perceive with their "moral sense." But the problems are structurally similar. While astronomers try to discern the real nature of the universe of stars and chemists the real nature of atoms as ordered in nature, ethics is an effort to discern rightness and wrongness as ordered in nature. The position is sometimes called the natural law position since, as with the physicist's law of gravity, moral laws are thought to be inexplicably rooted in nature.

Still another form of universalism or absolutism rejects both the theological and the empirical models. It supposes that right and wrong are not empirically knowable, but are nonnatural properties known only by intuition. Thus the position is sometimes called intuitionism or non-naturalism. Although for the intuitionist or nonnaturalist right and wrong are not empirically knowable, they are still universal. All persons should in principle have the same intuitions about a particular act, provided they are intuiting properly.

There are other answers to the question of what makes right acts right. One view—in various forms called noncognitivism, emotivism, or prescriptivism—which ascended to popularity during the mid-twentieth century, saw ethical utterances as evincing feelings about a particular act. A full exploration of the answers to this most abstract of ethical questions is not possible here.[1] Ultimately, however, if an ethical dispute growing out of a case is serious enough and cannot be resolved at any other level, this question must be faced. If one says that it is wrong to tell the truth to a dying patient because it will produce anxiety, and another says that it is right to do so because consent to treatment is a moral imperative, some way must be found of adjudicating the dispute between the two principles. Then one must ask what it is that makes right acts right and how conflicts can be resolved.

To Whom Is Moral Duty Owed?

Exploring what makes right acts right leads to a second question, To whom is moral duty owed? Especially in medicine the question of who it is to whom we have moral obligations is a crucial one. The problem is one of loyalty. The physician's duty traditionally has been to do what he or she thinks will benefit the patient. This obviously conflicts with others who are in medical need but do not happen to be the physician's patients. Closely related is the problem of how the physician should resolve a conflict between two patients both of whom need attention. The problem is not the physician's alone. Parents with a child who has special medical needs must decide whether they should devote time and resources equally to all children or preferentially to the one with the special need. Governments must decide whether they have a special duty to their own citizens to the exclusion of peoples in the rest of the world. All must decide whether children of future generations are to be taken into consideration in deciding about family planning, radiation levels, or genetic engineering.

The same problem of deciding to whom loyalty is owed arises in evaluating the status of the fetus or of the terminally ill and comatose. Can we count them as one with other creatures having a human genetic endowment, exclude them from the realm of the morally significant, or compromise by taking the position that they have some moral claim, but not that of other human beings? This problem arises in the cases of chapter 3 where the conflict between the individual and the society is the topic. It also arises in chapter 7 where abortion is the issue and in chapter 13 where the problem of the definition of death is posed.

What Kinds of Acts Are Right?

A third fundamental question of ethics moves beyond determining either what makes right acts right or to whom moral duty is owed to ask, What kinds of acts are right? This is called the problem of normative ethics. It questions whether there are any general principles or norms describing the characteristics that make actions right or wrong. In terms of the first question, what kinds of acts does God, society, or the person approve? What kinds of acts are in accord with nature or are intuited to be right? Two major schools of thought dominate Western normative ethics. One position looks at the consequences of acts; the other at what is taken to be inherent rights and wrongs. The first position claims that acts are right to the extent that they produce good consequences and wrong to the extent that they produce bad consequences. The key evaluative terms for this position, known as utilitarianism or consequentialism, are *good* and *bad*. This is the position of John Stuart Mill and Jeremy Bentham, as well as of Epicurus, Thomas Aquinas, and capitalist economics. Thomas, for example, argued that the first principle of the natural law is that "good is to be done and promoted and evil is to be avoided."

Since Thomas stands at the center of the Roman Catholic natural law tradition, he illustrates that natural law thinking (which is one answer to the first question of what makes right acts right) is not incompatible with consequentialism. The two positions are answers to two different questions. While many natural law thinkers are not consequentialists, they can be.

Classical utilitarianism determines what kinds of acts are right by figuring the net of good consequences minus bad ones for each person affected and then adding up to find the total net good. The certainty and duration of the benefits and harms are taken into account. Although in theory the utilitarian formula has the advantage of simplicity (actually determining benefits and harms is extremely difficult if not impossible) there are real problems with it. It is indifferent to who obtains the benefits and harms, although it recognizes that the same factor, such as money, medical treatment, or nursing care, may not be equally beneficial to all. Normally those who have the least are thought to benefit the most by the same amount of money. Those who are sickest, up to a point, are thought to benefit most from a physician's attention. But such may not always be the case, and according to this position, if money spent on a wealthy person can produce more benefit than the same amount of money spent on a poor person, the utility should be maximized. Thus, if the total net benefits of treating a relatively healthy but powerful figure are thought to be greater than those of treating a sicker Medicare recipient, the healthy and powerful ought to be given the treatment without further ethical debate.

The traditional physician ethics, oriented to benefiting patients, combines the utilitarian answer to this question of what kinds of acts are right with a particular answer to the second question raised, the question of to whom moral duty is owed. Loyalty is to the patient, and the goal is to do what will benefit the most. Traditional physician ethics is therefore a special kind of utilitarianism, avoiding many of the problems of classical utilitarianism. An experiment that does extreme harm to a small number of children but on balance produces greater benefit for society is morally acceptable according to classical utilitarianism. Another experiment that does little harm but no good to a hospitalized consenting adult and yet produces great benefit for society is immoral according to a strict interpretation of the ethic committed to patient benefit.

Over against these positions, which are oriented to consequences, the other major group of answers to the question of what kinds of acts are right asserts that rightness and wrongness are inherent in the act itself independent of the consequences. These positions, collectively known as

formalism or deontologism, hold that right- and wrong-making characteristics may be independent of consequences. Kant stated the position
most starkly.[2] It also appears in Hebrew moral law, in the doctrine that
man is endowed with certain inalienable rights, and in the view that
patient informed consent is required to promote self-determination even
if informed consent does not always promote the best consequences.

Different formalists have different lists of right-making characteristics
or ethical principles that they think are morally important independent of
consequences. The limitation of morally relevant consequences to the
physician's own patients is itself a formalist principle, since it is or at
least may be justified independent of the consequences. It may also be
justified on the ground that the total consequences are better if physicians pay attention only to the interests of their patients. Another
traditional position of physician ethics deviates still further from classical
utilitarianism. The principle of *primum non nocere* or "first of all do no
harm" is usually limited to the patient, as is the Hippocratic patient-
benefiting principle, but it gives special weight to avoiding harm over and
above the weight given to goods that can be produced. A similar special
weight is given to avoiding harm in certain Eastern ethics, in Aristotle,
and in some twentieth-century philosophers such as W. D. Ross. The
implications can be quite conservative: avoiding harm by not acting is
given more weight than acting to produce good. These problems of the
relation between classical utilitarianism, which counts benefits to all in
society equally, and traditional physician ethics, which focuses only on
patients and gives special weight to avoiding harms, are raised in the
cases of chapter 3.

Chapter 4 takes up problems of health care delivery and in doing so
poses probably the most significant challenge to the consequentialist
ethic. The dominant ethical principle of health care delivery is that of
justice. Taken in the sense of fairness in distributing goods and harms,
justice is held by many to be an ethical right-making characteristic even if
the consequences are not the best. The problem is whether it is morally
preferable to have a higher net total of benefits in society even if
unevenly distributed, or to have a somewhat lower total good but more
equally distributed. Put in terms of health, the question is whether it is
preferable to have better gross health indicators, such as average life
expectancy, even if it means discriminatory health care, as by excluding
the chronically ill poor, or to accept worse health indicators in order to
be more even-handed in the distribution of health care. Of course, health
indicators may increase if care is concentrated on the chronically ill poor.
If so, that would satisfy both the principle of utility and the principle of
justice. The utilitarian can be very sophisticated in taking account of
distribution. He argues that net benefits tend to be greater when benefits
are distributed more evenly (because of decreasing marginal utility).

Even so, he claims that the only reason to distribute goods, such as health care, evenly is to maximize the total good. The formalist who holds that justice is a right-making characteristic independent of utility does not require an item-by-item calculation of benefits and harms before concluding that the unequal distribution of goods is *prima facie* wrong, that is, wrong with regard to fairness.

Another characteristic that formalists may believe to be right-making independent of the consequences is the duty to keep promises or contracts. Kant and others have held that breaking a promise will at least tend to be wrong independent of the consequences, although many have held that on balance it may be right because of other overriding considerations. The utilitarian points out that breaking a promise often has bad consequences. If it were to become a usual practice, the act of promising itself would become useless. The formalist, although granting this danger, argues that there is something basically wrong in breaking a promise and that to know this one need not even go on to look at the consequences. The formalist might, with the utilitarian, grant that to look at consequences may reveal even more reasons to oppose promise-breaking, but such is not necessary to know that promise-breaking is *prima facie* wrong.

The patient-physician relationship is essentially a contractual relationship. There are implied and sometimes explicit promises. It would probably be better if more elements of the contract were made explicit. One of these promises is that information disclosed in the patient-physician relationship is confidential, that it will not be disclosed by the physician without the patient's permission. The principle of confidentiality in medical ethics is really a specification of the principle of promise-keeping in ethics in general. In Chapter 5 cases raising problems growing out of this ethical principle are presented.

Another ethical principle in addition to justice and promise-keeping that many formalists hold to be independent of consequences is that of truth-telling. As with the other principles, utilitarians argue that truth-telling is an operational principle designed to guarantee maximum benefit. When truth-telling does more harm than good, according to the utilitarians, there is no obligation to tell the truth. Physicians who hold the ethical principle that the physician's duty is to benefit the patient aggressively subscribe to this position. To them, telling the dying patient of his condition can be cruel and therefore wrong. In contrast, to one who holds that truth-telling is an ethical principle right-making in itself, the problem of what the dying patient should be told is much more complex. In chapter 6 the problem of what the patient should be told is the subject.

There are other ethical principles in formalist lists, such as gratitude, reparation for harm done, and self-improvement. Normative ethics, however, which questions the kinds of acts that are right, focuses primarily on the principles of maximizing utility, avoiding harm, preserving justice, keeping promises, and telling the truth. These are the issues in chapters 3 through 6.

The answer need not be a choice of one or the other. A position known as mixed formalism holds that both consequences and inherent right-making characteristics are relevant in deciding what kinds of acts are right. In effect, the mixed formalist adds the production of good consequences to his list of inherent right-making characteristics.

Any formalist, including a mixed formalist, who has more than one ethical principle, or right-making characteristic, must have some method for resolving conflicts among the principles. One method is a lexical ordering of the principles, ranking them from the most important to the least, so that the first on the list always takes priority. For those who claim that it is impossible to rank ethical principles, another method is to balance competing ethical principles when they conflict in a specific case. This requires an often intuitive system of weighting different principles. This is frequently unsatisfying when accurate weighting cannot be easily determined. The problem is no different, however, from that of the utilitarian or consequentialist who must assign weight to the different kinds of goods he envisions from various courses of acts even when those goods are qualitatively different. Utilitarians, formalists, and mixed formalists all have the problem of resolving competing ethical claims, unless they recognize only one ethical principle or one kind of good as morally relevant. This most find impossible to do.

How Do Rules Apply to Specific Situations?

There is a fourth question in a general ethical stance. It stems from the fact that each case raising an ethical problem is in at least some ways situationally unique. The ethical principles of benefiting, avoiding harm, justice, promise-keeping, and truth-telling are extremely general. They are a small set of the most general right-making characteristics. Application to specific cases requires a great leap. The question is, How do the rules apply to specific situations? As a bridge to the specific case, an intermediate, more specific set of rules is often used. The Ten Commandments are examples, as are the rules to obtain informed consent, to avoid abortion after twenty-four weeks or viability, and to get two physician signatures before making a psychiatric commitment. These intermediate rules probably cause more problems in ethics than any other component of ethical theory. At the same time they are probably more helpful as guides to day-to-day behavior than anything else.

The problems arise in part because of a misunderstanding of the nature and function of these rules. Rules may have two functions. They may simply serve as guidelines summarizing conclusions we tend to reach in moral problems of a certain class. The rule to get informed consent may, for instance, simply be a shorthand statement of the conclusion that things usually work out better from a moral point of view if consent is obtained. Some codes of human experimentation explicitly state that informed consent can be omitted or can be obtained orally instead of in writing if in the particular case it seems more appropriate. Sometimes a special procedure is prescribed for deviating from the rule, as when the opinion of another physician is required before the rule on written consent is waived. When rules have this function of simply summarizing experience in similar situations of the past, they are called rules-of-thumb, guiding rules, or summary rules.

In contrast, rules may function to specify behavior that is required independent of individual judgment about a specific situation. The rules against abortion of a viable fetus or against killing a dying patient are much more stringent than simply summaries of past experience used as guides in new situations. These more stringent rules are taken to be directly linked to right-making characteristics, so that they can be violated only with great trepidation if at all. Sometimes this kind of rule is called a rule of practice.

The conflict between those who take the rules more seriously and those who consider the situation to be the more critical determinant of moral rightness has become one of the major ethical controversies in the mid-twentieth century. It is sometimes called the rules-situation debate.[3] At one extreme is the rigorist who insists that rules should never be violated. At the other is the antinomian who claims that rules never apply because every situation is unique. Probably both positions in the extreme lead to absurdity. The rigorist is immobilized when two of his rules conflict. The situationalist is immobilized when he treats a situation as literally new with no help from past experience in similar if not identical situations.

Medical ethics has an acute problem with the rules-situation debate because medicine tends to be a highly individualizing activity. Physicians are at one extreme in society, wanting to treat every case as situationally unique and finding fixed rules inappropriate in resolving ethical dilemmas. At the other extreme are persons involved in medical ethics—the lawyers, clergymen, and patients themselves—who may find rules more helpful, having learned from their religious, occupational, and family groups that rules can be terribly important. If so, there will be conflicts in problematic cases over whether the rules should apply.

It may seem foolish to apply rules rigidly when each case obviously has its unique aspects. Beyond the reason of efficiency, the primary argument for the use of rules derives from the nature of man and his abilities in moral reasoning. If man is a fallible, limited creature, he may well make serious mistakes in determining afresh in each case what is morally required. Rules, if they have any purpose at all, reflect a long tradition of human experience with sometimes difficult moral problems. Consider the rule that one ought to stop when a traffic light is red. This is admittedly an inefficient rule in that time is wasted when no traffic is approaching on the cross street. The situational alternative would be to consider the particular circumstances at every red light and proceed when the coast is clear. If man were perfect in his ability to evaluate a situation, the second, more situational alternative would be preferable. But man is not perfect and so opts for the clumsier rule, which can be defended on the ground that it produces a greater good in the long run even though in specific cases it is wasteful.

A similar argument can be made over the rule about informed consent. As an alternative to this rule, physicians could be required to get informed consent for experimentation or medical treatment only in those situations where on balance they thought it necessary. Since there are great differences of opinion over when consent ought to be obtained, however, and there is reason to fear that physicians might not always judge correctly, society opts for a rule. Whether it is a stringent rule of practice to be followed even against the judgment of the physician or only a rule of thumb that can be waived for a good reason is still a major controversy in medical ethics.

Another component of ethical theory operates at approximately the same level as moral rules. Moral rights are those things to which one is thought to have a morally just claim. Claims of rights often have a slogan quality: the right to life, the right to health care, the right to refuse treatment, the right to determine family size. Rights are claims to a realm of freedom to act. They imply, but normally do not specify, correlative duties on the part of someone. They are thus closely related to moral rules, which are often generated in the name of protecting a claimed right. Rights are similar to rules in their level of specificity. They, like rules, often conflict with other rights and rules.

It is crucial to separate the issues of the rules-situation debate, which is the essence of the debate over how to apply rules to specific situations, from the issues in the question of what makes right acts right. The terms *universalism* or *absolutism* refer to an answer to the first question—that there is a universal standard of reference which is the basis for determining what makes an act right. The natural law position, which holds that right-making characteristics are rooted in nature, is one kind of universalism or absolutism. This position is often confused with legalism, which is an extreme answer to the question of how rules apply to specific situations. The two are independent and should never be confused. It is perfectly logical to be a universalist or absolutist in the sense of believing that there is in principle one correct answer to a particular moral problem, and still to be a situationalist in the sense of believing that every case is unique and thus no rules can apply. It is logically consistent to maintain that a case is unique and yet has one correct answer, whether in the nature of things, in God's judgment, or in a person's intuition of its nonnatural moral properties. It is also logical to hold the legalistic position of the rules-situationalist debate and still completely reject the position that in principle there is only one correct moral course. This would be the position of a social relativist in a totalitarian society. He could maintain that for X to be right means only that "X is approved by my society" and yet also believe that "my society holds to a set of rigid rules never to be violated." The unattractive features of rules—their rigidity and insensitivity to special situations—are sometimes opposed by arguing that rightness and wrongness are simply a matter of social or personal taste. This is to confuse the two problems. It may be that situationalism is preferable to rules and also that moral terms refer only to social or personal taste, but the two problems are separate. On the contrary, it may be that rules are important, particularly to protect those who are relatively powerless and have different values from those with power, as is often the case in the medical relationship. It may also be that universalism is more in accord with our understanding of the meaning of moral requiredness and makes intervention to promote moral justice more plausible. If both of these are true, if rules are important and universalism is more in accord with our understanding of the meaning of moral requiredness, they are true independently of one another.

The rules-situation debate does not lend itself to special cases grouped together. The problem arises continually throughout the cases in the volume. The final question, however, requires special chapters with cases selected to examine the problems raised.

What Ought To Be Done in Specific Cases?

After the determination of what makes right acts right, to whom moral duty is owed, what kinds of actions are right, and how rules apply to specific situations, there are still left a large number of specific situations which make up the bulk of problems in medical ethics. The question remains, What ought to be done in a specific case or kind of case? Medicine, being particularly oriented to case problems, is given to organizing medical ethical problems around specific kinds of cases. Since medical education is departmentally organized, it is not unusual for medical ethics courses and medical ethics volumes to separate the obstetrical, psychiatric, pediatric, and experimental pharmacology problems. Ethics too is sometimes divided into the problems of birth, life, and death.

The first two parts of this volume emphasize the overarching problems of how to relate facts to values, of who ought to decide, of health care delivery, confidentiality, and truth-telling. These are among the larger questions of medical ethics. Part three shifts to cases involving specific problem areas. Cases in chapter 7 raise the problems of abortion, sterilization, and conception control. Chapter 8 moves to the related problems of genetic counseling and engineering and of intervention in the pre- and perinatal periods. The next chapters take up in turn the problems of hemodialysis, transplantation, and allocation of scarce medical resources; psychiatry and the control of human behavior; human experimentation, consent, and the right to refuse medical treatment; and finally death and dying.

The answer to the question of what ought to be done in a specific case requires the integration of the answers to all of the other questions if a thorough analysis and justification is to be given. The first line of moral defense will probably be a set of moral rules and rights thought to apply to the case. In abortion, the right to control one's body and the right to practice medicine as one sees fit are pitted against the right to life. In human experimentation, the rules of informed consent pertain. Hemodialysis allocation has its own rules and guidelines. Among the dying, rules about euthanasia conflict with the right to pursue happiness; and the right to refuse medical treatment conflicts with the rule that the physician ought to do everything possible to preserve life.

In many cases the conflict escalates from an issue of moral rules and rights to the higher, more abstract level of ethical principle. It must be determined, for example, whether informed consent is designed to maximize benefits to the experimental subject or to facilitate his freedom of self-determination. It must also be explored whether harm to the patient justifies withholding information from the patient or whether the formalist truth-telling principle justifies disclosure.

The problem of what ought to be done in a specific case also requires a great deal of information other than the moral. It requires considerable empirical data. Value-relevant biological and psychological facts have developed around many case problems in medical ethics. The predictive capacity of a flat electroencephalogram may be important for the definition of death. The legal facts are relevant for the refusal of treatment. Basic religious and philosophical beliefs of the patient may be critical for resolving some cases in medical ethics. It is impossible to present all of the relevant medical, genetic, legal, and psychological facts that are necessary for a complete analysis of any case, but it is possible to present the major facts required for understanding. The reader will have to supplement these facts for a fuller understanding of the cases, just as he will have to supplement his reading in ethical theory for a fuller understanding of the basic questions in ethics.

PART ONE

MORALITY IN MEDICINE

CHAPTER 1

Values in
Health and Illness

Of all the problems in the field of medical ethics probably the most important and pervasive is identifying the ethical and other value dimensions of medical decisions. The fundamental premise of this book is that every medical decision has a value component. The first skill needed by one who takes medical and biological ethics seriously is that of recognizing the evaluative dimensions of cases which otherwise appear to be mundane and value-free. In some medical decisions, to be sure, the value choices may seem utterly trivial. One must have a blood transfusion *if* he *wants* to live—but the fact that some people, such as Jehovah's Witnesses, value other things more than continuing life in this world reveals that even when the values are so readily assumed, evaluations are still present. Many moral disputes in fact arise because the value alternatives are not recognized and spelled out.

Certain cases would not normally be thought of as raising crucial medical ethical questions. They are not the exotic cases—the transplant, abortion, cloning, and plug-pulling—which excite the curiosity of physician and layman alike. Rather, they illustrate the problem of finding the value dimensions in situations that otherwise appear routine, value-free, and innocent.

1 THE CASE OF THE BROKEN LEG

Kenneth Morrow was brought to the Lebanon Valley Hospital emergency room by the ski patrol ambulance. It was a compound fracture of the femur, the third one the emergency room had had in a week. Dr. Lester Olson, the orthopedist, was muttering about the monotony of setting leg bones as he scribbled the order for Mr. Morrow's pain medication on the chart, "propoxyphene compound 65 mg. qid.," and handed it to the nurse who was adjusting the tension lines. Propoxyphene compound is a nonnarcotic pain reliever containing aspirin plus a chemical structurally related to narcotics but supposedly lacking both their addictive properties and their potency in relieving pain. It is a common drug for moderate pain.

Mr. Morrow was semicomatose, beginning to recover from the anesthetic used to set the leg. He uttered a low, groaning sound, grasping subconsciously at the cast which was now in place on his leg. The moaning became louder as the anesthetic wore off and he recovered consciousness. Fifteen minutes later he was complaining to the nurse of the pain in his leg. She gave him a propoxyphene capsule, telling him it should take a few minutes to get relief.

As he recovered from the anesthesia, Mr. Morrow waited for relief. It did not come. By evening the pain of the leg was excruciating. He pleaded with the nurse, who gave him another propoxyphene capsule. "Something stronger—please! You must have something stronger," he begged. The nurse evaded the question, saying that propoxyphene was what the doctor had ordered.

Now beads of perspiration stood out on Mr. Morrow's brow. He felt as if he had to get up and out—to scream—to find some relief from the agony.

Finally the nurse phoned for Dr. Doug Barnett, the resident on call. The screaming, agitated patient was becoming too much for her to handle. The resident read the chart, muttered something about Dr. Olson's stinginess with the analgesics, and wrote the orders "methadone HCl 10 mg. IM stat."—a heavy dose of a potent synthetic narcotic to be given immediately. He left orders to repeat the dose in three hours if necessary and to check with Dr. Olson in the morning.

The next morning before the resident had finished his rounds, he was paged by Dr. Olson, who was furious at the use of methadone, especially at so high a dose. "Now Morrow will demand it for the next week," the orthopedist argued. "Do you want me to turn him into an addict just to relieve a little pain?"

The resident was defiant. "The man was in agony," he argued. "The physician's job is to relieve that agony. If modern medical science has given us the tools to intervene and we don't use them, then why bother becoming a physician?"

Dr. Olson was not convinced. "Who says the physician's job is to use every technical trick in the book just to make the patient happy? I took an oath pledging that I would do what would benefit my patient, not what would turn him on for the moment. The body is something very delicate, something sacred. Every time we stick some man-made chemical into it, we're tampering with nature. Tamper with that body as little as you can; it will take care of itself. The physician's job is to help nature take its course."

They were at an impasse. Dr. Olson turned and left the room.

A broken leg is normally thought to be a noncontroversial, straightforward medical problem. Yet in this particular case, which may be the single most significant case in the volume, the ethical and other value foundations of the choices become quite apparent. This broken leg differs from other broken legs primarily in the fact that such values are brought to the surface. Dr. Olson, Dr. Barnett, and Mr. Morrow agree that the patient is in pain, even severe pain. The physicians presumably agree that methadone is a more potent analgesic than propoxyphene or aspirin. The relevant medical facts of the case cause no problem. Yet a serious controversy erupts about the proper course of action.

Who is right? Perhaps both; perhaps neither. What all of the persons involved—the doctors, the patient, and the nurse—apparently fail to realize is that critical value choices are being made in even this most mundane medical problem. Decision-making, in medicine as everywhere else, is essentially an evaluative process. Although scientific medical information is essential in the choice-making, so are the values with which the alternatives are assessed. In some cases, to be sure, the values are so clear that for ordinary purposes they can be assumed. If so, certain alternatives are ruled out. Dr. Olson, Dr. Barnett, and Mr. Morrow are not interested in thousands of drugs that might have been used—aspirin, paralyzing agents such as curare, or a general anesthetic, which would have relieved one of the nurse's problems by silencing the patient. Even to rule out these alternatives, however, requires value choices. When those assumed values are questioned, as may be done by someone who would rather die than continue living in misery, then the so-called medical decisions based on those values are also questioned.

In virtually every medical situation more than one plausible alternative exists: experimental surgery or standard treatment, salt-free diet or diuretic, psychopharmacological agent or psychotherapy, scientifically trained physician or folk healer, and in this case, a more or less potent analgesic. If it is true that more than one plausible alternative exists at some point in the treatment of virtually every patient, then choices must be made based on some system of values.

In Mr. Morrow's case, one of the basic value alternatives is at stake. Is man, particularly medical man, to be the ruler over nature, making use of the technological tools created by his wisdom and cleverness in order to solve the problems of suffering and misery in the world? Or is man to be the servant of nature, helping nature take its course, as Dr. Olson maintains? Man's relationship with nature is one of the fundamental value orientations of human culture.[1] Any choice in the use of a drug, or even of a food with or without additives, will reflect this value orientation.

Every medical student is exposed to the concept of homeostasis, the notion that the body has a natural tendency to maintain a relatively stable state. Walter Cannon has become a father figure for medical students because of his testimony to the "wisdom of the body."[2] What these students often fail to grasp is that this view of the body as possessing an internal "wisdom" which should be tampered with only with fear and trembling is a philosophy of medicine, not simply a description of biological fact. It may lead to the value orientation of Dr. Olson or to the organic food advocate's position that man's intervention in nature's creation can be a dangerous and mischievous tinkering.

Dr. Barnett's value orientation reflects a radically different philosophy of medicine. Man—to use the Biblical formulation—shall have dominion over the earth and subdue it. Technological man of the modern West is man the maker—*Homo faber*. This philosophy of the use of rational organization to solve the problems of the world has produced the great medical miracles. Average life expectancy has doubled. Suffering has been relieved. What was once thought to be the inevitable force of an evil spirit is now swept away with a mere injection of penicillin.

But this same technology that has the power to save also has the power to destroy. Iatrogenic or physician-made illness now accounts for a substantial portion of hospital bed days. Even more significant is the emerging feeling that even if physical illness is not created by medical intervention, medicine has produced a depersonalizing, inhumane life-style.

Even among those whose orientation is generally interventionist, radical conflict over the goals of the intervention may exist. If the physician's role is to make use of modern medical technologies to solve the problems of mankind, he must decide to what end these technologies are to be used. One physician, a modern adherent to the Protestant ethic, may feel medical intervention is important to get the patient back to a productive life, to help him in his work. Another, whom Philip Rieff has called the "therapeutic man," may intervene to produce the psychological goal of "adjustment."[3] The drug use of the counterculture seems radically different from the Protestant work-oriented ethic. Yet it is still oriented to the same extreme, systematic pursuit of a salvation experience. Though its salvation is of a radically different, more present-oriented kind, this drug ethic may fairly be called "neo-Protestant." It is not enough to distinguish between value orientations in favor of or against medical intervention. Real conflicts may exist among those who are generally inclined to make use of medical technologies for the aid of human welfare.[4] The conflict between Dr. Olson and Dr. Barnett— between the value orientations that see the physician as subservient to or as conqueror of nature—underlies the crisis in modern medicine and virtually every choice made in the medical context.

Other value differences may underlie the conflict in this case. Dr. Olson may be more oriented to the long-term consequences of the possible addiction; Dr. Barnett to the more immediate problem of relieving pain. A different value orientation to time—a different weighting of the significance of past, present, and future—can be the unrecognized value conflict in many medical ethics cases. This is particularly true if the medical professional and the layman are from differing ethnic backgrounds which have differing orientations to time.

It may also be that the two physicians have different value frameworks in worrying about the addiction per se. While drug addiction is a problem having a medical component, there is controversy over whether or not its foundation is moral.

The final ethical problem growing out of this case of a seemingly morally neutral broken leg is the problem of who should decide. If the choice between propoxyphene and methadone, and indeed among aspirin, general anesthetic, and the "suffering-builds-character" attitude, is based on a value framework, the question arises who should be the choice-maker. Dr. Olson and Dr. Barnett share one perspective. They both feel that they have the authority to make the decision based on their own system of values. Mr. Morrow is a petitioner for relief. The nurse assumes that her role is to follow the "doctor's orders." This may be the greatest dilemma in medical ethics. It is obvious that technical knowledge is needed for decisions in the medical context. The more technologically complex medicine becomes, the more expertise is required to supply that knowledge. Mr. Morrow cannot possibly choose between propoxyphene and methadone on the basis of his own knowledge. Yet the two physicians' values relating man to nature are clearly not part of their technical expertise. They are value orientations that each human being possesses.

2   MASTECTOMY: RADICAL OR SIMPLE

The patient, Florence Dawson, was 38 years old, married, and childless. She had come to the physician, Dr. Bryan Marshall, in his private surgical practice on referral from her local physician in January 1974. Her presenting symptoms were tenderness and a lump in her breast. She also reported a weight loss from 127 to 119 pounds over the past eight months.

She had noticed the lump for several months before arriving at Dr. Marshall's office, but she had been so worried that several times she put off making the appointment. She knew of women who after breast surgery had never regained full use of their arms, failed to adjust, or experienced fits of depression. In addition, Mrs. Dawson had always been proud of her figure, and the thought of losing a breast was terrifying to her. Uncertain of her husband's reaction, she had not even mentioned the lump to him.

Mammography together with breast biopsy revealed a malignancy with a mass measuring 2 cm. in diameter in the upper, outer quadrant of the breast. Dr. Marshall tentatively classified the cancer as a low-grade malignancy, stage II, probably a fibroadenoma. However, because of signs of extension into the fascia, he was uncertain if it had grown locally in the confines of the breast or had spread to the lymph nodes. Staging, or classifying the stage of the malignancy, prior to surgery is an inexact science, and a preoperative conclusion that there is no involvement of the axillary nodes or lymph nodes of the armpit can be wrong 30 percent or more of the time. In as many as 60 percent of women diagnosed as having breast cancer, the cancer cells have spread to the lymph nodes. If there is nodal involvement, the risk of distant metastases increases greatly.

Dr. Marshall was faced with one of the more controversial choices in contemporary surgery. Traditionally a radical mastectomy would have been performed on Mrs. Dawson. This involves removal of not only the breast but also the lymph nodes and chest and upper arm muscle tissue. Now, however, three simpler procedures are also advocated, involving removal of only the breast without the surrounding muscle tissue, known as simple mastectomy, removal of only a part of the breast, or removal of only the original mass itself, called lumpectomy.

Dr. Marshall had followed the professional literature on the controversy over radical mastectomy versus the simpler procedures for some time. Dr. George Crile, Jr., a leading advocate of the simpler procedures, has reported a ten-year survival rate of 41 percent using a simple mastectomy and only 30 percent using a modified radical mastectomy. On the basis of his findings, he completely abandoned conventional radical mastectomies and became a strong spokesman for the simpler procedures. However, Dr. Anil Jain in a letter in *Ca—A Cancer Journal for Clinicians* has demonstrated that the difference between Criles's two groups was not statistically significant.

Seven major controlled trials have been undertaken to attempt to resolve the controversy. One in Cambridge, England, compared radical mastectomy and postoperative irradiation with modified simple mastectomy and irradiation on a total of 204 patients with stage II breast cancer. They found no significant difference in crude five-year survival and recurrence-free rates. Another trial at Guy's Hospital, London, however, produced different results. Of 370 patients, approximately half were subjected to radical mastectomy followed by irradiation, while the other half had an extended tylectomy, that is, a lumpectomy or local excision, followed by irradiation. They found that for patients with stage II tumors, those subjected to radical mastectomy had a significantly better ten-year but not five-year survival. They now treat all stage II patients with radical mastectomy.

Dr. Marshall had also recently read an article in *Medical Consultant,* a magazine sent at no charge to physicians, in which Dr. Guy Robbins argued for the radical procedure and against the simpler ones. He claimed no less than 30 percent of mastectomy patients with a primary lesion of 2 cm. or less in diameter had cancerous foci in other quadrants. "We know from harsh experience," he reported, "that such tiny foci are capable of killing at the sixth, seventh, or eighth year—or later." Radical mastectomy, he observed, challenges the physician because it is much easier to tell the patient she will not lose her breast. "It takes more time and trouble to explain why such a procedure involves a heavier risk of recurrence and why saving her breast now may mean losing it later—when surgery may be *too* little and *too* late!" He concluded: "those of us who do the radical procedure most of the time are doing so because the average patient lives longer that way. To contend that a surgeon can feel an involved node from the outside is ridiculous . . . Our data at Memorial Hospital and M.D. Anderson Hospital and Tumor Institute in Texas . . . have been analyzed by the most experienced biostatisticians available. They show that 'best is most' as to longer survival. I urge you not to sell your patients short by letting them become convinced to the contrary."[5]

Dr. Marshall was persuaded. He began preparing himself for the task of explaining to Mrs. Dawson that she must have the radical procedure.

———————

The mastectomy debate is one of the most confusing in contemporary clinical medicine. It is no wonder that the ethical and other value dimensions get lost in the statistical debate over surgical alternatives. A number of procedures are available: superradical, radical, modified radical, modified simple, simple, partial, and tylectomy. Some studies include radiation; others do not. The radiation levels are not always controlled. The size and stage of the tumor may or may not be controlled. Bernard Fisher, in the most recent review of the clinical studies, concluded that "those studies which have been concerned with the surgical management of breast cancer patients are not yet of sufficient validity to justify firm conclusions."[6]

The first value problem faced by Dr. Marshall is whose statistics to accept. If the aggregate data do not point firmly to one conclusion or another, how does he select the most probable answer? It is clear that competent surgeons are choosing both the radical and the simple procedures, and even the partial and lumpectomy procedures where the breast is spared. Dr. Marshall's problem can be called the condition of doubt. When in doubt about the scientific data, he must still make a choice between the more radical or the more conservative course of surgery. The choice is really one of whether he has faith that man's intervention tends to work or not, whether he is an optimist or a pessimist. This case is even more confusing since some argue that the more radical procedure, including node dissection, can actually spread the tumor by destroying one of the body's natural defenses. Advocates of more radical intervention consistently have less faith in the body's natural processes.

Even if one assumes that the only goal is to maximize the number of years of survival, the choice will depend greatly on the value orientation of the decision-maker. It hinges on one's faith in intervention or in more conservative courses. This is fundamentally a value or life-style problem, not one rooted in scientific or medical fact.

The value dimensions appear even more significant in view of the fact that Mrs. Dawson may not consider years of survival to be the only relevant consideration. She is worried about what the operation will do to her appearance. She is worried about not being able to use her arm normally, about how the operation will affect her figure, and what her husband will think. Suppose it were proved beyond doubt that the radical procedure would produce a 45 percent ten-year survival while the simple procedure would produce only a 40 percent ten-year survival. There is nothing illogical about choosing to live with a 5 percent greater risk of death within ten years. Whether or not the extra risk is worth it will depend on how the psychological and physical advantages of the simpler procedures are valued. To the vitalist, who considers years of physical survival to be the only or primary matter of legitimate consideration, the radical procedure is the properly valued choice. To one who values other elements of life even at the expense of a greater risk of earlier death, the simple procedure is more plausible.

If what is at stake is fundamentally a value choice between two plausible procedures, then it is difficult to see why Dr. Marshall ought to make the decision himself. Yet one recent informal poll among physicians reveals that this is the overwhelmingly preferred course of decision-making. A survey of 752 respondents in *Medical Opinion* revealed that 18 percent felt that a radical mastectomy should be done in every instance of confirmed breast cancer. Twenty-six percent said that in the absence of confirmed nodal involvement, simple mastectomy is probably sufficient. The largest group, 34 percent, said that the choice ought to be left to the individual physician. Only 7 percent argued that the patient should be given a choice, prior to surgery, if the tumor appears isolated. The remaining 15 percent had no opinion.[7] The survey reflects the confusion in the scientific literature. With the results so uncertain, it is not surprising that there is no consensus on whether there ought to be a radical or simple procedure. Although the survey itself confirms this confusion, most of the respondents appeared to treat the question as being in principle a technical rather than a value question. Most of them thought that the physician's judgment ought to be the decisive factor. Only 7 percent saw the matter as one for patient choice. Yet if the choice is in fact based on value orientation—if there is clearly no consensus based on the criterion either of survival or of whether an extra chance of survival is worthwhile—then it is hard to see why the matter should be resolved by the physician's rather than the patient's system of values. Whether or not the patient ought to gamble on the simpler procedure for the benefit of decreased physical deformity and increased psychological comfort, but at the possibly greater risk of death, is one that can only be answered by an appeal to what is valuable.

3   DRUG ADDICTION: CRIME OR ILLNESS

One serious problem in distinguishing the value dimensions of health and illness arises in the classification of certain conditions as inside or outside the medical model. More and more conditions are what may be called marginally medical. Obesity, homosexuality, heart attacks resulting from poor diet and exercise, so-called elective abortion, plastic cosmetic surgery, alcoholism, hair implantation, and drug addiction are all marginally medical cases. They are in some ways medical, but in other ways not. Some may be seen as criminal problems, such as drug addiction or alcoholism, others as arising from personal and social desires, such as abortion, plastic surgery, or hair implants, and still others as real health problems but arising from voluntary, irresponsible behavior, such as some heart attacks or obesity. Some persons see all of these as growing out of the foolish or irresponsible exercise of will power and thus as moral and possibly legal problems, while others see them as more nearly medical conditions where the "patient" is not really responsible for his behavior and "treatment" is appropriate.

One such policy debate has involved drug addiction. In 1955 a Joint Committee of the American Bar Association and the American Medical Association on Narcotic Drugs was charged with examining policies on drug traffic and related problems. Their interim report, published in 1958, has become one of the most important documents arguing that drug addiction is a disease. It called for an experimental outpatient clinic for the treatment of addicts.

Although the report was quite short, it was accompanied by a longer statement by Morris Ploscowe, director of the Narcotics Control Study, explaining the nature and characteristics of drug addiction:

> The law has largely acted on the premise, which is supported by some of the earlier writers, that drug addiction was largely a vice, which an effort of the will could conquer. Severe penalties were necessary to compel the will to make the effort to conquer the vice. Medical writers, on the other hand, have taken the view that drug addiction was a disease and that the drug addict was a sick person. For example, Ernest S. Bishop wrote many years ago: "The fundamental truth which applies to all cases of narcotic drug addiction is this—whatever may have been the circumstances of the primary administration of narcotic drugs, or whatever the physical, ethical or personal status of the person addicted . . . continued administration of the drug creates within the body of the person to whom the drug is administered a physical disease process . . . Every addict is sick of a disease condition . . . insufficiently recognized and insufficiently studied."
>
> Or as Dr. William G. Somerville put it: "Drug addiction is a disease, a pathological condition just as much as the psychoneuroses of any of the various toxic states."
>
> If the physiological and psychological need for the drug inherent in drug addiction is a disease, then it will be apparent from our discussion of relapse that it is a disease which is largely incurable by present methods and techniques. The course of the disease can only be controlled by the continued administration of the drug of addiction or some similar drug.[8]

The joint committee's conclusion that drug addiction is a disease produced a vitriolic reply from the Advisory Committee to the Federal Bureau of Narcotics, including an attack on the disease theory of addiction by Lynn A. White, the deputy chief of police and commander of the personnel and training bureau of the Los Angeles Police Department. White argued:

> Had the committee been unbiased and thoroughly objective, its conclusion would necessarily have been: "Had the Federal, State and local governments provided carefully selected, adequately trained narcotic officers in sufficient numbers; and with sufficient funds; joined with firm support from the prosecutors; and strong, vigorous action by the courts in their sentences and decisions; *the narcotic enforcement program in this Nation would have been an overwhelming success today.*"

The "Disease" Theory

The report appears to adopt the finding that opiate addiction is a "disease." It is somewhat surprising, particularly since the committee included men of the medical profession, that this "disease" theory was not explored in a manner typical of the medical profession's investigation of other diseases. It has long been presumed by the writer that inquiry into disease by the medical profession is accompanied by an objective investigation of:

1. What causes the disease?
2. How is it communicated or "carried"?
3. How is it cured?

(1) *What Causes The Disease of Narcotic Addiction?*—The cause of narcotic addiction is so well established that it did not deserve more thorough investigation in the report. The report, however, fails to mention that addiction is a *"permissive disease"*; that the sufferers, except for those few who acquire the disease through medical treatment, and the insignificant number who acquire the disease under conditions amounting to fraudulent overtures, become *narcotics addicts* by self-ministration; i.e., *with and by their own permission.*

Therefore, narcotic addiction (particularly after an addict has once undergone a "cure") may be considered as a self-induced or, more pointedly, *a "disease" resulting from self-abusive indulgence.* In this sense, it is not a true disease such as tuberculosis or diphtheria nor may those who become self-infected be considered unfortunate victims of a disease of contemporary society acquired innocently in the course of normal, moral pursuit of life.

(2) *How Is The "Disease" of Narcotic Addiction Communicated?*—It is difficult to assess the reasons why the committee ignored the contagion element of addiction. A cause of greater confusion though, is Ploscowe's naive observation . . . *"The only value* of jail or prison for the treatment of drug addiction is that the addict may be temporarily withdrawn from drugs during the period of incarceration." It ignores completely that while the addict is confined *he is not stealing* and more important—HE IS NOT INFECTING OTHERS.

Does the committee recommend a program under which the contagion may be contained?—No.

It recommends the establishment of an "out-patient clinic" where the "carriers" of the disease may obtain the "virus" which will be carried away to be used to "infect" another "uninfected" person, who in turn will become "infected," who in turn will present himself at the "clinic" to obtain more "virus" to "infect" another, ad infinitum . . .

(3) *How Is Narcotic Addiction Cured?*—The answer is well-known —deprive the addict of the drugs, and, historically, any other approach has been proved to be practically useless . . .

It has been this writer's personal experience with the many addicts he has known who have been "cured," more were "cured" by the "jail treatment" than were "cured" by the "hospital treatment." The "jail-cured" expressed it by, "I just got tired of having to 'kick' my habit 'cold'."

(Admittedly, the above is a subjective observation.)

Why did the committee fail to inquire into the important question—*After an addict is successfully cured does he return to society as a law-*

abiding citizen who has been fully rehabilitated or does he return to former criminal pursuits? . . .

The out-patient experimental clinic for the treatment of drug addicts

Had the committee recommended that arthritics be treated with cinchophen (a drug once widely used for arthritis; effective, but it destroyed the liver and the patient died), a conscientious investigator of addiction could not have been more startled than he is by the recommendation the Committee made . . .

Such a recommendation can only mean that the committee *intended, from the outset of the study, to make such a recommendation regardless of any evidence to the contrary . . .*

They have here, as they have throughout the report, totally ignored the fact that the *raison d'être* of our State and Federal Narcotic Laws is: "To protect the people of the United States from becoming a nation dependent on narcotic drugs."

NOT ONCE IN THE REPORT IS THERE MADE ANY REFERENCE OR RECOMMENDATION AS TO HOW WE CAN KEEP THE UNTOLD THOUSANDS, NOT NOW ADDICTED, FROM BECOMING ADDICTED THROUGH ASSOCIATION WITH PERSONS WHO ARE NOW ADDICTED!

Why is the committee so preoccupied with the belief that our narcotic problems are limited to the 60,000-80,000 addicts' comfort or discomfort; or whether "unrehabilitable addicts can be transformed into productive members of the community if their drug needs are met?" THESE ARE NOT THE PROBLEMS FACING THIS NATION! . . .

This Nation became great, not by coddling the evildoers, or pampering the morally weak and perpetuating their immoral appetites, but through vigorous action which removed them from our society—so only will we remain a great Nation.

In recent years we have indulged our young criminals and have given them a nice title to describe their little acts of misconduct; we have "rehabilitated" our prisons' inmates; and then worried and fretted when they again repeated their little depredations against innocent victims; such "thoughtful consideration" has been so successful in reducing crime, that our Nation is now the most lawless in the world.

With the committee's report at hand, we are again confronted with "do-gooders' " philosophies; obviously written by persons so concerned with the comfort of a few hopheads they would recommend a system whereby we would become, in time, a nation of drug addicts.

The time has come, if we are to survive as a nation, that we must return to the standards of morals and ethics of our forebears and again require adherence to the laws of our Nation by all. The clinic method of perpetuating the immoral weakness of a few is certainly not the road that will lead us back to a strong, vigorous, law-abiding nation.[9]

The British, however, had adopted a disease theory of addiction in the work of a committee of a distinguished medical authorities under the chairmanship of Sir Humphrey Rolleston. In 1961 the Interdepartmental

Committee on Drug Addiction under the chairmanship of physician Sir Russell Brain developed the disease concept further:

> Like the Rolleston Committee, we believe that addiction should be re-garded as an expression of mental disorder rather than a form of crimi-nal behaviour.
> We believe that every addict should be treated energetically as a medical and psychiatric problem. The evidence presented to us indi-cates that the satisfactory management of these cases is not possible except in suitable institutions. We are not convinced that compulsory committal to such institutions is desirable. Good results are more likely to be obtained with co-operative rather than with coerced patients. At a time when the compulsory treatment of the mentally sick is being steadily diminished we see no ground for seeking new powers of com-pulsion for the treatment of drug addicts.[10]

More recently the disease model of drug addiction has been challenged by radical commentators who see the medical interpretation of addiction as condescending, implying a lack of responsibility on the part of the ad-dict. The radical physician Richard Kunnes, for instance, has attacked both the medical and the criminal interpretations of addiction: "Heroin addiction is not a criminal problem, though criminals and crime are involved. Nor is heroin addiction a medical problem, though medical symptoms are produced. Heroin addiction is ultimately a political and economic problem created by, and controlled for, wealthy criminals with political connections, political officials with corporate and criminal con-nections, and corporate officials controlling the priorities of our soci-ety."[11]

Whereas prescribing a narcotic for a broken leg or surgery for breast cancer is normally thought of as a medical rather than a value problem, other problems that are normally thought of as moral or criminal may really be medical ones. This heated, often confused drug addiction debate, which has made bedfellows of radical representatives of the counterculture and the Federal Bureau of Narcotics, is symbolic of the conflict over marginally medical conditions. The radical critic of the disease model shares with the Los Angeles Police Department spokesman the view that addiction is willed behavior. However, they disagree vehe-mently over whether drug use is an affront to society so great that it ought to be made illegal. While the police department spokesman sees the addict as an "evil-doer," others see him either as choosing a plausible, valued alternative life-style or as making an appropriate response to a morally intolerable oppressive society. Both, however, see addiction as outside the medical model.

The defining of a condition as inside or outside the medical model carries with it important policy implications. People are not normally considered responsible for disease, although they may have an obligation to do what is necessary to overcome it. A disease is by definition something disapproved. To say that heroin use is a disease is to say that it is unacceptable. Also, to call a behavior a disease carries with it the implication that the sick person is not to blame. It may be that there are other behaviors for which people are not responsible. Social determinism, for example, is a theory that, among liberals, accounts for the behavior of the ghetto criminal. Such a theory is not as powerful in removing culpability, however, as is the medical model. A disapproved behavior is considered a disease particularly if it is thought to be "organic." Some conditions, however, may not be organic in their cause even if they are organic in their treatment. Thus, even if a biochemical cause of addiction is rejected, the fact that the addict can be treated with chemical agents convinces some that addiction is a medical problem. Because of the organic—biochemical, physiological, and pharmacological—nature of these treatments, to label a problem as a disease will have an impact on the decision as to the appropriate expert to correct the problem. It could be that the decision that addiction is a disease had already been made when the British appointed a committee of physicians to make policy recommendations in 1926. In contrast the joint ABA-AMA committee implied that addiction might be either a crime or a disease. That it might be a sin, a social deviation, or an acceptable alternative life-style does not appear to have been considered, nor would one expect it to have been in view of the origins of the committee.

The problem of labeling is fundamental in medical ethics. To call something a disease is to enter the realm of value judgments. If a special organic condition is desired, such as healthiness or intelligence, one does not call it a disease. Thus, to call something a disease is to make a value judgment. But is is also to make a policy judgment. It suggests that the possessor of the disease is not responsible for his condition, that he is not personally culpable for his disapproved condition. Other marginal conditions that are thought to be voluntarily caused, such as skiing accidents, lung cancer in smokers, or pregnancy, also create policy problems, for often they are not treated with the same urgency and priority as are conditions that are not thought to be the result of personal choice.

4 STERILIZATION AND THE 120 RULE

Maria Rivera, a 28-year-old born in Puerto Rico, was living in New York City where her husband worked as a serviceman for the telephone company. She had borne two children by Caesarean section, a girl now four and a boy two. She and her husband had decided that they definitely did not want any more children. She went to a New York City hospital clinic wanting to be sterilized. At the clinic she was told that it was the policy of the hospital that the sterilization could not be performed at her age unless she had five children. She asked the nurse about the policy and was eventually referred to Dr. Albert Goodfellow, assistant director of the Family Planning Service. He explained to her the alternative methods of limiting births: the pill, IUD, diaphragm, and condom. He was concerned about the fact that Mrs. Rivera had only two children and that she was rather young to be sterilized. "What would you do if something were to happen to your children?" he asked. "Do you really want to foreclose forever the chance of having any more children of your own?"

Mrs. Rivera explained to Dr. Goodfellow that she was aware of the risk but would never want to go through a Caesarean again no matter what. "God will take care," she said of her children. The other alternatives were just not acceptable. She could not stand the thought of taking a pill every day, and she had heard of friends who became tired after taking them. The thought of wearing an IUD was repulsive. The other methods, she had been told, were not reliable enough.

Dr. Goodfellow, when pressed, explained that the hospital's policy required that the age of the woman, when multiplied by the number of children she had borne, must equal no less than 120. "That is the policy at many hospitals in the area," he added. If a woman was 30, the sterilization would be approved after four children; if she was 25, after five children. "The procedure has some medical risks," the doctor pointed out, "and we don't want you taking those risks unnecessarily."

Mrs. Rivera could not understand the hospital's position. Sterilization in Puerto Rico has been widely known and accepted as a preferred method of permanent contraception for many years. Although she was Catholic, she was not troubled by the morality of the sterilization. None of her friends in Puerto Rico had been either. When she left the hospital, she did not know if it would be possible to scrape up the money to go back to Puerto Rico for the operation.

———————

It is not unusual to stereotype sterilization as an ethics problem in medicine. Certain traditions, including the Roman Catholic, have long objected to sterilization as a "mutilation" and as a morally unacceptable infringement on one of the primary ends of marriage. That issue apparently does not figure in this case, however. Mrs. Rivera, though Catholic, is not bothered by the moral objection. Dr. Goodfellow, a waspish Protestant, does not share the moral objection. In fact, if asked, he probably would say that he considers sterilization a perfectly moral procedure, pointing to the tubal ligations he performs routinely at the clinic. Yet he has reservations in this case. They are partially couched in medical terms: the inherent risks in the surgical procedure. But the basic difference in perspective between the physician and the patient is a more fundamental conflict in value orientation.

Whereas the physicians debating whether to give propoxyphene or methadone for pain relief disagreed over the proper relation of the human being to nature, Mrs. Rivera and Dr. Goodfellow disagree over an equally fundamental value orientation. The upper-middle-class Protestant ethic, which reaches its zenith in the medical profession, is aggressively future-oriented. The physician, after all, has devoted half his life to sacrificing for that day when he will be a practitioner of medicine. It is not surprising, therefore, that Dr. Goodfellow and his colleagues who set hospital policy are reluctant to cut off future options completely by cutting the fallopian tubes.

Mrs. Rivera, in contrast, is less rigorously committed to keeping future options open. She is worried about the present dilemma of raising two children on a meager family income and perhaps about the impact of a pregnancy on her relationship with her husband. The obvious moral problems of the specific case of sterilization do not constitute the significant value inputs into her decision or the doctor's. This does not mean that values are unimportant. They are. The significant values involved are much more subtle, bearing on the significance of present experience in relation to the future, the nature of the family, and the patterns of the subculture.

5 PRESCRIPTION WRITING: GENERIC OR TRADE

Twenty-six-year-old Beth Williams worked as a file clerk for a major insurance company to support her two children. From her salary of $6200 she paid a rent of $140 per month for her rent-controlled apartment. She had been on the waiting list for public housing for two years when she told the following story:

> I have been bothered by this ear infection for about a week. I have been vaguely sick with the flu for several weeks. The ear infection is probably related to or at least a result of lowered resistance. The trouble is in the ear canal, but my ear is oozing and the yellow crust looks awful. I wear a scarf and have changed my hair style so it is not so embarrassing, but then an infection has broken out on my chin. The pain in my ear has been unbearable so I finally called Dr. Foley.
>
> She looked at my ear and said she thought she knew what it was—a strep infection—but she wanted to take some tests. The tests will be back in two days now. She gave me a prescription for something called Achromycin. (I'm allergic to penicillin.) I asked her at the time to give me the cheapest thing that would do the job, but she said, "You don't want to take any chances when an ear is concerned." She was afraid

the cheaper drugs might not work as well. "It's just like refrigerators," she said, "You get what you pay for. Maybe that off brand will be all right, but why take a chance with a company you've never heard of?"

I went to Benton's Pharmacy this morning with the prescription, but the pharmacist said it would cost $8.50 for the seven-day supply. I told him I would get it filled this afternoon after I got paid.

Whether Mrs. Williams will have the prescription filled in the afternoon when she gets paid is anybody's guess. The conflict over generic name prescription-writing which lies at the base of this case is a well-known policy dispute, but the specific value components of the conflict are often unrecognized.

Although she may not think about it explicitly, Dr. Foley is probably acting on the traditional Hippocratic medical ethic that she should do what will benefit the patient. Her reasoning is that even though Mrs. Williams asked for the cheapest thing and a cheaper generic equivalent is available at a fraction of the $8.50 cost, it is a mistake to take chances. Reports that generic name drugs lack the potency of their trade name competitors circulate among physicians and pharmacists, although such reports seem to originate with the trade name manufacturers. Occasionally such differences are documented, as in a recent case of digitalis. Other charges against generic name drugs are that their disintegration in the gastrointestinal tract is not adequately standardized or that conditions of manufacture are not as sanitary. Documentation is difficult, but it is true that governmental inspections are not made often enough to assure quality control of all manufacturers. Some, including Mrs. Williams' physician, reason about drugs the way they reason about appliances. Because the trade name manufacturer has more to lose by producing products of substandard quality, one should play it safe by spending the extra money for the trade name product, at least until such time as standards are more carefully regulated.

Assuming for the moment that the physician's judgment is correct, the question remains whether the physician is doing what will most benefit the patient. If Mrs. Williams does not get the prescription filled in the afternoon, Dr. Foley probably is not doing the best for her—unless one takes the pessimistic position that drugs do more harm than good.

Buried among the technical, pharmacological judgments made by the physician about the relative safety and efficacy of the trade name and generic name products are a number of value judgments. Since the situations of the physician and her patient differ, it is reasonable to suspect that their values may differ as well. Possibly because of her income level, the physician is unimpressed by her patient's request for the cheapest product. For her, the admittedly small degree of extra confidence in the trade name product is worth the extra cost. Mrs. Williams,

g only $6200 as a file clerk, probably places a very different value
$8.50. She may also have a different value orientation of risk-tak-
...g. The gambler, who is optimistic about fate, may be more willing than
others to take chances. Mrs. Williams may also place a different value on
the corporate identity behind the trade name manufacturer and the
proprietary rights represented in their research and patent interests. She
may simply identify more with the generic name enterprise than the
physician does. Finally, even if $8.50 meant the same thing to her that it
does to the physician, which almost certainly it does not, she may have a
different set of priorities about how it should be spent. The physician is
uniquely oriented to medical problems, or she would not have opted to
become a physician. Mrs. Williams, however, may prefer to take the
hypothetical but slightly greater risk with her health in order to spend
the extra money on a movie, a contribution to flood relief, or a rock-and-
roll record. Who is to say which system of values ought to dominate?

CHAPTER 2

Responsibility
for the Decision

The recognition that value components exist in every medical decision leads to a second general problem in medical ethics: who should make the decisions. Before dealing with specific ethical dilemmas in such problematic areas as abortion, transplantation, euthanasia, and elementary health care delivery, one must come to grips with this procedural dilemma. The candidates for decision-maker are many. The relatively simple case is one where the physician and the patient have a difference of opinion on what constitutes the most reasonable or valuable treatment. However, the image of isolated patient interacting with isolated physician is a myth. The patient may belong to a family, whose members also at times figure as decision-makers. The physician may be affiliated with a professional group and a hospital staff, both of which sometimes claim to be the legitimate ethical authority. The physician has pledged loyalty to the profession and is guided by the moral precepts of that profession, as expressed both in the codes of Hippocrates and the American Medical Association and in the less formal, but probably more significant, social pressures which dictate behavior in the less than perfect world of reality.

While both patient and physician are involved in social networks that have a strong influence on their values, attitudes, and behavior, these networks are in turn part of an even larger system, a society with its culture. Laws set limits on the behavior of patient and physician alike. The physician cannot prescribe heroin in the United States; the lay person cannot self-prescribe a long list of taboo chemicals.

Absolutizing the authority of any one of these—the patient, the physician, the lay and professional social networks, and the larger society —would be a moral disaster. If society is to be less than totalitarian, the role of the individual must be preserved; if it is to be less than anarchical, some order must be superimposed from above. In the complex techno-logical society in which modern medicine exists, there must be some dele-gating of authority to those with technical expertise, but if there is to be any semblance of individual responsibility and dignity, the individual must retain significant control over the medical decisions that most directly affect his own welfare. The problem for medical ethics is how to allocate this authority for decision-making when there are conflicting roles and interests.

6 THE DYING INFANT AND THE NEEDS OF OTHERS

A four-day-old infant was currently on a respirator suffering from respi-ratory deficiency that was presumably, but not definitely, related to a diagnosis of trisomy-18, a genetic defect which for unknown reasons causes gross congenital malfunctions. A clinical conference was being held in an attempt to decide what should be done in the case. The partici-pants were the chief pediatrician, a psychiatrist, a social worker, a nurse, and a pediatrics resident.

Trisomy-18, the presence of an extra E chromosome, results in moder-ate to severe mental retardation, intrauterine growth failure, hypertonic-ity, anatomical malformations, particularly of the ears and fingers, cardiac and renal anomalies, rigidity of the body, and variable brain de-formities. Fifty percent of all cases result in death in the first two months; 13 percent live more than a year. There are reports of children reaching three and ten years of age and one report of three patients, all women, reaching adulthood.

The chief of pediatrics at the hospital reported at the conference that he had held several agonizing conversations with the father of the child, who had told him, "If you cannot guarantee my child will be normal, I don't want you to do anything for it." The chief of pediatrics, who was directly responsible for this case because of the nature of the medical and moral syndrome, shared the sympathies of the father. He reported hav-ing told the father, "I promise you that I will do everything in my power to see that your wishes are fulfilled."

The psychiatric consultant reported that he had also spent considerable time with the father. He said that he thought the father was in a phase of acute denial, but that in this case, guilt feelings could create psychiatric problems later if the respirator were turned off at the father's initiative. He pointed out, however, that there are reported cases of guilt on the part of parents who take an infant diagnosed trisomy-18 home from the hospital only to have it die under their care.

The psychiatric social worker reported that contrary to the psychiatrist's characterization of the father, she felt that, in general, the family would be put under extreme stress if the infant were brought home.

At this point in the conference a nurse who had been responsible for the care of the infant while it was in the nursery expressed her outrage. She said that the infant could not be allowed to die by the hand of man but must be given every chance to live. In fact, the nurse said, if no one else would care for the infant, she would do everything to try to adopt her and care for her herself. The Code of Ethics for nurses states: "The nurse's primary commitment is to the patient's care and safety. She must be alert to take appropriate action regarding any instances of incompetent, unethical or illegal practice by any member of the health care team, or any action on the part of others that is prejudicial to the patient's best interests." The code also specifies: "The nurse's respect for the worth and dignity of the individual human being extends throughout the entire life cycle, from birth to death."

Next in the conference a pediatrics resident called attention to the condition of another infant on the ward for whom she was directly responsible. This infant had a slight respiratory difficulty. The resident said that without the respirator the infant would probably have a fifty-fifty chance of some brain damage. She said that she would feel much better if the patient under her care were on a respirator. There were other respirators in the hospital, but all were being used with patients who had a serious and meaningful need for them.

———————

The case bristles with ethical problems. Should the baby be allowed to die under any circumstances? Are the parents the "owners" of their children? How are the needs of the other infant requiring a respirator to be taken into account? The prior question, however, is who should make these difficult decisions.

The potential decision-makers in this case are many. The father, the pediatrician, the psychiatrist, the social worker, the nurse, and the pediatrics resident concerned about another patient all have an interest. Other candidates, never mentioned in the case, are the hospital administrator, the medical board, and the state (through the courts). Still another person with a particularly close interest is surprisingly missing from the medical staff's discussion. One of the most crucial problems in medical ethics is to make sure that all those with relevant interests are involved in the decision-making. All too often medical decisions, perhaps because of their urgent and technical character, are made leaving out those who are most crucially concerned.

In order to know who the appropriate decision-makers might be, it is essential to know what questions are relevant. Certainly every medical decision requires a foundation in the relevant facts. Even here, however, values may be significant. Carefully trained physicians schooled in scientific method are influenced in their observation of what they take to be the facts by their values. While the scientific goal is often to eliminate values, at least at the stage of making observations and knowing the literature, no one, no matter how careful, is ever able to reach that ideal.

Values are even more significant in determining the factual foundation for medical decisions in another way. Determining the relevant facts is itself fundamentally an evaluative process. The psychiatrist's relevant facts may be quite different from the father's, or the pediatrician's. They may differ from the psychiatric social worker's. In this case both the psychiatrist and the psychiatric social worker, who presumably have expertise in observing facts of a similar kind, reach a different reading of the facts. The psychiatrist thinks that the father might later feel guilt if he decides to stop treatment of the baby. The social worker thinks that he might experience guilt if he takes the baby home and it then dies. It could be that they are really recording a slightly different constellation of facts as significant. The social worker may be more oriented to the domestic and familial scene, the psychiatrist to the isolated individual, perhaps emphasizing his psychohistory. Even if one decides that the medical and psychiatric facts are the significant ones—a decision which leaves out most of what is valued in human existence—disagreements will still exist over which medical and psychiatric facts are relevant.

Another kind of fact that could be significant in this case is the legal fact. What are the legal implications of turning off the respirator? Would the pediatrician be guilty of murder if he turned it off? Would he be guilty of treating without consent if he failed to turn if off? What is the legal difference between turning off the respirator and ordering it turned off, or simply watching it be turned off? What is the legal difference between turning it off and failing to turn it on? Or between turning it off on a dying child and turning it off on one who could continue living? These are questions with a substantive moral base. It is also relevant to decision-making to know what in fact the law requires. The physician or parent who acts without awareness of the legal status of his action might be morally certain, but practically he would be a fool. If these facts are relevant, then perhaps lawyers have some role in the decision-making, if not as choice-makers at least as informants.

Other kinds of facts that might be considered more crucial to this case than either the medical or the legal facts are the economic, familial, and social facts. To ignore them, as well as the role of those with relevant factual expertise in these areas, would be a mistake.

Even if one could settle the question of what facts are relevant—a question which itself requires a set of values—the facts alone can never lead to a decision. Every decision requires both a factual premise and an evaluative one, the minor and major premises of the argument respectively. The ethical and other value questions remain in this case even after the relevant facts are known. All the potential decision-makers could hold special ethical positions specifically because of their roles in the case. The father, for example, has a special obligation to his other children, the pediatric resident to the other baby in distress.

Special moral duties are thought to attach to special roles. Some physicians may have or think they have a special duty to "preserve life" or to "do no harm to the patient." Parents may have a special duty to care for their children's interests even if some other child somewhere in the world has a greater need.

Two possibilities exist if there is a perceived special duty of this sort. First, the general public may agree with those in the special role that they should have a special set of moral obligations. Second, members of the special group may tend to perceive and accept their special moral obligations while the general public does not accept them, even for those in the special role. In either case, direct, predictable conflict will result. If the lay persons, the parents in this case, do not accept the claim of special moral obligations assigned to the role of the physician, they will logically claim that those filling the role should be disqualified as biased when it comes to making the decision. If, on the contrary, they accept the importance of special ethical norms attached to the role but, as individuals who are not in that role, feel that they should act on different norms, then there will still be conflict. The parent may feel that it is a safeguard for the physician always to act to preserve life, but that from his own perspective as a nonphysician, not operating under that norm, the proper decision might well be different. The physician could make the same argument about the special value perspective of the parents.

One conclusion is inevitable. Expertise on the facts, or still less on one aspect of the facts, in no way necessarily makes one an expert on the values that are required to reach a decision. In fact, if expertise on one kind of facts carries with it a special set of ethical norms or a special interpretation of more universally shared norms, the expert may well make systematically skewed decisions. What is needed is some source of authority for the value inputs before determining who should make the decision.

The quest for expertise on values is a difficult one, involving an understanding of just what constitutes that expertise. In a complex technological society it is unlikely that even if such expertise on values could be found, it would reside in the same person who has expertise on the facts. There is no evidence that value expertise uniformly comes from long experience with a particular problem. In some cases, to be sure, those who have confronted a problem and have had a chance to reflect on it will be in a better position to see the ethical implication of alternative courses of action. Yet experience may bring monotony. The thousandth suffering, dying human being cannot be the same as the first. Whether the person who has seen the thousand dying patients is more or less sensitive to the needs of the last one than he was of the first one will depend on his own character, the nature of his setting, and countless other factors. On balance, it seems necessary to recognize that experience can inure as well as sensitize.

The quest for an expert on ethics may turn to other significant roles: the local clergyman, the judge, the legislator, or Plato's philosopher-king. Each has a special expertise. The clergyman may instruct the communicant about the position of his own tradition on some nuanced medical dilemma; the judge and the legislator can inform him of public opinion and group tradition. They may have some wisdom as well, but empirical evidence is difficult in these days. The philosopher is skilled in analyzing the implications of various classical ethical theories—of the attractions of utilitarian or formalist here, the dangers of legalism or situationalism there. But when it comes to the point of choosing a set of ethical and other values for deciding a specific problem, such as the plight of the baby dying of trisomy-18, it may be dangerous to assign ethical expertise to any of these roles.

There are two solutions to this problem of ethical expertise and human freedom. In the more authoritarian society, an effort is made to institutionalize wisdom. Plato's philosopher-king or the benevolent lord of the manor is granted the role of the wise man of society. Even in American society, which minimizes authoritarianism in ideal if not in fact, the Supreme Court judge is still thought of as a possessor of wisdom. He stands beyond the masses, presumably making judgments based on the Greek virtue of prudence.

The other solution is to abandon the search for the uniquely wise as such. The egalitarian society finds this alternative more attractive. To deny that one can readily identify the unique possessors of wisdom is not the same as to deny that values are rooted in a reality beyond individual and group taste. It is possible to hold that right and wrong, good and bad, are grounded in reality and still to maintain that no uniquely wise people have special skills in knowing the right and wrong. Thus, democratic theory is in part an epistemology, a way of knowing, in which no one individual's reading of ethical and other values is taken as identifiably superior to anyone else's.

These two extreme solutions—authoritarianism and radical egalitarianism—are in their pure form never the basis for medical decision-making. Several limitations are required, both in theory and in practice. At the theoretical level, it is not clear whether people always desire to base their decisions on the wisest and soundest values. Consider the case of the child learning how to spend his money. The parent may know that an expenditure is foolish, that the child will not value the purchase for more than a passing minute. But there is value in restraining even the benevolent authoritarian hand. Likewise in medical decisions. Even if signing out of a hospital against medical advice seems foolish not only to physicians but to lay persons who know of the case, we still think it crucial to protect the patient's individual freedom to sign out. The reason may be our belief that in the long run, in the majority of cases, the patient knows his own set of values better than anyone else. Or it may be our belief in the higher value of human freedom, even in those cases where we are confident that the individual is behaving unwisely. The choice of the proper authority for decision-making will have to reflect the value placed on human freedom.

At the practical level, it is not necessary to take a referendum to determine the most appropriate values for every decision. Nor is it necessary or even possible to consult with the patient to determine his values in every medical decision. Even if no experts in values can be identified and human freedom is considered fundamental, the ordinary, everyday decisions made in all contexts, including the medical context, can proceed on the assumption of many obvious and shared values. It is reasonable for the physician to assume that the patient wants to continue living, at least if he can continue living without significant physical or psychological suffering, unless the patient informs him to the contrary. Deciding who shall be the appropriate decision-maker must take into account the criterion of efficiency as well as of human freedom.

Finally, although human freedom is considered fundamental in the modern West, it is not absolute. Especially in cases where the patient is incompetent, other decision-makers are both justified and essential. In all but the most anarchical society, some limits are placed on human freedom. The society, as well as the community which is society on a more limited level, has a legitimate role, not only in protecting those who cannot protect themselves but also in setting limits—limits on the use of drugs, on sexual behavior, on the pronouncing of death—even if the case is currently being made that there should be no such thing as a crime without a victim. Society certainly has a role in setting limits on behavior affecting others: abandoning the helpless, medicating the insane, or consuming the scarce resources.

Deciding who will make the medical decisions and who will choose the values on which those decisions are based requires a full exploration of all these questions. It is not sufficient to know what the relevant facts are and who has the relevant technical knowledge. It is also essential to know what ethical and other values are at stake, what ethical expertise pertains to those values, and whether the real concern is expertise at all. It will then become apparent, as in the case of the father telling the physician he does not want treatment continued with the trisomy-18 baby, that there are many others whose involvement in the case is significant.

The Patient and the Physician

The simplest sort of conflict over whose values should dominate in making medical decisions is the conflict between the isolated individual physician and his isolated individual patient. Probably no case, however, can be reduced to this pure form of the patient-physician relationship. Moreover, the value inputs themselves are often not recognized because they are not brought fully to the surface.

7   BUT, DOCTOR, I'D RATHER HAVE SALT

Samuel Jordan, 64 years old, had been active for most of his life but was now in semi-retirement. He was in the midst of his annual physical examination when his physician found a blood pressure of 155/90, somewhat above the normal 120/80. The physician did not seem particularly alarmed, for the patient did not have a history of hypertension. He instructed Mr. Jordan that the only thing he must do was to cut his use of salt drastically, a standard recommendation for reducing fluid accumulation and thereby blood pressure. He told Mr. Jordan that this would surely help. The doctor would watch the blood pressure carefully in future examinations, and if necessary, there was a drug, chlorothiazide, that could be used. The drug would help to eliminate sodium and chloride, but he did not want to use it now because there were certain risks: nausea, vomiting, dizziness, occasional muscle cramps, and potassium loss.

Mr. Jordan returned home and began to follow faithfully the "doctor's orders." He soon found life very unpleasant, however, without the salt that he had used and loved for his sixty-four years. The next week he called the physician and said that in his opinion the possible benefits from the salt-free diet were not worth the miseries and that he wanted to begin taking the drug. The physician still had severe doubts about the wisdom of drug use at this point, suspecting that Mr. Jordan was simply not willing to make the sacrifice necessary for the good of his health, but she also recognized that some physicians would at this point go ahead and prescribe the drug. The physician contemplated what he should do.

----

1. Presumably the physician's value commitment is to preserving the patient's health. What values dominate the patient's position? How

can the significance of those values be compared to the value of health?

2. Are there any significant differences between the two over the relevant facts?

3. Suppose that the doctor knows of a colleague in town who routinely prescribes chlorothiazide rather than placing the patient on a salt-free diet. Should he refer Mr. Jordan to him, should he insist that Mr. Jordan continue on the salt-free diet, or should he simply withdraw from the case?

4. Suppose that the doctor is aware that some physicians would prescribe the chlorothiazide but is also confident that there are none who would do so within a convenient distance. How does that change the physician's options and obligations?

5. Suppose that the procedure upon which some patient insists is not a prescription to replace a salt-free diet but one to induce an abortion or to hasten death in what the patient thinks is a miserable existence. Assuming that the physician has strong moral objection, what should he do in these cases?

6. Are any others conceivably affected by the choice between the salt-free diet and chlorothiazide? How would it affect the decision-making if there were?

The Family

Although in the last case the only ones involved in the decision were presumably the physician and his patient, the patient could have had a spouse or other dependents, who would have had a relevant interest in his health. Often this is the case. The family plays a central role in many decisions made by or for the patient. The family of a child or a senile patient may be the most important lay people involved in the case. The family's interest is not limited to protecting their own economic and social welfare. The bonds between family members are typically close. Family members are given rights and responsibilities unthought of for those outside the family.

8 FAMILY CONFLICT OVER A LEG AMPUTATION

Sadie Nemser, a widow 80 years of age, had been a resident of the Jewish Home and Hospital for the Aged in New York City from May 1964 until August 22, 1966. She had a history of arteriosclerotic heart disease and had suffered at least three strokes and an equal number of attacks of pneumonia. On August 22, in a medical emergency, she was moved and admitted to Beth Israel Hospital, where she had been ever since. Her condition was diagnosed as "diabetic and arteriosclerotic gangrene . . . with infection . . . extensive gangrene of the right foot and heel with inflammatory reaction about both areas." The attending physicians thought an above-the-knee amputation was probably preferable but, in view of Mrs. Nemser's general condition, suggested amputation above the ankle. Dr. George Lowen, under whose care Mrs. Nemser was admitted to the hospital, expressed the opinion that "If delay ensues, further physical deterioration will surely occur. . . . If the deterioration is allowed to progress, death will follow."

Mrs. Nemser said she wanted no part of any amputation. She wanted to live, but she also wanted to retain her foot. An attending psychiatrist at Beth Israel Hospital examined her and reported that she was "not capable of understanding the nature of any permit for surgery that she might be asked to sign." As a result, neither the hospital nor the surgeon would proceed with the recommended operation unless consent was obtained from the patient's next of kin.

Mrs. Nemser had three sons who were her next of kin. Two of them, one a lawyer, were willing to consent to the amputation. The third son, Harold, a practicing physician in New York City, refused to approve the operation. Because of this disagreement, the case went to court.

On September 9, 1966, a preliminary hearing was held. Dr. Lowen filed an affidavit, again maintaining, "The recommended operation is distinctly a matter of the difference between life and death for Mrs. Nemser." The court appointed Richard Green as her guardian *ad litem* or for this proceeding and Dr. Abraham Franzblau as the court's psychiatrist. Dr. Franzblau discussed the case with Mrs. Nemser's two other medical consultants, Drs. Friedman and Schwartz, and with Mrs. Nemser herself. He also spoke to Norman, the lawyer son, and Harold, the physician son, and with the court-appointed guardian. He stated in his report:

1. Some difference of opinion exists as to:
   (a) whether the proposed operation is essential to prolong or save Mrs. Nemser's life;
   (b) the prognosis if it is done, or on the other hand, not done; and
   (c) whether the patient's mental status is such that she can understand the proposed procedure, and the significance of any consent that she might give.

2. Both of Mrs. Nemser's sons whom I interviewed appear to be motivated by love for their mother and a wish to see her life prolonged, free of pain and discomfort. Norman, the lawyer, is influenced by the opinions of the medical consultants whom he has brought in that a transmalleolar amputation would arrest the spread of the infection and gangrene, and prolong his mother's life. Harold, the physician, is doubtful of his mother's ability to tolerate anesthesia and surgery, and hopes that, treated conservatively and kept "clean," the gangrenous parts would slough off through auto-amputation. The disagreement between the brothers appears to be further clouded by long-standing

familial differences over the support and management of their mother, and over the question of the adequacy of her medical care up to the present episode.

3. There appears to be no disagreement among Drs. Friedman and Schwartz, that:

(a) The recommended procedure as proposed is not a life-saving measure, nor is it a medical emergency

(b) Its effectiveness is by no means assured

(c) The same condition may recur in the stump, after surgery, since such wounds heal notoriously poorly in diabetics

(d) There is no likelihood of ever applying a prosthesis or achieving ambulation in this patient

(e) There is very little possibility of proceeding ultimately to do the mid-thigh amputation, which is considered as a second and ultimately beneficial stage, in such cases

4. The patient is clearly unable to understand the situation or to render informed consent. (I agree completely with the opinion of Dr. Weiss as to her mental status.) *However, she is aware of her bodily integrity and wants no amputation of any part of her. She wants both to live and to retain her limb, and is not clearly aware of the conflict implicit in these alternatives.* Pressed to make a decision, she would be willing to leave it to the doctors, but she would not do so with a clear mind or perception. Her consciousness of pain is mercifully diminished by the partial oblivion which has intervened in her condition.

Accordingly, I do not believe that intervention on the part of the Court is indicated.

Richard Green, the court-appointed guardian, filed another report reaching the same conclusions. Both agreed that Mrs. Nemser was not capable of making for herself an informed judgment of whether the operation should be performed. Both, however, recommended that under the circumstances intervention by the court was not warranted. The judge was now faced with two sons demanding that their mother's life be saved, one son also requesting that the operation not be performed, in part because of the risks of the procedure itself and in part because he wanted to respect her wishes not to have her foot amputated, a physician who said it was a life-and-death matter, two others who were not convinced it was so, a psychiatrist and a lawyer claiming she was not capable of making an informed judgment but nevertheless believing she should not be ordered to undergo the amputation, and finally, a senile suffering woman who said she wanted both to live *and* to retain her limb.[1]

A significant point about this case is that it has gone to court. All agree, at least by implication, that the judge is the one who should make the decision. But to whose opinions should he give weight? And what does this imply for a case that does not reach the courts?

The case shows, first, that in spite of the fact that the hospital psychiatrist has concluded that Mrs. Nemser is incapable of understanding the nature of a permit for surgery and three physicians have apparently all recommended the amputation, one of them believing it is a life-and-death matter, they do not act on their own. The seek the permission of the next of kin and, ultimately, the court. Legally at least, and most would say morally, physicians do not have the power to determine that Mrs. Nemser will be treated. Even if they are convinced that she is not competent to judge for herself and the treatment is necessary to save her life, they still must obtain some kind of consent.

The case also shows that the physicians feel empowered to turn to the relatives for permission once they have judged Mrs. Nemser incompetent. This is a terribly important decision to thrust on the family, especially a family in disagreement on the care of the mother. Medical personnel routinely turn to relatives for permission to treat in such cases. Whether that can be justified, morally or legally, without a court determination of incompetency is questionable. What, for instance, if the physicians plus all three brothers agreed to the surgery? What if the physician son was not in the picture? Does this imply that physician and next of kin may overrule the patient's own wishes? Even those who would maintain that the next of kin is the most appropriate candidate for decision-maker in cases where the patient is not competent must grant that the assumption of that decision-making power can, in some cases, be abused. While all three brothers are apparently acting with their mother's best interest in mind, that is not always the case. Some consideration must be given to the process that transfers the decision-making authority.

Finally, the case shows how seriously Mrs. Nemser's admittedly muddled and perhaps confused views are taken. In what is probably a typical case, the physicians, the hospital, the sons, and especially the court take her own position to be very important. Although admittedly the physician feels that he has the authority to turn to the next of kin for an overriding consent, and this would probably be sufficient had not one of the brothers objected, still great respect is shown for the patient's position. Had she, in equal confusion and incompetence, been demanding that the leg be amputated, the result certainly would have been different.

Besides revealing certain things about the state of the law and of medical practice when the patient's decision-making competency is questioned, the case also reveals something about the ethical problem of who should have decision-making authority in cases when the patient is incapable of deciding for herself. By custom, if not by legal authority, the hospital and the court both turn to the members of her family. The family, the next of kin, has a central place in deciding, once the patient is not capable. This can create problems. Although no evidence exists in this case, in other cases relatives have made malicious or foolish decisions, perhaps with their own interests in mind. In addition, fear is often expressed that the psychic burden of making critical decisions is too great to force upon relatives. It is an even crueler burden to inflict upon family members who are already under the strain of having a loved one critically ill. According to this view, someone else, presumably the physician, should carry the burden of being the decision-maker.

But an argument can also be made for the importance of the family's role as agent for the patient when that patient is incapable of making decisions. The decision made for the no longer competent patient should approximate as closely as possible the decision that patient would have made had he been able to decide for himself. The decision should incorporate the value and belief system of the patient. Especially in a case such as this, where Mrs. Nemser is taken to Beth Israel Hospital in an emergency and has no long-standing relationship with the physicians, the family members are normally in the best position to know those values and to act on them. Still, family members may sometimes act maliciously or foolishly or the psychic strain may be too much and the family may become incapable of acting coherently. In such cases the backup of court intervention at the request of the physician, relative, or other person interested in the patient's welfare is always available. At least in situations where there is no dire emergency, some would argue that the family members must have a central role as agent for the patient in the decision-making.

The problem then arises of the patient who is a child or is mentally retarded, that is, the patient who has never been competent. It seems less plausible to argue that the next of kin should be the patient's agent because he is in the best position to know the patient's system of values and belief. Proponents of the central role of the family as agent for the patient may have a stronger argument, which applies equally well to cases where the patient has never been in a position to develop a set of beliefs and values of his own. The family is clearly one of the fundamental institutions of society. The bonds joining family members are among the strongest of the human species, even in the highly fragmented, mobile society of the West. It is they, after all, who gather at the critical times of sickness. Even if siblings have not communicated for years, they are often the first to respond in a time of crisis. At least in those cases where the patient is incapable of making his own decisions and where there is no clear evidence that the patient has expressed a wish about what treatment he would choose, the primary objective must be to do what is in the interest of the patient. The bond that joins family members is one of responsibility, including a mutual responsibility to protect one another's welfare. Unless there is evidence that this responsibility is not being fulfilled, the next of kin is in the most reliable position to act on behalf of the patient. It is their responsibility, as well as their right—or so the proponents of the role of the family in decision-making would argue.

This case, in which relatives of equal degree of kinship disagree, cannot be resolved by debating the importance of the role of the family, unless one is to conclude that the family has no role whatsoever. It would seem crass to appeal to a simple majority vote principle. Perhaps, therefore, in cases where disagreement is sharp and the decision is critical, as in Mrs. Nemser's case, elevating the decision to the more formal process of the court is the safest and most prudent course to follow.

The Hospital and the Medical Staff

As in the case of Mrs. Nemser, where the hospital along with the surgeon refused to proceed with the operation until the consent question had been settled, the hospital and its personnel have a stake in decisions in medicine. The fact that the physicians as well as the family members disagreed about what should be done suggests that there are still unresolved questions about the role of the hospital and the medical staff in the decision. One question involves the relation of the individual physician to the medical staff. Another concerns his relation to the official policies of the hospital where he has privileges.

9   THE HOSPITAL ABORTION PANEL

Anna Hiller was pregnant for the fifth time. She was terribly distraught. With four children ages five years down to fourteen months, another would be too much to handle on the meager income from her husband's work as a foreman in a paper plant. On May 4, 1971, as soon as she was sure she was pregnant, she went to the obstetrician who had delivered her other children, pleading, "Isn't there something that can be done?"

Dr. Melman was troubled. He agreed that another child would be a great hardship on the Hillers. Mrs. Hiller burst out in tears of desperation as she told Dr. Melman of a recent incident in which the two-year-old had knocked over a vase while the baby was screaming. Although she had always been a tense person, she had been reasonably normal both physically and mentally before the birth of the children. The marriage was fairly stable, given the stress that the couple was under.

The abortion law in the state of California at the time provided that abortion was legal only if there was a substantial risk that continuance of the pregnancy would gravely impair the physical or mental health of the mother, or the pregnancy had resulted from rape or incest. Impairment of mental health was defined as "mental illness to the extent that the woman is dangerous to herself or to the person or property of others or is in need of supervision or restraint."

Dr. Melman paused and then asked Mrs. Hiller if she thought that there was any danger she might harm or neglect her other children if she had another baby. Mrs. Hiller did not understand at first, then realized that she should say there was a danger. The problem, Dr. Melman pointed out, was that according to the law in California, the abortion committee at County Hospital, where he had hospital privileges, would have to approve the procedure. Since Mrs. Hiller was now in what they calculated to be her thirteenth week of pregnancy, the unanimous approval of the three members of the committee was required. Dr. Melman would recommend the abortion. The abortion committee was made up of Dr. O'Brien, a psychiatrist; Dr. Mills, an obstetrician; and Dr. Levenson, a cardiologist who had a special interest in problems in medical ethics.

On the morning of May 12, Dr. Melman presented the case. The vote was two to one against authorizing the procedure.

1. For what reason does the law require the abortion committee to be made up entirely of physicians?
2. How were the committee members probably chosen? How should such a committee be chosen, if it should exist at all?
3. Suppose that the one vote in favor of the abortion is cast by the psychiatrist. What relevant expertise do the committee members bring to the decision? From each of their fields of training what might be contributed to oppose the abortion?
4. Suppose that the psychiatrist, Dr. O'Brien, is Catholic. Should persons with religious objections to abortion be excluded from the committee?
5. Suppose that Dr. Levenson is Jewish. In view of the fact that orthodox Jews tend to oppose abortion, while Jewish physicians as a group tend to favor abortion more strongly than other religious groups, how should this information affect Dr. Levenson's appointment to the committee?

10   THE HOSPITAL'S RIGHT TO REFUSE AN ABORTION

Jane Doe became pregnant on February 4, 1973. She was scheduled for an abortion in a Madison, Wisconsin, clinic on April 4 but could not keep the appointment because of a severe snowstorm. Her personal physician then referred her to Dr. Herbert Santmire, who performed an examination on April 19. He determined, after consultation with the patient, that in his judgment the patient's pregnancy should be terminated in a hospital.

Practical conditions, such as time, distance, and expense, normally limited Dr. Santmire's practice to Green Bay hospitals, and he had practiced his profession at Bellin Memorial Hospital for a number of years. He therefore contacted St. Vincent Hospital, St. Mary's Hospital, and Bellin Memorial, the only Green Bay hospitals with suitable facilities, to request their use for the operation, but in each instance his request was refused.

The policy of Bellin Memorial, a private, nonsectarian institution, was to restrict abortions to cases where pregnancy would seriously threaten the health or life of the mother or would result in the delivery of an infant with grave and irreparable physical deformity or mental retardation, or cases where pregnancy had resulted from legally established rape or incest. The hospital was regulated by the state, received funding from the federal government under the Hill-Burton Act, and provided medical services to residents of Northeastern Wisconsin for both the state of Wisconsin and the United States government.[2]

---

1. Does a private institution, sectarian or not, have the right to act upon its moral judgment even when that action may infringe upon the rights of others as established by law?
2. What is the relevance of the fact that the hospital receives government funding and regulation? Would a public hospital have the right to refuse medical services it finds morally objectionable, such as abortion or sterilization?
3. If a hospital can refuse a procedure clearly stereotyped as ethically controversial, can it also refuse other procedures, such as prolonged intensive treatment of an elderly patient with multiple heart attacks, on the ground that such treatment is inconsistent with its values?
4. What is the relevance of the fact that there are no hospitals in the area willing to permit the abortion?
5. What if there was no physician in the hospital willing to perform the abortion? If a hospital can be forced to make its facilities available because there are no others, can an individual physician also be forced to perform a procedure in violation of his moral conviction when no other physicians are available?

The Medical Community and Society

In the most complex cases, those that probably best approximate the world of reality, neither just the medical personnel nor the hospital board of directors but many other candidates compete for a decision-making role. The hospital committee may not be made up entirely of medical professionals, as it was in the case of the California abortion committee, and disagreements can arise over the extent to which lay people should be involved in its work. The medical colleagues, the local community, and the larger society all have a role in decision-making in different contexts.

These broader social units can be seen, on the one hand, as tampering with the sacredness of the individual patient-physician relationship but, on the other, as providing a necessary check on the radical extremes of those with biased or otherwise specialized interests.

11   THE CHOICE OF A TRANSPLANT COMMITTEE

University Hospital was at the time one of the three major centers experimenting with cadaver kidney transplants. The transplant team had done 172 cadaver transplants. It had now achieved a rate of 48 percent functionally successful cadaver transplants at three years after the time of the transplant. Until this time its work had been considered experimental. Cases had been carefully selected, limited to adults who could give their reasonably informed consent for the surgery, and financed entirely by grants from the National Institutes of Health.

The transplant team, headed by Dr. Clark Churchill, felt that it was now ready to consider cadaveric kidney transplantation as a standard therapeutic procedure in cases where suitable living, related donors were not readily available. Dr. Churchill was worried about one critical problem, how to select recipients who could potentially benefit from the transplant from among the estimated 10,000 persons per year dying of kidney disease in the United States alone. After a staff meeting on the subject, Dr. Churchill prepared the following memo to the administrator of the hospital and the dean of the medical school with which the hospital was affiliated, about a proposed kidney transplant review committee:

Following our Renal Transplantation Coordinating Committee meeting of last Tuesday and the decision to make cadaveric renal transplantation a standard therapeutic procedure at University Hospital, we believe it is essential that a committee be established which we have tentatively named the "Transplantation Review Committee." Selection of the limited number of recipients from the vast numbers available will require careful screening. We feel, as the medical team directly responsible for patient care, that the individual surgeons should not have sole responsibility. We have prepared a list of potential candidates for the committee and urge you to make appointments as soon as possible, presumably in time for approval of the board meeting a week from Monday. A consensus was established on the first group of candidates for the committee. Attached you will find a minority report which, frankly, reflects a different philosophy for the committee. The majority of the renal team feel that the smaller committee, made up of the following persons directly involved in patient care, can work most efficiently and harmoniously:
1. Dr. Clark Churchill, head, renal transplant team
2. Dr. Sidney Duff, chief resident, nephrology
3. Dr. Michael Donaldson, pediatric nephrology

4. Dr. Gunther Lowenbaum, psychiatry

5. Rev. Malcolm Hortimer, hospital chaplain

The purpose of the committee, as indicated in our previous discussion, will be to select the candidates for kidney transplantation. Please see the minority report from Dr. James which is attached.

The minority statement on a transplant review committee, prepared by Dr. Vincent James, read as follows:

While the majority of the renal transplant team believes that the proposed committee of four physicians and the hospital chaplain will function efficiently and responsibly in selecting kidney recipients, I have reservations on two grounds. First I am not convinced that any committee should choose who shall receive cadaveric organs. Our committee considered four methods of allocation of cadaveric organs:
1. Medical need (predicted added years of survival)
2. Total benefits to be gained by the transplant (including contributions to family members and the rest of society)
3. Strictly first-come-first-served basis
4. Random selection

The selection among these mechanisms has not as yet been resolved. Only the second method, i.e., selection of the recipient on the basis of his potential value to his family and society, would require a formal committee mechanism. Some more limited choices might be required if the criterion were medical need or even if the principle were first-come-first-served, in case disputes arose about whether preference would be given on the basis of first to manifest symptoms, first to come under the care of the renal team, or first to have clear evidence of a transplant need.

I believe there is no need for a committee of the type proposed. Their one function would be to choose who would be most deserving of the needed organs. They are not in any particularly good position to make such judgments. Instead I believe that there should be a much broader committee whose primary purpose would be to set guidelines for the operation of the Renal Transplant Unit. Should they decide that some balancing of selection principles is required, then they should continue reviewing candidates on a case-by-case basis. I urge you to consider the following as possible committee members; I believe the role of the members of the transplant team itself should be very minimal:
1. Lewis Hayes, R.N., nurse from Psychiatry
2. Dr. Sidney Duff (assuming he disqualified himself from cases in which he was directly involved; his main function should be that of technical consultant to the committee)
3. A representative of the city's Kidney Foundation
4. Dr. Paula Meles, assistant professor of philosophy
5. Herbert Wolf, accountant in a local bank (who received a cadaveric graft in the hospital's experimental program)
6. George Milkovitch, regional Medicare/Medicaid assistant director

7. Florence Lewin, lawyer, American Civil Liberties Union
8. Walter Morgante, chairman, City Council Health and Hospitals Committee
9. Ernestine Samuel, NAACP Health Action Committee
10. Chairman, University Hospital Community Advisory Board (ex officio)

I strongly urge that the medical representation on the committee be kept to an absolute minimum. The dilemmas to be faced, including the choice of which criteria should be used for selection and who best meets those criteria that are not strictly medical, must be placed outside the hands of the renal transplant team.

12 AMPHETAMINE QUOTAS AND MEDICAL FREEDOM

George Walters, a 43-year-old, was seeing the physician for the first time. The primary reason for the visit was that his present 225 lbs. on a 5'9" frame made him grossly overweight. Also, Mr. Walters was worried about what he described as his inability to get anything done any more.

Mr. Walters, a believer in the Protestant ethic, had always been an aggressive insurance salesman. He used to spend his evenings calling on potential clients, but during the past few years he had simply been too tired to go out and make the house calls, so that now his insurance business had dwindled to a fraction of what it was formerly.

The physician, after a thorough physical examination, found no organic illness that would account for either the overweight or the continual tiredness. In response to the physician's suggestion that dietary control and exercise were the most appropriate treatments, Mr. Walters indicated that prior attempts at dieting had been unsuccessful. He asked if he could be given some "Dexedrine diet pills," having often heard that they not only helped in weight loss but also might help in overcoming tiredness.

At this point the physician expressed reservations. In the first place, he was not convinced that amphetamines were the most appropriate dietary treatment, although he was among those physicians who still believed that they had a positive clinical effect in weight reduction. Furthermore, it seemed implausible that the side-effect of the stimulation of the central nervous system would help Mr. Walters overcome his tiredness. The physician considered psychiatric referral, thinking the tiredness might represent a symptom of a more profound depression. Further conversations with the patient, however, turned up no corroborating evidence for recommending that he seek psychiatric help. The physician began to be convinced that, in this case, amphetamine treatment would be worth a try and would quite possibly benefit the patient.

However, there were other problems. Within the past year the Drug

Abuse Task Force had proposed and the County Medical Society had adopted a strongly worded policy statement that "amphetamine use should be greatly limited among physicians in this county." The society recognized only two legitimate uses for amphetamines: narcolepsy, and hyperkinesis in children. Although Mr. Walters was complaining of tiredness, the physician felt that the diagnosis of narcolepsy could not be made in the strict sense. He was concerned about the moral and perhaps legal pressure that might be brought by the County Medical Society if he wrote a prescription which in all likelihood would not accord with the policy of his colleagues in similar cases.

At the same time, the Federal Bureau of Narcotics and Dangerous Drugs had announced a second major reduction in amphetamine quotas for the United States. Mr. Walters, an intelligent man, was aware that amphetamines were not popular among either the medical profession or government policy-makers, but he had thought over the alternatives carefully. Since the use of the drug would help him to a more productive life, he felt that he should have the right to use it under his doctor's care. Thus, there were at least four potential decision-makers concerned with amphetamine use: the patient, the physician, the professional group, and the government.

1. Which of the four potential decision-makers should have a voice in the final decision, and on what grounds?
2. When the patient and his physician disagree about a course of therapy, what are the relevant considerations, and how should a decision be reached?
3. Under what circumstances, if any, does the state have the right to forbid the use of drugs by an individual? Why is it that the prohibition of the drug alcohol required a constitutional amendment because of infringing upon the freedom of the individual, yet for amphetamines and other drugs controlled by prescription, administrative agencies in the government can restrict the individual's use even without specific legislative authorization?
4. When a physician differs with his professional colleagues about the appropriateness of a treatment, especially when the disagreement is rooted in differences about values in the choice of a treatment, how should such a conflict be resolved? What regulative authority, if any, should be placed in the hands of a professional body?
5. How does regulation by a professional group differ from regulation by a government agency?
6. Is there a constitutional or moral right to self-medication? To the use of drugs when necessary to be productive or to fulfill other felt moral obligations? For any other purpose?

7. Should a patient have the moral right to know of differences in attitude among professionals about the use of drugs?

13 THE PHYSICIAN AND COMMUNITY CONTROL

"Health care for the people! Goldberg must go!" was the cry from the picket line outside the Washington Hospital Pediatrics Department. The pickets included most of the young pediatricians at Washington Hospital, a city hospital on the city's south side serving a community of 400,000, primarily blacks and Puerto Ricans. The hospital had been built in 1874, and its 384 beds now lined the walls of antiquated, graying wards.

No one questioned Dr. Daniel Goldberg's competency as a pediatrician. Community and staff discontent, however, had led to demands for his resignation. The Young Lords (a radical group of young Puerto Ricans), the Black Panthers, and other groups claiming to represent the community were demanding better medical care and community control of the hospital. Black and Puerto Rican militants had formed the People's Health Alliance to fight for a hospital more responsive to the people's needs. The interns and residents had developed a reputation as political activists. In the Pediatrics Department all but four of these junior physicians had formed what they called the Pediatrics Group. Two female residents and two foreign-trained physicians had not joined the group. Although themselves predominantly Jewish, members of the Pediatrics Group were supporting demands of the Young Lords and the People's Health Alliance for a black or Puerto Rican head of the department. They argued that Dr. Goldberg, who was a Jew, was insensitive to minority group interests.

Washington Hospital was under the administrative control of Jewish Medical College. The protests were directed in part at the domination of the hospital by the medical school and at the use of the hospital as a training ground for physicians who would later move to suburban Jewish communities to practice medicine. Dr. Goldberg, who currently earned $54,000 (his colleagues said he could easily earn twice that much in private practice), had been chairman for the past nine years, building the staff and services with innovative outpatient programs. He had fought with the city for more funds to upgrade the services and readily admitted that the quality of care was still far below what the community had a right to expect.

After several months of internal meetings and protests, the Pediatrics Group had set up a picket line demanding more radical changes. They were staffing the pediatrics ward and clinics only on an emergency basis with the assistance of the People's Health Alliance. In addition to their own demand for a new department chairman, they were supporting the demands of the community group for a wage increase for hospital workers, more home care, a community-staffed nursery for children of staff and patients, a 24-hour "grievance table," and "total self-determination of all health services through a community-worker board."

A Lay Advisory Board had been in existence at Washington Hospital since 1966. Appointed by the hospital director, it included representatives of the area churches, the community chest, and poverty agencies, as well as seven members appointed to represent the community. The board had met only once in the last year. During the crisis over Dr. Goldberg's position they had not met at all, but several members had publicly supported the demands of the community groups. The People's Health Alliance had protested the appointment of the Lay Advisory Board by the hospital director, who was a black, arguing that only "safe" appointments had been made.

In an interview Dr. Goldberg said, "Politics and medical care don't mix. I'm for greater community participation, but not at the expense of chaos in health care for the children of the community."

---

1. Is the appointment of the head of a pediatrics department a medical or a sociopolitical decision? Can ethnic identity be a legitimate criterion for selecting a person for such a position?
2. What ethical problems are created by the working arrangement between the Washington Hospital and the medical school? What should be the medical school's proper role in department head appointments if it is to maintain an administrative role in Washington Hospital?
3. What is the proper role for a community board in such decisions? Should it be only advisory or should it have more direct administrative authority?
4. If the community is to have a role in such decisions, how should the spokesmen for the community be selected? Which of the following criteria would be most acceptable: residence or employment in the hospital community, membership in community agencies, membership in the community at large, and representation of special interests such as youth and the elderly?
5. What ought to be the role of unofficial social and political groups in the community, such as the Young Lords, the Black Panthers, and the People's Health Alliance?
6. Try to formulate a set of working rules for a community board of a hospital, indicating its composition, function, and limitations.
7. How ought such a community board relate to the hospital's board of trustees, the medical board made up of all the senior physicians, the hospital director, the department heads, the nursing staff, and the housekeeping staff?

PART TWO

PRINCIPLES OF
MEDICAL ETHICS

CHAPTER 3

Duty to
the Patient
and Society

One of the most significant issues in medical ethics is the conflict between
the physician's duty to the individual and to society. Although other potential decision-makers may experience this conflict, the strain exists most
dramatically in the role of the physician, or of the medical professional in
general. The patient has his own set of interests and responsibilities,
which occasionally may raise a conflict between his duty to an individual
and to society or to some particular group. But the physician faces such
ethical dilemmas with greatest regularity. This does not mean that the
physician must always be the one to resolve the dilemma; the solution
may rest with the legislature, for example, or the physician's employer.
Even then, however, it is the physician's role that usually produces the
moral dilemma.

   Historically the Western physician has seen his duty in highly individual terms. In the Hippocratic oath the physician pledges to do what he
thinks will benefit the sick. Hippocratic ethics not only permits but
requires exclusive attention to the needs of the individual. When the physician Rieux in Camus' *The Plague* is questioned about the intensity of
his commitment to his suffering patients, he responds: "For the moment
I know this; there are sick people and they need curing. Later on, perhaps, they'll think things over; and so shall I. But what's wanted now is
to make them well. I defend them as best I can, that's all." Ludwig
Edelstein, a historian of medicine, observes of Greek and Roman
medicine that grew out of the Hippocratic commitment, "one feature
sharply distinguishes pagan humanism from the Christian attitude and

that of the nineteenth-century humanist reformers . . . pagan ethics lack any recognition of social responsibilities on the part of the physician.''[1]

This unique commitment to the individual patient which emerged early in medical ethics is closely related to individual freedom in decision-making. The primacy of the individual is essential to the claim that one's duty is to an individual rather than to society as a whole. Early society displayed a collective consciousness in which duty to the individual could not dominate. In Greek society the notion of the individual began to evolve. That transition manifested itself very early in medicine. The tribe was subordinated to the individual, at least in the guild ethics of the medical craft.

Although Judaism and Christianity have always viewed man as a social animal, they have also contributed greatly to the emergence of the individual. From them came a radical monotheism which subordinates earthly sociopolitical forces to a transcendent power. The doctrine of the resurrection requires that souls cannot be interchangeable. Each human has a uniqueness, which is essential for the conviction that lives are not interchangeable in calculating goods and harms. God communicates to individuals, both in the prophets and in the religious mysticism that is the precursor of modern individualism. Especially in its later Calvinistic and sectarian forms, the covenant of God with man assumes that man is an individual. This set the context for the secular individualism of the contract theories of Locke and Hobbes and for the doctrine of natural rights which places the individual before the social aggregate.

Yet this foundation of egalitarian individualism which is the basis for insisting on the primacy of individual freedom and self-determination in medical decision-making differs from the principle that the physician has a duty to the individual that supersedes any duty to society. The duty of the physician may be a corollary of the individual rights of the patient, but it need not be. Duty to an individual can be extremely paternalistic, as shown by the duty of the parent to the child, the archetypal case of paternalism. In this sense the principle of individualism does not imply a radical egalitarianism of the natural rights tradition but simply a subordination of the interests of larger social units to those of the individual. The Christian ethic of neighborly love may imply this special duty to individuals. The good Samaritan did not stop to calculate the long-range consequences for society of alternative courses of action. His obligation, like that of the parent, was to take care of the individual's immediate need, not worrying about the needs of the broader society.

In the nineteenth and twentieth centuries the dangers of this kind of individualism, which gives primacy to individual needs, were discovered. It is probably wrong to consider the doctrine of laissez-faire economics as truly individualistic. For Adam Smith, the invisible hand would guide individuals to do what was best for society. Nevertheless, the de facto or instrumental individualism of *The Wealth of Nations* led to something less than what was beneficial for either the individual or society. The social utilitarianism of Bentham and Mill as well as of the public health movements had an individual conception of the units of good. Still, social utilitarianism once again discovered the primacy of the social aggregate with the claim that the morally right is that which produces the greatest good for the greatest number—a principle radically at odds with the Hippocratic ethic of individual patient benefit. Marx, perhaps drawing on the social dimensions of his Jewish heritage as well as on Hegel's organic theory of society, developed more fully the theory of the primacy of the general welfare. As a result, individualism today is paradoxically the moral foundation of Western society and the evil depriving man of a larger social vision.

The conflict has not escaped medicine. The backbone of medical ethics is the physician's duty to his patient. To subordinate the interests of the genetically suffering infant to the cost-benefit analysis of a government accounting office is crass utilitarianism. Yet all would insist that the psychiatrist seeing a homicidal maniac report him to government authorities so that he can be suppressed, even if it is not in his interest to be suppressed. Especially in a day when the physician is in the employ of institutions, governments, and even private industries, the conflict between the duty of the physician, or anyone else involved in medical decisions, to the individual and his duty to others had best not be resolved by simplistic rules.

The Individual and Society

Every time the physician undertakes research other than for the benefit of the subject, every time he decides that he must violate the patient's confidence to disclose a diagnosis of venereal disease as required by law, every time he participates in a public health campaign for rubella inoculation, he is subordinating the interests of his patient to those of the larger society. Aside from these classical cases, where the physician is forced to choose between serving his individual patient or the more general interests of society, the problem can arise in a more ad hoc fashion, sometimes where least expected.

14 SOLDIER, PHYSICIAN, AND MORAL MAN

The Article 90 court-martial charge read: "In that Captain Howard B. Levy, U.S. Army, Headquarters & Headquarters Company, United States Army Hospital, Fort Jackson, South Carolina, having received a lawful command from Colonel Henry F. Fancy, his superior officer, to establish and operate a Phase II Training Program for Special Forces AidMen in dermatology in accordance with *Special Forces AidMen (Airborne), 8-R-F16, Dermatology Training,* did at the United States Army Hospital, Fort Jackson, South Carolina on or about 11 October 1966 to 25 November 1966, willfully disobey the same."[2]

Capt. Levy, a physician, had arrived at Fort Jackson in July 1965 to take over as chief of the Dermatology Clinic. The aidmen he was to train would work as medics with the Special Forces (Green Berets) in Vietnam, providing them with dermatological skills that would be used, among other things, to win support of local residents for the American cause. His troubles began almost immediately. The Saturday after his arrival he read in the morning newspaper that ten blacks had been denied voter registration. He joined the civil rights group campaigning for voter registration. In September of that year he wrote a letter to Sergeant First Class Geoffrey Hancock, a black soldier known by Capt. Levy to be in Vietnam but not known to him personally. He wrote: "Geoffrey who are you fighting for. Your real battle is back here in the U.S. but why must I fight it for you? The same people who suppress Negroes and poor whites here are doing it all over again all over the world and your helping them." The letter showed up later in Capt. Levy's court-martial with the charge that he had written it with the "intent to interfere with, impair, and influence the loyalty, morale, and discipline of the military forces of the United States."

By October 1966 Capt. Levy had reached the conclusion tht he must refuse to train the Special Forces in dermatology. According to the brief filed in his defense, Capt. Levy maintained that the medical training being given to the Special Forces Aidmen was prostituting medicine for political and military purposes. He quoted Colonel Richard Coppedge, former Chief Surgeon for the Special Forces' Warfare Center who had originated the aidman program, as calling it "a political use of medicine; certainly its effects are political . . . The motives of those who engage in it may differ." Co. Coppedge saw nothing "incompatible really in the humanitarian aims of this program and the political aims of the program and the military aims of the program."

The Staff Judge Advocate, summarizing Col. Coppedge's testimony at the Army court-martial, said:

> The purpose of the Special Forces medical aidmen training at the time of its institution in 1954 was primarily geared to the type of situation where the Special Forces would be deployed behind enemy lines to assist in the organization, training, supply, and direction of guerrilla forces. With the advent of the Vietnam war the mission of the Special Forces changed somewhat; there were more counterguerrilla forces than there were guerrilla forces. It became recognized that the struggle was in many respects a social war in which social instruments such as

medicine would have to be utilized. So "we sought to use medicine as a means of approaching the enemy and imposing our will on his." This is a peculiarly American approach and is opposed to the Viet Cong approach which is more likely to be terroristic . . . the one great "in" that you have is this medic because people are short on doctors and trained medical personnel in there; that the thing to do is sort of push a medic up there in front and let him get the confidence of these people by treating them; usually it starts off—sometimes it starts off very slow, but the word gets around. More and more people are coming for this treatment; certain dependency is sometimes involved; then, of course, this lays the way open now for the rest of the team to come in and organize them in their primary mission which could be border surveillance; it could be CIDG strike force; it could be regional forces, popular forces.

Capt. Levy made two arguments in his defense when charged with disobeying the order. First he argued that the order to train the Special Forces was illegal because to do so would require him to participate in the war crimes of the Special Forces in Vietnam. He also argued that the order was illegal because it forced him, as a physician, to violate medical ethics. To support this second position, he cited several authorities. One was the Hippocratic oath: "I swear . . . that by my precept, lecture and every other mode of instruction, I will impart a knowledge of the art to . . . disciples bound by a stipulation and oath, according to the law of medicine but to no others . . . Whatever . . . I may see or hear in the lives of men which ought not to be bespoken abroad, I will not divulge, as reckoning that all such should be kept secret."

Another authority cited was Dr. Jean Mayer, a nutritionist and professor: "I would say that the whole thrust of progress has been to separate the functions of the doctor and his auxiliary from . . . the destruction of life and property . . . It is an ethical judgment and it is one which is based on the whole thrust of what professional men have [tried to make medicine] for the past twenty-five hundred years."

Capt. Levy also cited Dr. Victor Sidel, another physician and professor:

I believe that in order to be a good and ethical physician he must refuse to obey an order which he believes violates his medical ethics.

The decision I believe must be made on medical grounds rather than on political grounds if the medical profession is to be able to help the people.[3]

This case raises the question of how the physician's obligation to society compares with his obligation to those who are directly affected by his practice of medicine. It also raises the question of whether the physician is obligated by universal moral requirements or by the morality of his profession. The two arguments Howard Levy uses in his defense are quite different. The first, that to carry out the order will be to participate in a war crime, argues on the state's own terms. Any citizen, including a military officer, has the right, indeed the duty, to resist an order which is itself illegal. In using this argument, Levy makes no appeal to his duty "as a physician." He is taking exactly the same position any soldier ought to take if he is convinced that an order will require him to commit a war crime. The justification is one that the state, or at least the United States, recognizes as a legitimate defense.

The second argument, however, takes the different position that, in order to be a good physician, he must refuse to obey an order that he believes violates his medical ethics. Here Capt. Levy would appear to be arguing that, as a physician, he has a special duty to protect the eventual recipients of his medical teaching, a duty that the ordinary soldier would not be expected to have or even to recognize. The Hippocratic Oath is meant to bind only physicians.

If it is the case that the professional ethics of the physician requires a different moral behavior than the general public morality, what is required of the physician? If the court decides that participation in the Vietnam war is not a war crime and if at the same time the medical profession reaches the consensus that using physicians to train Special Forces violates the ethical standards of the profession, is Capt. Levy bound by the more public judgment, the judgment of the profession, or neither? Is he, as a citizen, bound to serve society's interests, including a refusal to participate in war crimes, or is he, as a physician, bound by a special responsibility to those who are directly affected by his medical skills?

There is a third alternative. In addition to being a citizen-soldier and a physician, Capt. Levy might also see himself as a member of the broader human community. If he still believes that training Special Forces is a crime against humanity, even though the state has reached the conclusion that it is not, how ought he to act? If he believes that ethical requirements are universal in the sense that they extend beyond the particular society of which one happens to be a member, he might take the position that he has a moral obligation to refuse this particular order in this particular situation, that is, to be civilly disobedient, in the name of a higher moral authority. He might feel he has a moral duty beyond that of being a good physician and even beyond that of being a good citizen. The choice among these three alternatives provides a basis for ethical conduct.

15 CERTIFYING STERILIZATION FOR THE PUBLIC GOOD

Bill and Helen Dean lived with their three children in a modest three-bed-room apartment in Victory Towers Housing Project in a large Midwestern city near the Mason-Dixon Line. Bill had recently gotten a job driving a truck for a grocery wholesaler for $137 a week. Helen had held a clerical job part time for the past three years, since their youngest child started kindergarten. She usually earned about $65 a week.

The city, which had built and managed the housing project, was now giving the tenants the chance to buy their apartments. The price for the Deans' apartment was $24,500. The city would provide mortgages for those who qualified financially and had a 10 percent down payment. The Deans had saved almost $1500 and believed they could borrow the additional down payment from her brother. They met with the city loan officer, who told them that the payments, including principal, interest, insurance, maintenance, and taxes, would be $230 a month. That was $30 a month more than what they were paying in rent, but they were terribly eager to own their own apartment and "have something to show for their monthly payments." Although it would be difficult to scrape up the extra money, they were willing to make the sacrifices. If necessary, Mrs. Dean would take in some typing on her own.

The loan officer seemed concerned about their income, feeling that Mr. Dean's income by itself was just too low to justify the mortgage. After inquiring about their plans for a larger family, he said that he needed assurance that they would have no more children, since additional children would probably impair Mrs. Dean's earning power. The couple assured him that they were going to have no more children; three was hard enough. Mrs. Dean was 32; their oldest child was 12. Since Mrs. Dean had been able to go back to work, life had just become financially tolerable; they could at least put food on the table. There was no way they would have more children. If she became pregnant again, she definitely planned to get an abortion.

It soon became apparent that when the loan officer said he needed to be sure they would have no more children, he really meant it, for he wanted a doctor's certificate that Mrs. Dean had been sterilized. Mrs. Dean did not think too much of women's liberation, but she had heard of women's complaints about not being able to get loans from banks. The more she thought about it, the more outraged she became. "I've told them we'd have an abortion," she said to her husband, "Isn't that good enough? I don't know what it is, but I just can't stand the thought of never being able to have any more children. Besides, I don't see any reason to waste the money, time, and misery on the operation."

She had not seen the obstetrician, Dr. Joyce Hilliard, since their youngest child had been born. Dr. Hilliard was one of the few woman doctors she knew of. She thought she would understand if she asked her to sign a statement that she had been sterilized. Since she was definitely not going to have any more children anyway, it was almost the same thing. She puzzled whether to ask Dr. Hilliard for the favor and wondered what her response would be.

———————

Requiring special standards for women to obtain mortgages is an ethical and public policy issue of increasing controversy. In order to get to the medical ethical problems raised by the case, however, the focus should be on the request Mrs. Dean is considering of her physician. The question is whether, assuming the cause to be just, medical authority can be appealed to for support even if it requires occasional outright dishonesty.

The first medical ethical problem is Mrs. Dean's, whether she is justified in using the institution of medicine for ulterior purposes. The question is not as simple as it may seem, especially from the medical consumer's perspective. Mrs. Dean has no particular commitment to the profession of medicine; she has taken no oath of loyalty; she has no code of moral medical conduct. If she is to be restricted in any way from making her request, it must be from her own ethical convictions, not from those of the medical profession. She may realize that the dishonesty she is considering is generally disapproved. She may realize that repeated actions of the kind might jeopardize her own access to health care or even the institution of medicine itself. But whatever her decision, it must be based on her own moral framework, her own concept of whether it is justified to use medicine for what one believes to be a moral purpose.

Dr. Hilliard's dilemma, if she is asked for the certification, is somewhat more complex. If she begins with the traditional ethical principle of medicine, that the physician's duty is to do what she thinks will benefit the patient, then many of the problems may be avoided. If her duty is exclusively to the patient and the only patient-centered duty is to benefit her, then she only need determine whether getting the mortgage is beneficial in the long run. She may decide that she thinks the sterilization is more beneficial, or that teaching honesty is more beneficial, but the ethical problem is restricted.

Dr. Hilliard may be worried, however, about other ethical obligations. She may feel that she has an obligation to society as a whole. Public funds may be jeopardized by her false certification. She knows that she and her physician colleagues often serve as society's agents in such tasks as performing school health examinations, testifying about the danger of a mental patient, and giving life insurance physical examinations. It thus may be naive to argue that the physician should never act to serve the interests of society. If Dr. Hilliard is willing to grant that in at least some cases the physician must act for the general welfare rather than for the benefit of the individual patient, she must decide how such distinctions are to be made.

Dr. Hilliard may also feel an obligation to the medical profession or to medical science in addition to her duty to the patient and to the general society. If it became widely known that physicians falsely certified medical conditions whenever they thought it benefited their patients, physician certifications would soon be useless. Even if physicians falsely certified medical conditions only when they thought it was for a moral cause, such as to keep a draftee out of an immoral war, the credibility of the profession would be jeopardized. More fundamentally perhaps, physicians, as scientists, have a respect for objectivity in diagnosis and prognosis and a respect for medical knowledge per se which militates against the prostituting of the physician's skills for ulterior purposes. They therefore have a particularly strong reason for not cooperating in any falsity in the name of justice, just as they have an equally strong reason for cooperating because of their value commitment to benefiting the individual patient and ignoring the interests of the broader society. These two moral forces pushing in opposite directions might mean that Mrs. Dean and Dr. Hilliard would reach different conclusions about the proposed scheme. They could do so because they have different perceptions of the medical role and different ethical frameworks for making moral decisions.

Even if Dr. Hilliard decides that the requirement of certification is so morally outrageous that it must be opposed, two very different courses of action are open. First, she might simply sign the certificate, circumventing what she considers to be the city's immoral request in a private and individualized manner. Or she might refuse to sign it and work with Mrs. Dean to take more public action. She might attempt to get a court determination that discrimination on the grounds of sex is unconstitutional. She might take political action to make it politically uncomfortable for the public officials requiring the certificate. Such a step would take the physician completely out of what is normally thought to be the medical role. Obviously, as a citizen, the physician has as much right and duty to take political action as anyone else. But some would claim that when a moral problem is encountered in the medical role, the physician must respond in that role as well. The individualism of the medical professional might incline the physician to favor the more private response, the quiet signing of the certificate. In more and more areas, however, the problem of corporate social responsibility is raised, as when a professional medical association tries to decide whether to take a public stand on a social issue indirectly related to health.

16   PROFESSIONAL POSITIONS ON PUBLIC ISSUES

The April meeting of the County Medical Society had the largest attendance of any meeting in memory. Three physicians had introduced a resolution calling for the group to take an official position that the United States should immediately withdraw its military troops from Pacifica, a Latin American nation the United States had supported with military and economic aid since the military junta was threatened by a left-wing countercoup three years ago. The three physicians were Dr. Michael Cohen, a psychiatrist; Dr. Mary Brown, an internist at the neighborhood health clinic; and Dr. Frank MacMillan, a resident at City Hospital who had recently joined the County Medical Society under a special arrangement giving the medical residents membership privileges while they were in the county.

The opposition was heated. Dr. Brian Northman, past president of the county society and one of the most respected internists in the community, led the debate. He argued that never before had the society taken a stand as an organization on political matters of this sort. He granted that the members as individuals should write their congressmen. He said he could not understand why Americans were always meddling in local fights all over the world anyway. But he argued that it would be a disaster for medicine in the county if the physicians as a group began taking political stands.

Dr. Juan Hernandez, a staff physician with the Fayette Medical Group, agreed. The County Medical Society was made up of individuals, he argued, who had very different opinions on the war. As physicians, they had learned that every person is unique. To take a public, corporate position would be unfair, especially on something not related to health.

Dr. Brown spoke first for the resolution which her group had introduced. She argued, first, that the invasion of Pacifica by United States forces was very much a matter of health. Americans and Pacificans were being killed and maimed by the hundreds because the presence of American forces permitted fighting at a much more intense level than would otherwise have been possible and prevented a rapid victory for the insurgents. Second, she argued that the military government in Pacifica had been grossly irresponsible in failing to provide essential medical care for the people of the country, a need the new government would serve. Third, physicians were being drafted to serve the American troops in Pacifica.

Dr. Cohen then explained that, as a psychiatrist, he was becoming concerned about what the war was doing to the mental health of the residents of the county. He pointed out that his younger patients were alienated from their parents, from the institutions of society, and from society itself. He was treating more cases of depression than ever before. One mother had been in a prolonged depression since hearing that her son was missing some eighteen months ago. The war, he argued, was presenting a serious health problem in the county.

Between those who opposed the intervention in Pacifica in particular and those who opposed American internationalism in general, there was clearly a substantial majority opposed to the military action. The real split was over whether the County Medical Society had any business taking an official position on something so remote from medicine and so remote from the county.

---

1. Does an organization have an identity, a personality, of its own, which makes an official position something more than simply the sum of the views of its individual members?
2. Does a medical organization, whose members are committed to the health of individual patients, have any right or any reason to take official stands in public on social issues indirectly related to health?
3. Is it more plausible for a medical organization to take such a stand if the issue is shown to be related to health, as Dr. Brown and Dr. Cohen argue? If so, how is a social issue related to health? According to the United Nations, health refers to total well-being. Does this mean that every social issue is really a health issue?
4. Would a local professional medical organization be more justified in taking a public stand on a local health issue, such as a city health ordinance on lead paint or sanitation inspections of local restaurants?
5. If physicians have a unique perspective on social issues, should not their views be heard and identified as the medical perspective rather than simply as the perspective of citizens who also happen to be physicians? Is that unique perspective an artifact of medical specialization or a relevant expertise that the public should consider?

17 THE PHYSICIAN AND COMPULSORY PUBLIC SERVICE

Congressman Gerald Crawford was considering introducing a bill which, if passed, would become national policy. The abstract of the bill read:

> Every physician educated in any medical school receiving federal funds shall, after his graduation and one year of supervised hospital experience but before being licensed for practicing medicine in any state, serve for two years with a National Health Corps. Physicians so serving shall be compensated at the civil service rate of GS-8 ($11,029-14,341 per annum). The National Health Corps shall be established by the Public Health Service as an agency to supply needed medical services to any municipality, county, state, or federal health facility unable to obtain needed medical services. The objective shall be to serve those sectors of the population now unable to obtain adequate health services.

Congressman Crawford subsequently gave an address in which he defended his proposal:

In the richest country in the world it is appalling that the health of our citizens is so abysmal. The fact is that 140 of our counties in 26 different states now have not a single nonfederal physician, and that number has increased by 42 counties in a nine-year period. Now just short of half a million of our citizens have no physician they can turn to in their entire county. Medicaid and Medicare are a good beginning, but are useless to those who cannot find a doctor who will give them attention in the first place. The only answer is a National Health Corps. It is the least the doctor can do. He has a unique talent, a lifesaving talent. We cannot tolerate the hoarding of that resource for the few who can afford it, for those who are fortunate enough and rich enough to live in those attractive areas where physicians like to congregate. Health care can no longer be handed out according to the whims of the market place. Each of our citizens has a right to life, liberty, and the pursuit of happiness. But these are hollow words unless that citizen also has the right to health care.

I ask you, how can we tolerate government subsidies for educating that special group in our society with the highest income of all occupational groups? How can we subsidize the physician who will practice in suburban splendor when those in the central cities, on the farms, and in the desolate hills scratch out a living without a penny of government help?

Some have argued that medical students should work off those huge subsidies for their education as the teacher works off a loan—a 10 percent forgiveness for every year of public service—or that the medical students should be given the chance to pay back the subsidy out of their earnings if they wished. That would be an improvement over the present system, but I ask you, who would be the ones to end up buying their way out of public service? We cannot afford to set up another program where the rich can avoid paying their debt to society as they did in the Civil War. Being trained as a physician is a great honor. It also creates public trust. It is not enough to have the poor and the uniquely devoted paying their debt to our physicianless masses. It is not enough to let off those who are attracted to lucrative specialties where they can earn enough in six months to pay back the entire cost of their education. If we are going to invest in the education of a select group of our nation's young, the least they can do is pay back their debt to society with two years of service to those who are suffering.

The claim of Congressman Crawford is that the physician has a debt to society, not simply to individual patients. He sees health care, if not health itself, as a fundamental right of every citizen, and the investment made in the form of support for medical education as a sufficient justification for requiring public service to fulfill that right.

Many in the medical community would find the congressman's proposal offensive. It violates the principle of individual freedom in practicing medicine which the profession has treated as sacred. It violates the principle that the physician's duty is to his individual patient. But these claims are hard to reconcile with the claims of the physicianless and of those who have supported the physician's education. Moreover, the physician can hardly cite his duty to his individual patient at a time when he has not yet entered private practice and has no patients of his own.

The congressman's argument contains two different claims. One is that because society has provided something for the medical student, it has a right to expect something in return. Society expects public service from teachers who were supported by education loans while in school. Society expects West Point graduates to serve in the army for a minimum period. From this perspective the congressman is really arguing that the government has struck a bad bargain, that it deserves something more specific in return for its investment. If so, however, it is hard to see why medical students should not be allowed to buy their way out of the bargain, either by paying their full tuition or by repaying the full loan at the going market interest rates.

The second claim is more radical and at the same time more consistent with the ethical tradition of medicine. Health care, the congressman argues, is a right. It can no longer be reduced to considerations of the market place.

Being given the opportunity to gain the lifesaving knowledge and being licensed by the state to use that knowledge generates a public trust—an obligation to serve the people who are the source of the special opportunity. If such is the basis of the National Health Corps, then it is no more sensible to make public service optional in a time of health crisis than it is to make military service a matter of choice in a time of military crisis. If the congressman's idea of two years of service indeed makes sense, this is its most convincing defense. The program would mean that those who are wealthy and self-serving would not be able to escape their public responsibility.

There may be pragmatic arguments against the congressman as well as more principled arguments of individual freedom for the medical practitioner. Coerced physicians may make poor physicians. Those who are not willing to serve ethnic, poor, or inconvenient populations may not serve them well when forced to do so. Certainly the advocates of the National Health Corps would have to plan for such pragmatic problems. But the underlying question raised by the case is whether the role of the physician includes within it, in principle, the obligation to serve the medical needs of the general public or simply the needs of those chosen to be patients.

In some instances, of course, it is hard to tell whether the physician is being asked to serve society or simply to serve his patient, even if the patient does not realize it. Such is the dilemma faced by the psychiatrist who learns that his patient may commit a violent crime.

18   THE PHYSICIAN AS DRUG REFORMER

Oscar Edmund was a 22-year-old black man with S-S hemoglobinopathy or sickle cell anemia, a genetic disease affecting the red blood cells primarily of blacks. His brother had died two years ago at age 18 from the same disease. Over the past twelve years Mr. Edmund had made over three hundred visits to the Mount Zion Hospital outpatient department, including the emergency room, generally with a complaint of pain or for a follow-up visit. He had been admitted to the hospital with the diagnosis of "suspected sickle cell crisis" more than thirty times in the past few years, with an average of six times per year.

Typically, Mr. Edmund complained of severe, unremitting abdominal pain and believed he was in a sickling crisis, a periodic acute attack. Generally his physical examination, laboratory, and radiographic evaluation upon each admission showed no change from previous admissions or his outpatient records. The usual treatment plan included intravenous fluid and alkali therapy, intermittent oxygen, and an analgesic (meperidine 50-100 mg. I.M. every 3-4 hours). These hospitalizations generally lasted three or four days, but soon after discharge Mr. Edmund would reappear in the emergency room complaining of pain. The physicians there now suspected that Mr. Edmund was addicted to meperidine, a synthetic narcotic. He denied using street narcotics outside the hospital but was often discharged with a supply of oral narcotics to "tide him over," despite his claims that they were inadequate.

Mr. Edmund was now readmitted with a history, physical exam, and lab values similar to previous admissions. His doctor, Dr. Norman Moore, an intern new on the ward, had never seen him before but knew of him by word of mouth and from reading his chart. He believed that the patient was an iatrogenic narcotic addict, that is, addicted through medical use of narcotics, and that rather than being in a real sickle crisis, he merely wanted shots of meperidine. The nurses who took care of Mr. Edmund on each admission agreed. Doctor Moore decided that he was going to detoxify or withdraw Mr. Edmund during this admission "once and for all." He pointed out that, since studies of patients with sickle cell anemia have found that when there is continuity in the physician-patient relationship, hospitalization is required only one or two times per year for true crises, Mr. Edmund "must be faking it."

Dr. Moore wrote orders for tapering doses of methadone in an attempt to withdraw the patient. He instructed the nurses not to tell the patient what medicine or how much he was receiving. When he later visited Mr.

Edmund, he was writhing in pain and pleading for pain relief. Dr. Moore informed him that he had just received a "pain shot" an hour earlier and would have to wait three more hours for another. The patient began to cry unconsolably, but Dr. Moore was firm, stating, "We just can't go on making addicts out of these sicklers, because the law won't allow us to send them home with a syringe, and they'll be forced to support their habit on the street or come into the emergency room every day for shots. What else can I do?"

This case raises still another way in which the physician can be put in the role of servant of society. Dr. Moore's response to the sickle cell patient presents three major conflicts. First, is Dr. Moore's sole responsibility, as the Hippocratic Oath tells him, to do what he thinks is in the interest of the patient, or does he have a responsibility to the larger society to protect it from the horrors of street addicts? Second, this case poses a conflict about attitudes toward the use—particularly the addictive use— of chemical agents. Much like the broken leg case, the resolution of the problem presented will depend heavily on whether one sees daily use of a drug as enslaving and dehumanizing or, on the contrary, as therapeutic and liberating. Third, different emphases on the importance of patient freedom, as opposed to patient well-being, will lead to very different answers to the physician's dilemma.

Robert Murray, a professor of pediatrics and medicine, has cared for many patients in sickle cell crisis. In commenting on this case, he takes the position that the physician's task is to do what he thinks will benefit the patient even if that means ignoring societal interests: "Dr. Moore must fulfill his obligation to help the patient survive and also preserve his well-being. To do so in this case means compromising certain medical and societal values. It also means compromising the patient's freedom." Murray, however, is uncomfortable in sacrificing patient freedom, even though he realizes that full commitment to the Hippocratic principle may require it. He even justifies a solution which would maintain some patient freedom by showing that treatment requires it: "It is well known that individuals cannot be permanently freed from addiction without their cooperation, so this doctor's efforts will ultimately fail." Murray is committed not only to the patient-benefiting perspective but also to the view that addiction is "bad." He is therefore convinced that it is in the patient's interest to be withdrawn from drugs and is willing to compromise with a maintenance program administered in a medical setting, as shown when he analyzes a physician's attempt to resolve this case:

With respect to this conflict, a physician might go through the following stages of thought:

1. For a physician not to relieve pain associated with a disease is "bad."

2. The patient became addicted to the drug in the process of relieving pain.

3. It is "bad" for a patient to be addicted to a narcotic.

4. Since being addicted is "bad," the physician responsible for it must withdraw the patient from the drug.

5. Although withdrawal from a drug causes the patient pain, the addiction will terminate.

6. The patient, once withdrawn from the drug, may have future episodes of pain, again requiring the drug, and the process may start all over again.

The simplest resolution of this conflict is merely to accept the patient's "bad" addiction as a consequence of the illness and continue to administer the drug, since at least it will prevent further pain. But this method still leaves an element of risk. The patient, although between episodes of pain, might still be in need of and in search of drugs and, in seeking them, become a street addict. Attempts to withdraw a drug from a patient are always fraught with a need for the physician to make value judgments, and there is the risk of causing much immediate suffering to the patient.

Recently another treatment alternative has been added—the maintenance of an addicted person on a drug such as methadone—which does not produce the euphoric effects of morphine or heroin, but does prevent the painful side effects that come with withdrawal from a narcotic agent. This circumvents, in large measure, the occurrence of street addiction and keeps the patient in close touch with the physician who can administer medical care in the event of pain crisis. In this instance, one drug addiction has been substituted for another, but it is (at least conceptually) "better" because it allows the patient to function in a self-supportive way. For the physician it may be the easiest alternative, and the patient still has a modicum of freedom.[4]

What is striking in Murray's position is that there is no hint that the physician has any obligation to protect society from the dangers of having an addict on the streets. It is not so clear that Dr. Moore has the same attitude. The question is whether he finds it horrifying to produce an addict because of the tragic impact on the patient or because of the impact of putting an addict on the street. If the morally right course of action is that which will produce the greatest good for the greatest number—as the classical utilitarians believe—then it is bizarre that Dr. Moore would ignore these significant social impacts of his decision. If Dr. Moore feels that he can justifiably ignore these social consequences, either he must reject the initial premise—that the morally right course of action is that which will produce the greatest good for the greatest number—or he must show why in his special role as a physician in the long run the greatest good will be served if he considers only what he thinks will be in the best interests of the patient to the exclusion of all other interests.

Another commentator has interpreted this case quite differently. Alan Soble, a philosopher with training in pharmacology, rejects both the Hippocratic patient-benefiting ethic and the classical utilitarian position that the total social good is decisive. He also holds a radically different view on the importance of individual freedom. Finally, he differs from Murray over how evil drug addiction is. This leads to a position that Mr. Edmund should be given the drug because, in general, use of narcotics should be legalized and at least tolerated if not actively embraced. He even suggests that Dr. Moore should take advantage of the opportunity to be a drug reformer:

> Assuming that Dr. Moore's diagnosis is correct and he is serious about helping Mr. Edmund avoid the street market, his plan is counter-productive in that it is likely to cause precisely what Dr. Moore wants to avoid, especially if Mr. Edmund is detoxified against his will. Living in the environment that he does, it is a delusion to think that Mr. Edmund, after detoxification, will remain nonaddicted "once and for all." Furthermore, an injustice occurs if Mr. Edmund's addiction was originally, or always, iatrogenic.
>
> The continued treatment of Mr. Edmund with narcotics (under the ingenious guise of sickle cell anemia pain) would contribute toward the realization of a de facto maintenance system. By not doing so, the young intern's decision failed to utilize an opportunity to be a "drug reformer" of the current medical system from within.
>
> But it is surely simpleminded to assume that Dr. Moore's diagnosis is correct. His evidence leading to the conclusion that Mr. Edmund "must be faking it" is not so crystal clear as to leave no room for doubt. In Dr. Moore's perspective, being addicted is not a sufficient reason for the administration of narcotics, but he is still faced with the insuperable difficulty of determining whether, in fact, Mr. Edmund does experience frequent sickle cell anemia pain.
>
> I would conclude that as long as Mr. Edmund is addicted it does not matter whether his pain is real or feigned; in either case he should receive the drug. There is an epistemological problem for me only when the patient is not addicted. It may well be the less risky procedure to administer the drug . . . I believe that this difficulty can only be resolved by the legalization of narcotics.[5]

The relation between the individual and society, attitudes toward drug addiction, and the importance of patient freedom are not the only issues posed by this case. Dr. Moore instructs the nurse not to tell the patient what kind or how much medicine he is receiving. He at least implies that the patient has received an effective dose of a "pain shot."

It may be that the physician's duty is not adequately defined either by the formula of doing what the physician thinks will benefit the patient or by that of doing what will serve the greatest good for the greatest number. Viewing the patient-physician relationship as one of a contract is the major competitor to the Hippocratic perspective. The contract perspective is also a major interpretation of the individual's relationship with society. If there are implicit contracts both between the physician and the patient and between the physician and society, new obligations may be added to the picture. The contract perspective leads to holding consent as a crucial element in the patient-physician relationship. Certainly Mr. Edmund has not consented to the narcotic withdrawal. While consent might be irrelevant under the Hippocratic norm where the physician's task is to do what he thinks will benefit the patient, it becomes fundamental if the contract is the basis of the relationship.

The physician may also have a contract with society. He may be under some obligation to fulfill its laws. If that is the case, there can be no final resolution—even a moral resolution—to a case where clandestine withdrawal, drug maintenance, and becoming a drug reformer are the alternatives unless it is known what the laws of the jurisdiction require. This does not mean that it is always morally wrong to violate the law, but only that the individual's contractual relation with the state must be morally relevant.

The Individual and the Group

In some cases neither the whole society nor the individual patient is the one competing for the physician's loyalty. Rather, a specific group of people or a specific corporation makes a claim on the physician that conflicts with the patient's best interests. With the advent of "company physicians" or physicians on the payroll of institutions, public and private, such conflicts are predictable. The question raised is to whom the physician owes allegiance, to whom he or she is morally obligated.

19 THE PSYCHIATRIST AS DOUBLE AGENT

A first-year medical student was having a severe emotional crisis. He went to a private psychiatrist, obviously on the verge of a complete breakdown. He was agitated, anxious, and uncertain whether he could handle his studies, although his college record was brilliant and he showed outstanding intellectual capacity.

He was in acute distress and seemingly in the process of disintegration. The psychiatrist, trying hard to avoid hospitalization, started intensive psychotherapy. The student was already at a point where it looked as if he would have a schizophrenic break: reality testing was impaired, ideas of reference were occurring, and a hypomanic mood with grandiose ideation was forming. To relieve the pressures on him, the psychiatrist recommended that he take a medical leave of absence from school. He wrote a letter for the student saying that he was treating him for "emotional problems" and recommending a medical leave. The student dropped out at the end of the semester in good academic standing.

The next fall the student attempted to return to medical school but was refused readmission, even though the psychiatrist had written another letter, as the physician in charge of the treatment, that he was now medically able to continue his studies. The school gave no reason for not reinstating him except that he was not considered suitable. He then began to apply to other medical schools, at his psychiatrist's suggestion, and was refused in every case.

Before seeing the private psychiatrist, the student had consulted the school psychiatrist, who had diagnosed him as a latent schizophrenic. When other medical schools wrote to his former school, the reason given for the discharge was a medical leave with latent schizophrenia. It is known that about half of those with schizophrenia in remission will have another breakdown. In the case of this student, who was planning to become a surgeon, there was a real risk to future patients. The combination of a grandiose self-appraisal with the power of the surgeon could cause serious harm.

The private psychiatrist recognized that there might be psychiatric conditions that would interfere with a career in medicine and therefore might be grounds for exclusion from medical school. The problem, as he saw it, was whether the school psychiatrist was seeing the student in his role as psychiatrist or in his role as part of the school administration, and whether these two roles could be separated. He questioned whether it is acceptable for a physician on the staff of a school or a business corporation simultaneously to serve as the agent both of the organization employing him and of the patient who is enrolled or employed in that organization.

The conflict between the school psychiatrist's obligation to the medical student and his duty to the medical school and society seems clear, even if it is not obvious to the psychiatrist himself. Whether the psychiatrist is acting to benefit the medical school or the general society is a more subtle problem. Since the medical school probably sees its role to some extent as serving the public, the two benefits may be confused, although in this case the interest of the general society is less than it would be, for example, in cases where public funds, military goals, or public safety were at stake. Whatever the interest of the general public in escaping the potential dangers of a schizophrenic physician, the psychiatrist probably also feels a somewhat narrower obligation to the medical school. Valuable faculty time and funds are invested in medical student training. The reputation of the medical profession and the school are at stake. The psychiatrist is an employee of the medical school. He may be used to giving psychiatric tests to entering students with no objections being raised. It is thus awkward to argue that he has no responsibility to his employer.

This notion of a physician having a duty to his employer conflicts dramatically with the traditional obligation of the physician, including the psychiatrist, to serve first the interests and needs of his patient. One argument could be that the school psychiatrist's duty is only or primarily to the student, the individual patient in need of medical assistance. This position is taken by psychiatrist Willard Gaylin in commenting on the case:

> Certain roles, because they serve needs of such essential importance, have been granted extraordinary privilege and priority. The physician, perceived as preserver of life, has traditionally been a man of great privilege and has pledged himself to honor that privilege with responsibility. In order to sustain a relationship in which one individual places his very life in the hands of another, there must be some assurance that the relationship will be governed by its primary purpose: that is, the good of the patient, the preservation of his life, the protection of his well-being. The physician is under oath to "do no harm." It is the basis of trust on which the profession of medicine has survived.
>
> Any infringement on the inviolability of his contract threatens the whole medical structure. Of course nothing in life is inviolate, and there will always be times when the physician will break his word to his patient for higher responsibilities. We will quarantine the contagious, commit the psychotic and confine the dangerous.
>
> A young student, recognizing mental illness for himself, consults the physician assigned by his school to serve those needs. On making the diagnosis the school physician refers him for outside help, and, indeed, he is helped. Then he wishes to continue his career. In the judgment of the treating physician, the patient is qualified to go on with his professional work. Yet he is refused readmission, despite the fact that it is of the nature of most medical leaves to allow for return. Further, it is apparent that a kind of black-ball by diagnosis has been effected. Schizophrenia, a broad category of disease, in psychiatry carries the same often unwarranted dread as cancer in general medicine. Knowing this, the private physician guarded this diagnosis. Had the student only seen the private doctor, he would have been readmitted. The student's problems arose because he assumed that the the school psychiatrist was indeed a psychiatrist, bound by the codes of conduct, oath and ethics of his general profession.
>
> Were I an admission officer in a medical school I would discourage the admission of schizophrenic applicants. On the other hand, there is also no question that among the schizophrenic patients I personally

have seen have been successful medical students, not to mention
political leaders, psychoanalytic candidates, judges, educators, doctors, lawyers and merchant chiefs. Schizophrenia is no asset in any of
these professions.

If the physician has a great responsibility to his patient, he also has a
responsibility to the future patients of this would-be physician.
Nonetheless, the young man in the case approached the school psychiatrist for care, not for professional guidance. Because of cases
similar to this, I have repeatedly advised all of my patients and friends
to make sure that their children never consult school professionals,
whether they be psychiatrists, psychologists, internists, or what have
you. I have seen too many cases where the school psychiatrist has
adopted the manner of personal physician, but seen his responsibility
as an employee of the institution. And that is precisely the problem.
Unless a physician's role is clearly defined as primarily serving the
needs of the individual patient rather than the needs of the employer,
the trust on which all medicine rests, particularly psychiatric medicine,
will be destroyed.

Every occasion when it is decided that responsibility to a greater
good must supersede responsibility to the patient is a violation of the
medical contract with the patient. It must not be called otherwise. We
must not rationalize the dilemma by asserting that we are fulfilling our
responsibility to our patient. We are not. We are granting a higher
priority to other responsibilities. Never should this violation of
contract be a matter of diffidence or routine, as is too often the case
with "company" physicians. To use the diagnostic skills of the
physician to the detriment of the patient, albeit for a larger good,
should be a decision made with the personal agony that always
accompanies a moral dilemma. I wonder if the school psychiatrist in
this case suffered much when he committed his casual diagnosis to the
public record.[6]

Gaylin's argument for the obligation to the student is a strong one. Yet
even he concedes that some duty is owed to the school or to society in
general. Daniel Callahan, a philosopher, has also commented on this
case, arguing that the psychiatrist's obligations extend beyond the
individual patient:

This case raises questions at two different levels, one general, the other
more specific. At the most general level, I have long been troubled by
the problem of whether there can be ethically correct decisions within
settings which are inherently unjust or immoral, i.e., in those
situations where certain kinds of ethical dilemmas would not ordinarily arise but for the fact of distorted or corrupt institutions. In the era
of slavery, for example, acute ethical dilemmas used to arise (for some,
at least) over the most moral way of separating children from parents
when all were to be sold at auction. Obviously the very institution of
slavery was immoral. But does that entail that each and every decision

made within the *given* context of such an institution was also and equally immoral, regardless of what the decision was?

I will leave that question hanging for the moment. But it has direct bearing on how one might judge the actions of the various parties in the case at hand. On the face of it, the procedure used in judging the question of readmission for the student was unjust. First, it is highly doubtful that, when the student initially went to the school psychiatrist, he was informed that "anything you say to me may be held against you," which was exactly what turned out to be the case. Second, it seems clear that the school psychiatrist acted as the agent of the school at a final, critical moment—the moment of decision about readmission. Third, and worse still, the school psychiatrist acted in effect as the agent for all medical schools, creating a very nasty kind of black-ball system. Fourth, since the case clearly implies that the student, on the advice of his private psychiatrist, initiated the request for a leave, and took that leave voluntarily, it seems to me thoroughly unjust that he should be subjected to special conditions in order to regain his place in the school. He had already won his admission to the school. Finally, it is evident that the school provided no formal review mechanism for its procedurally arbitrary decision, and nothing remotely approaching due process.

But did the school make a wrong ethical decision in this particular case? My phrasing of the question implies that a distinction can be made between an unjust system of making decisions and the moral correctness of any given decision within the context of that system. Given the specifics of the case, I think the action of the school can be defended, though hardly praised. Let us charitably assume that, when the student's readmission case came up, those making the decision were at least sensitive enough to recognize that it would be a great blow to the student, a blow made all the harsher by the black-ball system which then ensued. But I would also assume they felt, appropriately enough, that they had obligations not only to the student but also to his potential future patients. The notion of a surgeon incipiently subject to "grandiose self-appraisal" is hardly reassuring. Even if there were only a risk (though not a negligible one), the consequences for his patients could be enormous. And I would suppose that, given the fact that there are many qualified candidates for medical school (who are not latent schizophrenics and who could be taken but for lack of space), they may well have reasoned that there was no *need* to run the risk to future patients. In a situation where a hard choice had to be made, they chose to worry more about the potential harm to patients than the harm caused by thwarting the student's medical ambitions. It is a defensible choice and, as in many hard cases, that may be all that can be achieved.

Let me return to the question I left hanging in the opening paragraph. My answer is "no": correct ethical choices *can sometimes* be made in unjust contexts. But the larger ethical question remains that of the unjust context, which requires correction. I am hardly a devotee of the increasing tendency in our society for all institutional disputes to be taken to court. But in this instance I wish the student had done so. He may not have been admitted in the end, but others might have been the beneficiaries of a system forced to give up arbitrary exercises of power; and the school psychiatrist might have been forced to protect the confidentiality of his relationship with other students.[7]

One special aspect of this case may help to resolve the problem. If it became widely known that school psychiatrists might report their findings to administrative authorities with the power to remove a student from school or to keep him from re-entering, the result would be a disaster. No intelligent student would seek psychiatric help from the school health service. School authorities would learn even less about the psychiatric needs of students and the psychiatric risks to the school and the public. The psychiatrist's actions could then be self-defeating, even if his objective were to serve the school and the public rather than his patient. This argument, which could be used to oppose the psychiatrist's disclosure, is nevertheless based on the conviction that the physician's duty includes serving the school or the public as well as the patient. While focusing on the long-range consequences of the practice, the argument assumes that the physician's obligation can be to others than the patient, even though its conclusion appears similar to that reached by Gaylin.

Another unusual aspect of this case is the impact of the psychiatrist's example on the medical students. Suppose that the psychiatrist took a position similar to Gaylin's, that only rarely should he violate patient confidentiality to serve the interests of others. Even if he felt that the present case was one of those rare times when such a violation is justified, he must also recognize that as a medical school employee, he is a role model for the future physician. The argument can be made that it is impossible to train physicians to a role of normally serving patients when the model held out to the student in the staff physician demonstrates a differing set of commitments.

To ban altogether the institutional employment of physicians, however, might be more contrary to the interests of the students or employees served by institutional physicians than is the present admittedly ambiguous situation. Another alternative is to maintain the present confusion of responsibilities, but also to warn each patient before establishing a relationship with a physician that the conflict exists and that what the patient discloses might be used against him. This might have the same effect as banning the institutional physician completely. Still another alternative is to insist that the physician in the employ of an institution serve the individual patient exclusively and ignore the conflicting interests of his employer. In public institutions such as schools, this might be feasible. Even here, however, it may be unrealistic to think that an employee can so completely divorce himself from his employer's interests. Even if this is possible in public institutions, it clearly is not so in private, commercial businesses.

20   THE COMPANY PHYSICIAN'S DILEMMA

Joseph Fogarty had worked as a machinist for DeVito Asbestos Company for thirty-one years. For many years he had experienced shortness of breath which had recently worsened. Beginning in 1962, the company had employed a physician to give each employee a physical examination every three years. Mr. Fogarty had had three physical examinations by the company physician at the time that he saw a private doctor about his breathing difficulty. The private physician informed him that he had asbestosis, a fibrotic reaction of lung tissue to the irritating effect of the asbestos fibers. In addition to respiratory difficulty, asbestosis substantially increases the risk of lung cancer.

Mr. Fogarty discovered that the company physician had found advancing signs of asbestosis during the first examination but had failed to advise him of the fact or to refer him to a chest specialist. The physician did not deny the presence of the asbestosis, but argued that it would have been useless to refer him to another physician or to have him change his work at a point after some twenty-two years of exposure to the asbestos fibers. He pointed out that there is a long latency in harm caused by the asbestos fibers and that the plant had taken major steps to reduce the fibers in the air at the time the physician was hired. He also argued that he would simply upset Mr. Fogarty by telling him of the untreatable condition. He maintained that his only obligation was to report the results of the examination to Mr. Fogarty's employer. Mr. Fogarty's private physician agreed that substantial damage had already been done at the time of the first medical exam, but maintained that Mr. Fogarty should have been advised at that time to avoid further exposure to the fibers and that in any case he had a right to be informed of the diagnosis.

This case poses a more interesting ethical dilemma if the company physician really believes that no great good will come to Mr. Fogarty by telling him of his asbestosis and that, in fact, psychological harm might be done. It is conceivable that such a position can be held in good faith, although it would presumably be a minority view. If he does believe that no medical use can be made of the diagnosis of asbestosis, two questions remain. The first is whether a company physician has an obligation to reveal a diagnosis, even if it might produce psychological stress, when no medical use can be made of the information but the patient might reasonably want to know it.

The second, more directly relevant question is whether the physician's conflicting loyalty to the corporation is any way related to his judgment that no good and possibly harm might come from the disclosure. Especially if that conclusion is a minority opinion in medicine and Mr. Fogarty's private physician does not share the opinion, there is reason to suspect that it may have been influenced by the physician's loyalty to his employer. Certainly the conflict in this case between the duty to the employer and to the patient is intense.

The dilemma arises because at the same time that businesses and other institutions are taking progressive steps to provide health care for employees, they are also creating the conflict of interest faced by the asbestos company physician. Banning the employment of physicians by companies that expose employees to health risks does not seem to be the answer. Yet if the physician is an employee of the company, it is reasonable to expect that this conflict will emerge from time to time.

Part of the problem might be resolved by requiring corporations to provide primary health care for employees not through company physicians but through privately arranged physicians of the employee's own choosing. This would eliminate the conflict of interest in the role of the physician, but at the expense of many of the advantages of the asbestos company's arrangement. Company physicians can be alerted to occupational hazards and receive specialized training to care for them. By connecting health care with employment, patients are also able to communicate and perhaps even to express their collective voice through a union.

Even if some aspects of the dilemma could be resolved by using privately arranged physicians at the company's expense, the more perplexing problem remains. Should physicians enter into arrangements to sell their services to business? Can they justifiably owe their allegiance to someone other than the patient? It is not uncommon for business to use physicians to screen prospective employees for medical and psychiatric risks or for insurance companies to pay physicians to minimize the company's risks. Even if there is no pretense that the patient's interests are to be served and even if the patient understands exactly the nature of the relationship, is it acceptable for the physician to sell his services for these purposes? The question is to whom the physician owes his loyalty.

The Individual and Other Individuals

An even more difficult challenge to the principle that the physician's duty is to the individual patient arises not when a specific institution or corporation but when another identifiable individual competes with the patient. The conflict between the duty to the individual and the duty to society is finally reduced to a conflict between loyalty to individuals.

This problem of loyalty conflict is one of the most pervasive in medical ethics. It normally arises in the role of the physician, even though, as in the legislative proposal for compulsory physician service in a national health corps, the decision-makers may be persons other than the physicians themselves. But the conflict can also arise in many other roles, such as the parental.

21 THE PHYSICIAN AS CHILD PROTECTOR

Sarah Green was an unmarried 20-year-old who had been a heavy user of heroin for three years, shooting up from ten to twenty bags per day. She supported her habit by prostitution and other activities.

On September 22, 1972, after a pregnancy with no other complications, she gave birth to a premature male infant weighing only 4 lbs. 2 oz. with an estimated gestational age of thirty-two weeks. The immediate postnatal period was marked by signs of mild respiratory distress syndrome complicated by infant heroin withdrawal. Although his first seventy-two hours of life were tenuous, the infant, christened Reginald, recovered and began to gain weight slowly in the intensive care nursery.

After her discharge from the hospital Ms. Green at first visited the child regularly but appeared awkward and ill at ease around the bewildering array of incubators and electronic monitors. After several days she ceased to visit Reginald spontaneously and came only when asked by the social worker or the pediatricians taking care of her son. The presence of a large cultural gulf between the professionals and Ms. Green aggravated the erratic, anxiety-marked relationship between her and the nursery staff, and consequently also her son. Ms. Green's less and less frequent visits became an issue when plans for Reginald's eventual discharge began to be discussed on ward rounds each morning.

As the time of his discharge drew nearer, the pediatricians became increasingly apprehensive about discharging the infant to a mother whose concern seemed so ephemeral and whose drug habit seemed to occupy the majority of her waking life. A debate developed as to whether or not Ms. Green was capable of being a "fit mother." One of the nurses said that an aide had told her that on one occasion after the mother had been called up and asked to come in to help feed the baby, she had "nodded off" with the baby on her lap and seemed to be as "high as a kite."

Rising apprehension by the pediatric staff led to their asking the medical social worker to investigate the home situation. For the first time, contingency plans to have the child placed with the Children's Protective Services Agency were considered. The social worker reported back several days later that Ms. Green had "sensed what was up" and had, on principle, refused to let the social worker into her home, stating that she had a "right to privacy." The social worker added that she was beginning to sense a paranoid reaction of the part of Ms. Green, who had screamed through the locked door, "You'll have to kill me before I'll let you take my baby away!"

Two days later a "hold" was placed on the baby and the Children's Protective Services Agency was asked to find a foster home for him pending a more thorough investigation of Ms. Green's suitability to serve as the mother for her child.

22   THE PARENTS' DILEMMA
WHEN CHILDREN'S INTERESTS CONFLICT

Dr. Marilyn Janis came to Clara Clifford's bedside with her husband, Paul. There were signs of distress on the physician's face. Mrs. Clifford had given birth to a girl the day before and now Dr. Janis began slowly to explain the problem to the Cliffords. The baby had an open myelomeningocele, a congenital opening in the spine with a projection of the spinal cord and its meninges into a pouch of skin protruding from the infant's back.

Until recently about 80 percent of babies with myelomeningocele died. Now surgical intervention can save the baby's life 70 to 75 percent of the time. Even when the baby's life is saved, however, serious physical and often mental problems remain. According to one recent study, Dr. Janis explained to the Cliffords, only six percent of those who survive can walk without the aid of braces. The chance of incontinence is great. She also told the parents that if the baby lived, there was a good chance that her intelligence would be affected. In one study of 79 children with myelomeningocele, only 22 had IQ scores above 110, while 31 had scores in the range 90-110 and 16 had scores below 70. Dr. Janis pointed out that of those who survive, the chances are about fifty-fifty that they will have only minimal or moderate impairment, that they will be able to walk with braces, or possibly even without them, and that they will have above normal intelligence. Finally, she told the Cliffords of one family in which a baby had been born with myelomeningocele who had received the operation. Even though there was a moderate handicap, the baby had brought a great joy to the family.

The Cliffords had three other children, ages two through six. Mr. Clifford worked as a pressman in a small printing plant, earning $14,500 a year. Mrs. Clifford had held several jobs—as receptionist in a real estate office and file clerk in a business firm—before she was married, but now had a full-time job taking care of the children. The physician indicated that she thought the chances of survival for their baby were good. She had sensation down to the L-4 level of the spinal cord, which was not as low as Dr. Janis would have liked, but indicated a good chance of only moderate disability. There was no indication of hydrocephalus and no neural plaque, both good signs. Even so, she pointed out, the Cliffords should expect a lifetime of extensive medical treatments and physical therapy.

Some parents might decide at this point that it was in the baby's interest not to survive. The Cliffords recognized that life was going to be difficult for the baby if she survived, but they could not bring themselves to believe that for their baby's own sake she would be "better off dead." They were horrified, though, at the thought of the impact on their other three children. The medical expenses would completely change their lives. They had been planning to move within the next two years from the two-family house where they lived. They looked forward to the time when they could afford weekend outings, perhaps even a vacation, which had been impossible since they were married. More than that, they were worried about the social and psychological impact on the family. The oldest boy was beginning to read. He desperately needed help from his parents on arithmetic, as the teacher had urged them during a recent parents' conference.

After Dr. Janis left the Cliffords alone in the hospital room, they discussed what they should do. For themselves, Mr. and Mrs. Clifford were willing to sacrifice. But, they argued with themselves, could they really impose that burden on their other children?

These two cases present the problem of trading off the interests and needs of one person, who is first thought of as the patient, for the needs of some other specific person to whom obligations are also owed. The two cases differ in at least two ways. In one case the physician must choose to whom he owes allegiance; in the other case the parents must choose. Often it is said that the physician's moral obligation is solely or primarily to his patient, while the parents have equal obligations to all their children. The question arises whether this implies that the physician seeing Ms. Green, who first identifies her as his patient, has no obligation to Reginald, whereas the Cliffords have a duty to consider the needs of their older children as well as the new baby with myelomeningocele.

A second contrast between the two cases is that while both Ms. Green and her baby have medical needs, only the Cliffords' newborn baby does. Some might suggest that Ms. Green's physician makes a moral mistake in identifying only the mother and not the baby as the "patient." One could argue that the physician has an obligation to consider the needs of the "other patient." Even if that case were made, however, it would have no bearing on the decision-making problem of the Cliffords. Even if physicians should consider the medical needs of one while excluding the nonmedical needs of another, it must be wrong for parents to give unique priority to medical needs to the exclusion of nonmedical needs. The question is whether this implies that the Cliffords have not only a right but a duty to trade off the interests of one child for those of others.

The underlying philosophical problem is the interchangeability of goods from one person to another. Classical utilitarianism holds that the morally correct action is the one that will produce the greatest good altogether. In order to determine which action is morally right, the net good for each person in the society for each plausible course of action is summed up. The major criticism of this ethical tradition is that it fails to take into account both who receives the goods and how the goods are distributed—except for the likelihood that more good is produced in total when goods are distributed rather evenly. Risking the lives of a few in a medical experiment is acceptable according to utilitarianism so long as it is likely that, on balance, more good will be done, even if that good takes the form of a smaller individual good for many more people.

Both physicians and parents normally believe that goods are not completely interchangeable. The physician has a special obligation, a contract, with his patient. Parents have a special obligation to their own children. If this is true, two moral problems remain. For the physician, the question is to avoid individualistic ethics. Especially in situations where the interests of one patient conflict with those of another, it is not helpful to say that the physician's duty is to his patient. For the parent, the question is how to serve the children's interests equally when those interests conflict.

There are some possibilities of avoiding the moral dilemmas. If mother and child have different physicians, some conflict might be avoided. That, however, would make the medical role an adversarial one. If decent social support were available for the Cliffords, they would not have to choose between the baby and the other children. Short of such ideal resolutions, some solution must be found, even if it is only the best of poor solutions. Some mean must be found between the hyperindividualism of focusing only on the isolated patient and the utilitarianism of casually trading off the interests of one for the interests of another.

It is possible to have a social ethic, an ethic considering the relations among people and among institutions, without resorting to a utilitarian indifference to how goods are distributed. Promises or contracts may create a complex set of obligations. A principle of justice may require a special distribution of benefits and harms. In the case of Ms. Green and Reginald, one resolution would be to treat both mother and son as the physician's patients and then conclude that Reginald's interests are more weighty or more legitimate than his parent's. That would probably justify the intervention to begin the process of taking custody away from Ms. Green. But with or without considering Reginald as a patient, the physician may conclude either that Ms. Green's interests have a greater claim or that, despite his feeling that intervention to protect the baby is called for, it is best in the long run that the physician not intervene into the mother/child relation. He may conclude that the imposition of his own values about how a child should be treated smacks of a paternalism which will do more harm than good, more wrong than right. In this event he would conclude that the intervention is not justified.

In the case of the Cliffords, intervention cannot be avoided. They are in the parental role, like it or not. They could have reasoned that it is in the baby's interest, as well as in the other children's, not to intervene with treatment. Or they could have concluded that it is in the other children's interests, as well as the baby's, to intervene. They apparently did not reach either conclusion, however. Instead, they were forced into deciding what is a fair or just distribution of the family's limited resources. Certainly special needs justify some special commitment of those resources to the sick family member. Yet the same principle of fairness must set some reasonable limit on how much the other children can be harmed for the good of the sick one. In the Cliffords' case, if not in Ms. Green's, a direct conflict of interests exists because a specific duty exists to all the children.

CHAPTER 4

Health Care Delivery

The right to health, or at least to health care, is becoming a major ethical issue in medicine. Health care is not evenly distributed in American society. In a period when the walls cry out for social justice, the hospital and the physician's office can no longer remain silent. A full medical ethics must include a social ethic of health care delivery. Not every problem in medical ethics is a problem because the case itself is ethically exotic. Drug experiments on helpless babies, decisions to inject potassium in the veins of a helpless paraplegic, manipulation of the human genetic code—all these are important ethical issues, but in each it is the medical condition or the proposed remedy which poses the ethical dilemma. In questions involving health care delivery, the medical conditions are much less provocative. The patients in these cases could have almost any medical problem. The specifics are not important. What is important is how these patients ought to be treated by the health care delivery system or whether they ought to be treated at all.

As with the moral problem of a conflict of loyalty, health care delivery requires an ethic to overcome both the irrelevancy of an individualistic ethic and the crudeness of calculating total benefits and harms, which ignores the question of who receives those benefits or harms. One answer is to turn to other ethical principles that may supplement the utilitarian ethic of maximizing the total good. In addition to the Hippocratic principle that the physician's duty is only to his patients, many believe that the principles of justice, freedom, trust, honesty, and promise-keeping are required. The moral problems of ordinary health care delivery often hinge on these principles and on their relation to efforts to maximize the health of the individual patient or the society as a whole. The ethical problems of confidentiality are really problems of keeping implied or explicit promises, of fulfilling a contract between patient and physician, even in the face of what in retrospect appears to be overwhelmingly bad consequences. The dilemma of whether to tell the dying cancer patient of his bleak prognosis when the physician believes it would be upsetting for the patient is a problem in the conflict between the principles of truth-telling and doing good.

Some of the most serious ethical problems in medicine today are those of justice in health care delivery. A closely related issue is the right to health care. Other conflicts involve efficiency in health care delivery as opposed to patient freedom and dignity, and professional or collegial trust as opposed to patient needs.

Justice in Health Care Delivery

The Hippocratic physician pledges to benefit his patients and to "keep them from harm and injustice." Aristotle pointed out that "justice" has more than one meaning. On the one hand, one who is law-abiding is called just. On the other hand, in a much more restricted sense, one who is fair in the way he distributes things is called just. In the broader sense, justice simply means moral rightness. As applied to human character, this kind of justice, according to Aristotle, "is complete virtue and excellence in the fullest sense." In other words, "In justice every virtue is summed up." The Greek term translated as "injustice" in the Hippocratic oath really means "wrongdoing." The oath seems to use the term in this broader sense.

Often, however, "justice" refers to the way something is distributed. This is a much more limited meaning. To be just is to be fair in distributing goods or harms. In this narrower sense Aristotle spoke of the just as being equal or proportional or "fair." He then introduced the great problem in the history of moral philosophy which is at the heart of the ethical dilemmas of health care delivery: "If the persons are not equal, their (just) shares will not be equal; but this is the source of quarrels and recriminations, when equals have and are awarded unequal shares or unequals equal shares. The truth of this is further illustrated by the principle 'To each according to his deserts.' Everyone agrees that in distributions the just share must be given on the basis of what one deserves, though not everyone would name the same criterion of deserving: democrats say it is free birth; oligarchs that it is wealth or noble birth, and aristocrats that it is excellence."[1]

The problem of justice in distribution, which is the only sense in which the term is used here in these cases, is even more complicated than

Aristotle claimed. He recognized that different people hold to differing claims for a just or fair distribution. But the possible criteria for a just distribution are even greater than he envisaged. Some things, like votes, are thought to be fairly distributed in one manner, while other things, like medical services, might be distributed fairly in another manner. In fact, to distribute health equally certainly does not permit distributing health resources or even health care equally. To speak of a just or fair distribution requires identifying the thing that is to be distributed as well as the way it is distributed. Abstract arguments about distribution on the basis of need rather than merit or ability turn out to be vacuous.

Aristotle suggested free birth, wealth or noble birth, and excellence as criteria for justice. Certainly there are more. In some, if not all, cases health care delivery would be considered outrageously unjust if it were distributed according to either birth, wealth, or excellence. To be sure, health resources are often distributed as if wealth, social status, and ethnic identity were the most relevant considerations, but few would defend these criteria as morally justified. At least nine other criteria for a just distribution have been used to defend health care delivery policies. Some of them are quite plausible, others less defensible. By these criteria, health care should be distributed:

Equally
According to need
According to desire
According to ability
According to merit
According to usefulness to society
According to desire to serve society
According to what society owes
According to an objective measure

Specific medical services needed by all, such as immunizations, might fairly be distributed equally. Every human being has an equal claim to these services without regard to any objective or subjective differences among people. Even here, however, relevant differences may exist, such as exposure to risk. The clearest case where the distribution is thought to be fair when every person gets the exact same amount is the right to vote. The principle of one person, one vote, implies that all persons are equally entitled to the vote without regard to differences which obviously exist. These differences are thought to be morally irrelevant with regard to the vote.

Access to health care clearly should not be distributed so that each person gets the same amount. Perhaps it should be distributed according to need. Distributing health care according to need would have as the objective, whether or not it could ever be fulfilled, the distribution of health equally. Some would argue that health care should not be distributed according to need but according to ability. They would not leave to the toss of a coin to decide whether a physician attends first an artist, a scientist, a community leader, or a familyless peasant. Distributing according to merit is the subjective side of distributing according to ability. Both merit and ability differ from usefulness to society.

All three criteria are very problematic as a basis for a fair distribution of health care, but all have their defenders. Distributing according to willingness to serve others is once again the subjective analogue of usefulness to others. Distributing according to what society owes is really the principle of retributive justice, of being fair in making up for past wrongs. The moral question here is whether oppressed groups should be given special compensatory medical services so that health statistics for these groups rise to the level of the general population.

Nourishing food might be thought of as justly distributed according to body weight rather than equally to each human being, although someone would certainly ask whether it is fair for the three-hundred-pounder to get proportionally more than the malnourished, underweight child. This is the meaning of the criteria of distributing in proportion to some objective measure.

Normally the distribution of necessities such as health care is not considered to be fair if they are allocated according to desire. There are special cases, though, where this might be fair. Distributing according to desire is thought fair when limited amounts of two interchangeable goods are available for two equally deserving people. Suppose two chronic nephritis patients were being treated in a facility where there was one available hemodialysis machine and one available cadaver kidney. If one wanted a transplant and the other wanted dialysis, it would be thought both fair and wise, other things being equal, to distribute the scarce resources according to the desires of the two patients.

23   THE PATIENT AND THE PHYSICIANLESS POOR

Dr. Harrison Dorman was leaving his Westchester County private office, where he practiced internal medicine, just in time to drive to New York City for a 3 P.M. meeting of the senior staff of the Outpatient Clinic at Williamson General Hospital. Dr. Dorman was an adjunct professor and one of five senior attending physicians in the Ambulatory Care Department, which was responsible for the Outpatient Clinic. Williamson General Hospital was the main teaching hospital for one of the city's medical schools. In addition to serving as a referral center for many of the most complicated medical cases in the area, Williamson General served as the primary health care source for an inner-city area of 52,000 people, primarily low-income black and Puerto Rican. The Outpatient Clinic was an embarrassment to the medical school as well as a source of friction in the community. While private patients at Williamson General rested in cheerful private rooms and overstuffed leather chairs lined their waiting-room walls, the Outpatient Department was a dingy, overcrowded, mass-production medical assembly line located in the building next door. Over the years as the clinic's role as primary health care provider grew, a series of "examining rooms" had been created by placing seven-foot-high folding partitions in the corridor of the first floor. On any given day between one and two hundred patients sat in rows waiting their turn to see a physician. Babies crawled on the floor. Lunches were brought in brown paper bags because patients feared losing their place in line if they left for food.

The meeting was a critical one for planning a completely new outpatient facility. As Dr. Dorman was leaving his office, he had a phone call from the hospital. He started to indicate that he was not available but then, thinking the call was about the meeting, decided to take it. The call was from the resident on the internal medicine service in the private section. Doris Kern, one of Dr. Dorman's private patients, had taken a turn for the worse. She was coughing and complaining of diffuse thoracic pain. She had been hospitalized for the past two weeks with broncho-genic carcinoma. Yesterday she had undergone surgery for the removal of the lobe of the lung containing the cancer. The resident later thought he noticed a slight sign of possible infection. He had given an injection of meperidine for the pain, and now the surgical dressing needed to be changed. He was prepared to change the dressing, but Mrs. Kern had pleaded to have her "own doctor do it." Dr. Dorman, annoyed because it would prevent him from attending the meeting, said that the resident could do the job at least as well. They recognized, however, that Mrs. Kern was under a great deal of stress and that she would be much more comfortable if Dr. Dorman came in to change the dressing. The resident wanted to know if Dr. Dorman could come to see her at once.

As Dr. Dorman left his office, he noticed the framed copy of the Hippocratic oath on his waiting-room wall. "I will follow that system of regimen," it read, "which according to my ability and judgment, I consider for the benefit of my patients, and abstain from whatever is deleterious and mischievous."

The problem faced by Dr. Dorman resembles the ethical conflicts where the duty to benefit the individual, often the patient, is pitted against the duty to benefit society more generally. What is striking in such cases is that if one were to follow the ethic of patient benefit, the physician would have not only a clear right but an actual obligation to ignore the needs of the anonymous clinic patients. The ethic of social consequences would counter this individualism by arguing that the good which Dr. Dorman can do by attending the clinic meeting might in the long run produce much greater benefit in toto than the more immediate and personal good he can do to Mrs. Kern. This is particularly true if Mrs. Kern's physical needs are being dealt with competently by the resident and if there is a crucial need for the rapid building of the clinic.

This rebuttal to the patient-benefiting ethic appeals to the consequences of the alternatives, but thereby opens the door for abandoning patients or even directly abusing them if a good case can be made that on balance society will gain. To avoid this problem, an alternative standard could be the just use of medical resources, in this case Dr. Dorman's time. It appears that Mrs. Kern is comparatively well off and has access to medical care far beyond that available to those who might use the clinic. If the criterion for a just distribution of health care efforts is need, then failure to fulfill Mrs. Kern's request for attention might be justified. If ability to pay is the basis, then a rather different outcome might result. An appeal to the keeping of a patient-physician "contract" might also defend Dr. Dorman's attendance to Mrs. Kern on a quite different moral principle.

24 HOME HEALTH CARE AND INPATIENT LOYALTY

Brown City Hospital had just received notice of the funding of an experimental program in integrated geriatic health care. It was an ingenious proposal designed in part to provide additional funds for the desperately understaffed geriatrics program. The thesis of the project was that geriatric patients have a complex set of medical, social, and psychological problems requiring integrated attention by physicians, psychologists, social workers, and nursing staff, all of whom need special skills and aptitude to deal with the elderly. Until now geriatric patients had had to shift for themselves, moving in the hospital from department to department to meet their needs. This was particularly difficult for the elderly. The grant was considered both an experiment providing health care for geriatric patients and a new source of funding for medical services.

The senior staff of the geriatrics program included geriatric specialists from psychiatry, internal medicine, surgery, and public health, in addition to personnel from nursing and social work. They were meeting to begin planning the details of the new service. Brown City Hospital served an inner-city community of 300,000. Since geriatric patients presently in the hospital were being cared for by separate clinics, it was difficult to estimate the size of the population of patients actually being served who would qualify for the new program. It was clear, however, from waits of four to six weeks for appointments that the present patient population could be served much more effectively.

A major policy problem arose during the meeting. Dr. Joel Winters, an internist, and Dr. Roberta Hays, a psychiatrist, advocated a new geriatric clinic at the hospital. They argued that their first responsibility was to meet the needs of those who were already using the hospital's services. They claimed that those who had sought out the hospital were likely to be in the greatest need. More important, they held that a special obligation existed to improve the health care of those who were already in the Brown City Hospital patient population.

Dr. Martin Dover, the public health epidemiologist, and Ms. Wilma Ryder, the social worker, defended another approach. They felt that the program, to be truly innovative, must emphasize home health care. They argued that there was even greater medical need among those who were not yet in the hospital's patient population, who were too sick or too immobile to come to the hospital for help. They made another argument, however, which extended beyond the empirical question of who could be helped the most. They argued that because it was a city hospital, they had an obligation to all the elderly sick in the hospital's catchment area. Their special obligation was not to those who were already getting care from the hospital but to those who were not yet being served. They conceded that home health care might be less efficient. Much time of medical personnel would be spent on travel. They defended the program, however, first by arguing that the quality of care would be better in the patient's home, and second by maintaining that home care, even if less efficient, was owed as a special duty to those not now getting medical attention.

There are several ways to structure this debate between the two groups in the geriatric program staff. Their primary disagreement appears to be a simple, empirical one. They disagree over which course of action would produce the most health and happiness for the community. Both groups are arguing morality based on the expected consequences. Even though it appears that this is an empirical issue, however, such may not really be the case. It is interesting that the psychiatrist and the internist are the ones who believe that the most good can be done by seeing patients individually and in the hospital setting, while the public health physician and the social worker believe that more good can be done if patients are seen in the familial setting in the context of their day-to-day living. Both the public health physician and the social worker have made vocational choices implying that the social context is more important, while the psychiatrist and the internist are involved in specialties where the presumption is that the individual is an autonomous unit whose problems are more individual. Thus, even the disagreement over consequences may be rooted in the underlying value orientation of the members of the staff.

It appears that their real disagreement, however, is not simply over which course would most improve the health statistics of the geriatric population of the community. Drs. Winter and Hays maintain that they have a special responsibility to those who are already in the patient network, those who are already involved in some patient-physician relationship with the hospital staff. They are defending the traditional physician ethic of patient benefit. The argument of Dr. Dover and Ms. Ryder, however, runs counter to that principle. They argue that there is a special duty to the physicianless. Their position, if analyzed, focuses on what is just or fair. Those already in the hospital, so the argument goes, are already being provided some medical services. Although these services are not ideal, they are meeting at least some of the needs. If fairness requires meeting the needs of those who are not now receiving any medical attention, then there is a duty to go beyond the hospital walls and provide home health care. This is true, at least within certain limits, even if it means compromising the care given to those who are already within the hospital sphere. The argument from justice requires at least two assumptions: that need rather than ability or usefulness is the proper basis for a fair distribution, and that those not getting care who could be served in the home health care program have needs at least as great as those who would benefit in the new hospital clinics. The resolution requires both empirical and ethical evaluations.

25   COMPENSATORY JUSTICE AND CLINIC LOCATION

The city, one of the largest in the Midwest, had just received approval of a $4,000,000 federal government grant for family planning clinics. Twelve city hospitals, spread throughout the city, made up its main health resources. In addition, two private hospitals and four facilities sponsored by churches served the area.

Councilman Carter Lyons led off the debate in the City Council. The city health commissioner had just reported the Health Department's recommendation that because of need, the clinics should be established only in the four hospitals serving the two urban renewal areas. Per capita income in the area was one-third that of the semisuburban outer areas of the city. The four hospitals were admittedly old, overcrowded, and poorly staffed. They depended on interns, residents, and a large number of foreign medical graduates. The health commissioner argued, however, that the limited clinic funds should go to the area where there was the most need.

Councilman Lyons rose to demand that all hospitals in the city be treated equally. It was only fair, he argued, that every taxpayer should benefit from the government grant. He pointed out that if only the urban renewal area hospitals received the funds, those patients might be stigmatized. He believed that the only way to have a just system of health care was to have all citizens receive the same services. On the national level he was for national health insurance. He even held privately that such insurance should be made compulsory, so that every person would be treated as an equal without regard to social class, race, or economic status.

Councilman Joseph Vassello, who represented the conservative working-class north side, rose to defend the health commissioner. He did not often agree with the commissioner, but in this case he found that the need was indeed greatest in the four hospital areas. He pointed out that the illegitimacy rate in the areas served by those hospitals was twice that of the rest of the city. This, he argued, was one area where the city could save itself some money while helping those in need.

To this, Councilman Tom Brown responded with passion. Councilman Brown represented the south side urban renewal district. He began by noting how rare it was for the council's only black councilman to find himself agreeing with Councilman Vassello. He did not agree, however, with the implications of the councilman that the area should be singled out because it was a source of trouble for the city. He defended the targeting of the family planning grant funds into the four hospitals, but not for Councilman Vassello's reasons. In fact, he thought it strange that the areas which had the lowest per capita school expenditure of any area in the city, the lowest street maintenance budget, the smallest branch library, and the worst hospitals were suddenly so concerned about making sure the black community got its share. He then asked the commissioner if a really effective family planning program would not require high-quality maternal, family, and child health programs. The commissioner, stumbling, said he thought it probably would. "Then," Councilman Brown replied, "we'll be delighted to support the commissioner's proposal. We've got it coming."

The allocation of family planning clinic funding introduces the question of justice in a very direct form. Each of the participants in the City Council debate apparently opts for a different criterion for a just distribution of those funds. The health commissioner, representing one liberal position, makes his case on the basis of need. He does not spell out, however, exactly what the urban renewal area needs, whether it be family planning assistance, health care, or general support of schools, roads, and social services. The argument on the basis of need could be quite different depending on precisely what is being distributed.

Councilman Vassello's position is first put in terms of need as well, though he apparently does not share the rest of the commissioner's position. The tone of the councilman's remarks implies that he may have in mind usefulness to society as his criterion. If this is the basis of the distribution, the targeting of the urban renewal area may indeed stigmatize, as Councilman Lyons suggests.

Councilman Lyons is holding out for another liberal criterion of justice. He wants the resources to be distributed equally. Everyone, according to this position, should have equal access to the newly funded program. He makes a good case that this would work against class-based health care, but at the same time he ignores the needs growing out of the social history of the community.

Councilman Brown is very conscious of that social context. He argues in essence for compensatory justice. Distribution must be such as to make up for past wrongs. The same argument for racial and gender hiring quotas has become a matter of controversy. A similar decision was recently made in China where rural peasants are given special priority in health care delivery.[2]

26 A HEALTH CARE DELIVERY EXPERIMENT

Three years ago the Neighborhood Comprehensive Child Health Center, designed especially to provide pediatric care, was funded in the severely economically depressed Judson Heights area by the Children's Bureau of the Department of Health, Education, and Welfare. Although almost all of the previously existing private doctors had fled the area, it was not devoid of medical care. The outpatient department at City Hospital was nearby, but waiting was often long and uncomfortable and care might be impersonal and fragmented. The only other doctors were practicing in offices in the newly established Medicaid centers, which were generally open only from about 9 to 5 which, because of the reimbursement pattern, often required patients to see multiple doctors and return for frequent visits without clear necessity, and which, it is alleged, provided care of questionable quality.

The Child Health Center provided excellent service to the children of the defined geographic area, but the parents of those children were having a difficult time getting medical care for themselves. The staff thought it would be valuable to provide some medical care for the parents as well as for the children. But all of their medical staff were pediatricians. After a long struggle, they convinced a federal agency to place two internists in the project.

This move made it possible for the center not only to care for the children but also to offer some care to the adults. Since the center had fewer internists by far than pediatricians, there was no way that it could provide care in a blanket fashion to all of the parents and all of the children being cared for. The question was how to choose the parents for the project, whether to admit them on a first-come first-served basis, to care for only the sickest adults, or to allow adults in a certain geographic subsection of the area devoted to children to take advantage of the care available. What the staff decided was to define a research project in which in some random fashion they could assign the opportunity for care to one group of adults and not to another group. Over the course of two or three years they might thereby determine whether it made any difference in the care of the children if their parents were also being seen at the same time by the same medical team. Nobody has ever demonstrated, although many have long claimed, that if an entire family is under care from the same doctor or team, then the whole family, including the children, get better medical care than if the children alone are being treated. It is an article of faith of family practice medicine that a doctor seeing everyone in the family improves the medical care, but this has never been formally demonstrated.

The Child Health Center then faced the question of how to allocate randomly and how to get permission for patients to be randomly allocated to this scarce, new, high-quality care in the neighborhood. They decided that the best scientific basis for the random allocation was to label each book in the defined geographic area as either *A* or *B*. Census data on the blocks was used to ensure that the *A*'s and *B*'s were matched on characteristics like racial distribution and medial family income. Those children newly arriving at the center from blocks labeled *A* would have not only themselves and their siblings registered but also their parents. Those who came from blocks labeled *B* would have only the children of the family registered. This plan was felt to be superior to alternating the assignment to the two groups as patients registered at the clinic, because alternating could lend itself more easily to abuse. A person manning the registration desk who knew that the next registrant was going to receive care for the entire family might be inclined to choose Mrs. Jones rather than Mrs. Brown on the basis of personal prejudice. The block assignments were supposed to be unknown to the registrar and the community until someone actually came in with the address. In short, the blocks in the area were to be randomly allocated. The first 200 families newly registering at the center from blocks in group *A* were to get parental as well as child care; the first 200 from blocks in group *B* were to get child care only. Both groups of children were to be closely followed for two years to determine the nature of the differences, if any, in the patterns, outcomes, and satisfaction with care. The research design was highly praised and handsomely funded by an appropriate government agency.

The research proposal was taken for approval, on the one hand, to the

Community Advisory Board of the Child Health Center and, on the other hand, to the Committee on Human Research of the hospital with which the Child Health Center was affiliated. The community board raised no objections. The Committee on Human Research, however, asked how the project fit in with their requirement that anybody who was being experimented on must be adequately informed and give consent. After discussion, the committee decided that as long as the director of the project fulfilled two requirements, the experiment could be approved. First, the director had to get consent from the community. In this connection the approval already obtained from the Community Advisory Board was felt to be adequate. Second, the patient had to fill out the usual—nothing more than the usual—consent form for treatment, which carries the statement that data on patient care are sometimes used for research purposes. The committee decided that any specific announcement to the patient that he was getting only child care or parent care as well on the basis of a prior randomization of their block faces might prejudice the experiment and would not be necessary.

Only after the study began did problems arise, when people came to realize that some families were being given the opportunity for treatment at the center whereas other families were not being offered this privilege. Some who were not offered the service felt annoyed and angry. One of the house staff claimed that a few parents in the *B* group had asked: "Why can't I get care? I know that Mrs. Smith down the block who also came into the project about the same time I did is getting care."

Also, a group of young physicians reintroduced the argument about justice. They held that the services of the internists should simply go to those families most in need. Senior physicians replied that they did not know any way of deciding a priori who had the most need. Taking those adults who presented themselves as the sickest probably would not really reach the ones most in need. They might simply be the ones who either most perceived the need for care or were most skilled in manipulating social institutions to meet their own needs. Since resources were inadequate to care for everyone, such a policy itself might sow dissension and lead to injustice.

The Right to Health Care

Another set of moral problems is closely linked to the question of justice in health care delivery. The slogan "the right to health" is beginning to have a significant impact on the discussion of ethics and health care delivery. It summarizes the deeply felt conviction that all people ought to have access to health care independent of their financial or social means.

A "right," as defined in ethics, is something to which one is thought to have a morally justified claim. In contrast with a "duty," it refers to something to which one is entitled, rather than something one must do. Rights imply, but normally do not specify, obligations of others. The language of rights is therefore permissive language. Affirming a right means recognizing someone's claim to behave in a certain way or to obtain a certain good if he so desires.

Rules, such as "Thou shalt not kill," must be distinguished from general ethical principles, such as justice or promise-keeping. Rules are more specific, more ad hoc, while principles are more abstract and can be brought to bear on a wide variety of situations. A right is more like a rule in its level of specificity. The right to health care is therefore a summary statement of something rather specific to which one is thought to be entitled. Although the claim of a right to health care is more specific, the underlying moral basis is close to the more abstract claim of justice applied to health care. To say that one has a right to health care is to say that it is only just or fair that such care be provided. Thus the debate about the right to health, or more appropriately the right to health care, is really a variant on the debate about justice and health care delivery. The same sorts of problems arise. The critical question is how to apply the right to health care, particularly when someone else also claims a right to health care or to another conflicting right. The problems will become more critical as the right to health care is more generally recognized.

27 THE COMMITTED PATIENT'S RIGHT TO CARE

In this class action, originally filed in behalf of patients involuntarily confined for mental treatment purposes at Bryce Hospital, Tuscaloosa, Alabama, this Court on March 12, 1971 . . .

The patients at Bryce Hospital, for the most part, were involuntarily committed through non-criminal procedures and without the constitutional protections that are afforded defendants in criminal proceedings . . .

In the matters presented to this Court by the parties, there seem to be three fundamental conditions for adequate and effective treatment programs in public mental institutions. These three fundamental conditions are: (1) a humane psychological and physical environment, (2) qualified staff in numbers sufficient to administer adequate treatment and (3) individualized treatment plans. The report filed by defendants with this Court, as well as the reports and objections of other parties who have studied the conditions at Bryce Hospital, demonstrates rather conclusively that the hospital is deficient in all three of these fundamental respects . . .

The dormitories are barn-like structures with no privacy for the patients. For most patients there is not even a space provided which he can think of as his own. The toilets in restrooms seldom have partitions between them. These are dehumanizing factors which degenerate the patients' self esteem. Also contributing to the poor psychological environment are the shoddy wearing apparel furnished the patients, the non-therapeutic work assigned to patients (mostly compulsory, uncompensated housekeeping chores), and the degrading and humiliating admissions procedure which creates in the patient an impression of the hospital as a prison or as a "crazy house." Other conditions which render the physical environment at Bryce critically substandard are extreme ventilation problems, fire and other emergency hazards, and overcrowding caused to some degree by poor utilization of space. In addition, the quality of the food served the patients is inferior. Only fifty cents per patient per day is spent for food, and sanitation procedures with regard to the preparation and service of food, commonly recognized as basic health practices and utilized at other such hospitals, are not followed at Bryce.

The second fundamental condition needed for effective treatment is a qualified and numerically sufficient staff. It is clear from the reports of Bryce's expert consultants that Bryce is wholly deficient in this area, both as regards its professional staff and its nonprofessional staff. More psychiatrists, Doctor of Philosophy level psychologists and qualified Medical Doctors are not only a medical but are also a constitutional necessity in this public institution. Special staff is needed to place the custodial patients still residing at Bryce . . . The nonprofessional staff is poorly trained; nurses' aides, for example, are required to have only a tenth grade education. Also there is no effective "in-service" training program for, or even any regular supervision over, the nonprofessional staff. The nonprofessionals are spread very thinly; thus, they are overworked, creating not only an inadequate situation for the patients but extreme stresses for individual aides. Both Bryce consultants agree with amici and plaintiffs that additional aides and activities therapists are a necessity.

The third necessary condition for an effective treatment program is individualized treatment plans. Bryce is also deficient in this area. Although every patient has been classified as to treatability, the records made on each patient are inadequate. Minimum medical standards require that periodic inquiries be made . . . [with] a view toward providing suitable treatment for them. Yet, at Bryce the records evidence no notations of mental change. They consist generally only of notations of the times and amounts of drugs given and participation in the Patient Operated Program, the Token Economy Program or the Level Program. Bryce's own consultant advises that treatment is geared primarily to housekeeping functions. The three main programs which have been implemented motivate the patients to some activity and do effect some degree of socialization, but at a minimum level. What programs there are do not yet seem to be operating effectively, partly because of the untrained staff members supervising them.

All the objections raised by amici and by plaintiffs generally are supported by the reports of Bryce's consultants. There seems to be a consensus of opinion among the experts that the treatment program at Bryce Hospital continues to be wholly inadequate.[3]

The first question raised by this case is whether it poses an ethical problem at all. The case is one of patients involuntarily committed through noncriminal procedures. The court record makes clear that such patients have a right to treatment: "When patients are so committed for treatment purposes they unquestionably have a right to receive such individual treatment as will give them a realistic opportunity to be cured or to improve . . . Adequate and effective treatment is constitutionally required because, absent treatment, the hospital is transformed 'into a penitentiary where one could be held indefinitely for no convicted offense.' "[4]

Dr. Stonewall Stickney, the commissioner of mental health in Alabama at the time, later spoke in his own defense:

Our biggest problem along about the middle of the case was how to lose gracefully. The only way we could win was at the expense of the patients, because we felt we had pretty well exhausted our efforts to get sufficient money from the legislature or to sufficiently impress the governor so that he would insist on adequate funds.

We felt our only hope was to bring this to court, so we more or less surreptitiously took sides with the court, and only defended what we thought was truly defensible. We did not defend anything that was not defensible, which led the governor and some of our other critics to say that we rolled over and played dead.

Over 90 percent of the standards that were ultimately set were stipulated to by the department in advance of public hearings. I am not sure how widely known that is, but it indicates that we were refusing to be the bad guys and villains that the adversary process requires us to be. But it didn't work.[5]

The real problem, then, is what the mental health commissioner and the judges ought to do when they realize more funds are needed to provide constitutionally required medical care, but the funds cannot be obtained from the state. The one legal remedy seems to be to release the patients. The argument is that such patients can be held involuntarily only when treatment is offered. When treatment is not offered for involuntarily committed patients, they must be released. Although release is legally required, the question is whether it is best for the patients. Is release better than being held under current conditions? Assuming that it is, is release ethically acceptable when psychiatric care is needed?

Or suppose that the involuntarily committed patient refuses the treatment thought best by the medical staff. The question then is whether that patient has a right to the next best treatment. This was the situation in *Donaldson* v. *O'Connor,* a Florida case of a Christian Scientist who refused drug treatment and then wanted psychotherapy. Donaldson sued not only the institution but also the physicians who refused to provide the requested treatment.[6] Many have argued that only the institution should be responsible for such a refusal.

The right to treatment in cases such as the Bryce Hospital one is based on the claim that once a person is committed, he has a constitutional right to treatment or else must be released. What does this imply about the right to treatment if one is not involuntarily committed but voluntarily seeks, say, basic physical medical care? If the patients are released from involuntary confinement, do they no longer have a right to treatment? Or if a patient at Bryce Hospital at some point refuses psychiatric treatment, would that jeopardize his right to treatment in the future? If a patient refuses medical treatment of a physical problem, would that jeopardize the right to future treatment?

28 PATIENT NEED AND PUBLIC RESPONSIBILITY

Arnold Miller was a sick and lonely 67-year-old. Two years ago he had begun treatments at Southeastern University Hospital for a malignant melanoma. The treatment was experimental—a form of immunotherapy which had shown promise in animals but had never before been tried in humans. The Southeastern University Cancer Clinic researchers were optimistic.

Mr. Miller was given a year to live when he entered the clinic's experiment. Six months ago he had decided that he could no longer resist the invitation of his only daughter to move to a northeastern town so she could care for him. He longed for a final chance to see her, her husband, and his grandchildren. He hoped that he could continue the treatments in the city where his daughter lived.

When he arrived, he found there was no place where he could get the experimental treatment. In fact, physicians at the world-famous Borkmann Cancer Research Center told him that they were not convinced the treatment was worth testing. They encouraged him to seek alternative therapies at their center. Mr. Miller complained to Southeastern University. The researchers tried unsuccessfully to find some hospital where Mr. Miller could get the experimental treatment. None would cooperate. The researchers then suggested that Mr. Miller fly back to Southeastern University for the biweekly treatments and try to get Medicare to pay for the transportation charges.

Mr. Miller's application for reimbursement reached the desk of Dr. Abraham Sudnill, regional officer for the State Health Department. He soon became convinced that the transportation costs could not be paid for an unproven experimental treatment. He consulted with four oncologists in the city, all of whom agreed that the experiment was speculative and might be keeping Mr. Miller from possibly useful alternative therapy. The air fare and ground transportation bills were averaging $71 per trip. Mr. Miller had submitted bills for thirteen trips over a six-month period and was planning to continue the treatment indefinitely. Even though Mr. Miller was not charged for the treatments themselves, his Medicare bills were going to cost the state over $1800 a year.

When Dr. Sudnill disapproved the payment, Mr. Miller asked that it be referred to Dr. Gilbert Hanson, deputy commissioner of health for the state responsible for Medicare administration. Dr. Hanson had been trained as a political scientist. Now acting as a public servant, he was in a quandary. He realized that Mr. Miller had already lived twice as long as the doctors had thought he would. He wondered whether it could really be that the treatment was helping. He wondered what would be the impact on Mr. Miller and his family if the treatments were canceled. Even if they were useless, Mr. Miller retained hope because of them. Yet Dr. Hanson was reluctant to override Dr. Sudnill's judgment. He respected his regional officer's competence and did not want to create disharmony in the Health Department. He also did not want to squander $1800 of the state's health money.

––––––––––

Mr. Miller's case reveals how dangerous the appeal to social consequences can be. It is inconceivable that society has much to gain from the treatment of this particular cancer patient. His treatment is expensive and controversial, and even though there is the possibility of a slight prolongation of life, the experiment is doomed to fail or at most will extend the patient's life at great expense. One could argue that society has an interest in establishing the principle that the individual should be respected. Life, liberty, and the pursuit of happiness are an integral part of the American value system. But to introduce that argument is to appeal to individual rights and to the duty of society to the individual. The moral question is whether Mr. Miller has a just claim to societal support in the form of that particular type of health care.

The argument from the principle of justice is also a tricky one in this case. That Mr. Miller has a medical need seems clear. Less clear is how his need for this particular kind of care compares with the need of others who are competing for the same funds. The alternatives for Mr. Miller are either getting the recommended treatment from a northeastern hospital or staying in his southeastern state and continuing the experimental treatment as a lonely, dying man, perhaps with the support of his daughter who would then have to give up her obligations in the northeastern town to come to help her father. It may be that the decision about need is a relative one, which can only be applied when both the possible sources of medical funds and the needs of others are known.

Other criteria for a just distribution of health care funds might well lead to a different conclusion. The implications for this case would differ if health care were distributed according to ability to pay or according to usefulness or merit. Dr. Hanson may have no business making calculations of what is just at all. If not, he faces the question of how to avoid paying every Medicare bill submitted to him. If so, he has to determine what principles to use in deciding what is just.

Adjudicating the worth of a claim to care requires complex value judgments. Yet such value judgments cannot be avoided. The problem is particularly acute in a case such as Mr. Miller's where it is questionable whether the need being fulfilled is a medical or a sociopsychological one. If Mr. Miller's alternative is to get the same treatment but be lonely in the process, one could argue that it is the loneliness which is being treated. This is one example of a much larger class of marginally medical problems which are increasingly being brought into the medical model. Others include drug addiction, abortion without specific medical indication, obesity treatment, plastic cosmetic surgery, hair implantation, and psychotherapy.[7] When treatments are seen as elective, or when the medical problem is brought on by what appears to be voluntary behavior on the part of the individual, other serious ethical and public policy problems emerge, even if in general there is an agreement on the right to health care.

29   PAYING FOR SMOKERS' MEDICAL CARE

Joseph Adamson, an economist, was employed as consultant to the Assistant Secretary for Health at the Department of Health, Education, and Welfare. In the context of the imminent enactment of legislation for national health insurance, Mr. Adamson had been asked to make a policy recommendation on details for funding the insurance. The National Antismokers Protection League had petitioned HEW with the claim that it is unjust for nonsmokers to pay the costs of health care required for smokers as a result of their smoking. The league proposed that a health tax be charged on smoking materials. The exact amount of the tax should be determined by assessing the increased national costs of health care attributed to smoking. The league argued that while it is the right of every citizen to health care financed by the government, that care should be limited to medical needs for which the individual is not personally responsible. The league granted that there are many areas where personal behavior contributes to health care costs, such as diet, exercise, and driving habits. They claimed that any proposal to tax health-risky behavior in order to transfer health care costs to those engaged in the behavior must meet two qualifications: there must be a good, predictable relationship between the behavior and the health effects, and the behavior must be easily subject to tax.

The tobacco industry had filed a brief opposing the cigarette health tax. They argued that there is no absolute proof that smoking increases health costs. They also argued that to claim that smokers are responsible for their behavior is unfair since many learn it in childhood from their parents or develop the habit as a result of early personality development. Finally, they called it unfair to tax some health-related behaviors that happen to be easily regulated while others that do not happen to be so easily regulated go untaxed.

30 BLACK LUNG DISEASE AND NATIONAL HEALTH INSURANCE

The Harris County Coal Company operated ten small mines in West Virginia with an average of thirty miners each. National health insurance had just been passed by Congress providing government-financed health care for all, with a provision that the insured pay the first $50 in any given year. Within the past year it had also happened that a number of techniques were developed to minimize the impact of coal dust on miners, who develop black lung disease from prolonged exposure. The problem was that the most effective prevention techniques were expensive. They required both massive ventilation systems and costly hourly monitoring of the air quality throughout the mine. It was estimated that the full prevention program would cost $750 per miner. The union had demanded that the program be initiated by the company, but recognized that these small-scale West Virginia mines were marginal operations. The added cost, according to management, would close the mines. By coincidence, a government study had just shown that the predicted cost to the government for treatment of the black lung disease from the mine under present conditions would also be about $750 per person prorated over all mine workers.

Serious policy questions were raised for the government. Should it require the mine to install the black lung disease prevention program in order to protect the miners as well as to promote the public interest by lowering the cost of national health insurance? Should the mines be allowed to pass the cost along in the form of a pay cut?

The mine management proposed another plan, giving the miners a choice of either working in the mines with the prevention program installed and taking a $750 pay cut, or working in the mines in their present condition without taking the pay cut. Those working in the mines without the prevention program would not be covered for black lung disease in the national health insurance program.

———————

These two cases anticipate the problems raised by the right to health care in national health insurance policy planning. Both the smokers and the miners are clearly in need of medical care. In contrast with Mr. Miller, the cancer patient being flown some distance to get an experimental treatment, the problem in these two cases is not whether the treatment is justified. Rather it is who should have the correlative obligation to pay for the treatment. In both cases the problem arises because of the belief that choices can be made by the individuals who may become sick.

In the case of the smokers, their behavior is viewed, rightly or wrongly, as being within the realm of voluntary control. The problem is whether it is just to require the state to pay for conditions brought on by voluntary acts. The right to health care is normally thought of in terms of more traditional illnesses. One of the primary characteristics of illness is that it is normally thought of in traditional terms. And one of the primary characteristics of illness is that it is normally thought of as being outside the realm of voluntary control.[8] The individual is not responsible for his condition, though he does have an obligation to cooperate in trying to overcome it. This is not the way in which smoking and some other illness-producing behaviors are normally viewed.

In this case good personal intentions may be relevant in determining a just distribution of society's resources. Merit is associated with voluntary behavior and, in an egalitarian society, is minimized in considerations of justice except in special cases. One such case is when two individuals are thought to be equal in their natural gifts and social opportunities and yet one chooses a more meritorious course. In a society worried about individual needs, medical or otherwise, and about inequalities in natural endowments and social opportunities, merit is a minimal consideration in determining what is just. Yet at the same time society believes that, other things being equal, the individual should pay the price for costly or foolish behavior undertaken solely to satisfy his whims or tastes.

This is apparently the position of the National Antismokers Protection League. Its members recognize that need is still an important consideration in designing a just health insurance. They could have, but did not, ban all smokers from insurance coverage. They must have considered that need is a relevant criterion even in cases where the need results from unwise voluntary choice. But that need does not justify, according to their view, the use of society's resources to meet it, at least in those cases where the behavior can be readily identified and easily taxed. Their position is one that combines the criteria of need and responsibility or merit.

The opposition makes an empirical argument that the correlation between the smoking behavior and the medical need has not been proved, and then makes two arguments from justice or fairness. The first is that it is unfair to treat those who do not choose to smoke voluntarily the same way that voluntary smokers are treated, which rests on the empirical claim that conditioning results in involuntary behavior. The second argument is that it is unfair to treat this kind of injurious behavior to health differently from other kinds that are not readily taxed. The problem of national health insurance coverage of medical conditions thought to be brought on voluntarily will be a serious problem in years to come. It is a problem of what is just or fair.

In the insurance case of the Harris County Coal Company and its miners, justice can conceivably be based on desire. At least that appears to be the criterion of justice behind the coal company's proposal. Based on the facts of the case as presented, the coal company does not have a great deal to gain from either of the two alternatives they propose. Either they reduce salaries $750 per person for those wanting the safer conditions, or they continue without the equipment and pay the workers their existing wages. Perhaps no real situation will ever arise meeting all of the conditions of this case. It requires that the workers can readily choose between the two alternatives. It requires that all agree the company does not have the responsibility to pay for the improvements out of its profits. It requires, as the smoking tax proposal does, that risks are readily quantifiable and behavior is identifiable. In this case the miners in the riskier mines are separated from those in the safer mines and paid for the risk taken.

If all of the conditions are met, the remaining problem is whether individuals should be permitted to trade medical benefits for other benefits they desire more. The miners who would opt for maintaining their wages while continuing to work in the plants without the new safety equipment are in essence choosing to spend $750 on something they prefer more than medical protection. It may be that society wants to treat some health care, like social security, as not only a right but an obligation. Compulsory minimal health care would presumably be based on the conviction that certain envisaged needs are so great that society cannot morally tolerate ignoring the need once it is established. Or some social or governmental benefits may be thought to be simply a right rather than an obligation. Consider a hypothetical society that guarantees to each citizen a minimal wage from which a few very elementary items are required to be purchased: a basic diet, at least for children, minimal housing, clothing, social security, and health maintenance services. That society may include a total minimum wage somewhat beyond the total purchase price of these required minimums. The additional certainly would not provide for luxuries, but would give some personal freedom to purchase a life-style according to one's tastes. In such a society, the goods that could be purchased beyond the basic requirements for living would be viewed as interchangeable goods. One person might buy desserts with his dinner, another an extra room on his basic housing, another flowers for his garden, still another some medical services beyond those that society requires.

A society that values both freedom and justice will provide enough to meet the basic needs, which is only just, but will also permit freedom to choose alternative goods to the maximum extent possible. It would be considered both fair and freedom-enhancing to permit the greatest possible trade-off among goods that one might choose. The just distribution among these interchangeable goods would be according to desire. It would certainly be foolish to give every person exactly the same amount of dessert, extra housing space, flowers for the garden, and medical services. If any case at all can be made for the Harris County Coal Company's proposal, it would have to rest on the conviction that insurance against black lung disease is not something so essential that it, like social security, is required against the individual's will and that the miners can justly trade off their additional medical protection for something they would prefer to purchase with the $750.

Efficiency and Patient Dignity

Of all the moral problems in medicine, perhaps the most common is the simple one of depersonalization, insensitivity, and commercialization of what is normally thought to be a very personal need. Such cases are not emphasized in this book because they are not really ethical dilemmas but rather ethical outrages. If a perpetrator of these acts is challenged, however, he may defend his behavior in the name of efficiency in health care delivery or on the ground that compromise is necessary to save lives and meet desperate medical needs.

The conflict in such cases is between respect for patient dignity on the one hand and efficiency on the other. Sometimes it is costly to treat a patient with dignity. One of the objections to obtaining informed consent from patients is that it is costly in time and psychic energy. Or to justify excessive waits before appointments the argument is made that leaving adequate time in the daily appointment schedule would make health care more costly. It would be an inefficient squandering of the physician's valuable time.

As in any situation where ideals conflict with the reality, the question when dignity is pitted against efficiency is how much deviation from the ideal is tolerable and when. The idealist will say that when human personality is at stake, no compromise is tolerable. To accept inadequate examining rooms or crowded waiting rooms is dehumanizing to the patient. Yet the realist will say that when human life is at stake, compromise of ideals is essential. It is precisely because the stakes are so high that a compromise is acceptable.

31   THE DOCTOR SAYS IT WILL BE A FEW MINUTES MORE

Cynthia Cavill rushed to pack her three children—Gregory, age seven, Billy, age four, and Patty, eleven months—into the waiting taxi. They were late for their 3 o'clock appointment with the pediatrician. Annual visits for Gregory and Billy and a routine exam for Patty were on the agenda. They ran up the stairs to the second floor office, arriving with a minute to spare. Walking into the small but crowded waiting room, they stood at the glassed-in receptionist's compartment until she returned. They were told to take seats until they were called. Only one seat was available.

Billy had been cranky during the taxi ride. He escalated the confrontation once he was in the physician's office. The summer temperature was in the high eighties, making tempers short and trips to the drinking fountain in the hall a major diversion during the wait. After fifteen minutes the receptionist came into the waiting room but called for a woman and two girls who were sitting across from them. This meant that Gregory and Billy could have chairs of their own. Mrs. Cavill counted three other clusters of mothers with children. She dreaded what was to follow.

After another ten minutes, which included a trip to the bathroom and an altercation over a toy car, Mrs. Cavill was exhausted. At 3:32 another mother-child team was called for and still another brood emerged from the corridors of the inner office. Candy brought for such an emergency, as Mrs. Cavill had grown to anticipate the wait, were now producing a drool onto two jerseys which were fresh only an hour ago. At 3:52 the receptionist finally called for Gregory. Mrs. Cavill gathered up the baby's things, Billy, and the excess candy and accompanied Gregory into the examining room. When Gregory was settled, she returned to the waiting room until it was Billy's turn. At 4:18 when there had been no further appearance of the receptionist and no emission of examined children, Mrs. Cavill approached the glassed-in office and through the opening asked when her other children would be seen. She was at her limit. She was to meet her husband at 5:30 at his plant so they could share a ride home.

The receptionist disappeared to find out what the problem was. She returned at 4:23, saying to Mrs. Cavill, "The doctor says it will be a few minutes more." He had an emergency earlier in the afternoon and was running behind. Mrs. Cavill wondered if he always had emergencies on the days of their appointment, but was grateful that he kept the children healthy.

32 BLOOD MONEY

The growing need for blood and blood products in the United States had led medical suppliers to seek sources overseas. United Blood, for instance, recently opened a facility in one of the poorest Central American nations and now exported 10,000 liters of blood plasma to the United States monthly. The company was criticized for dealing with the country's notorious dictatorship and for removing protein-rich plasma from undernourished people; but United Blood pointed out that its operation made a sizable contribution to the national economy. About half a million dollars was paid annually to plasma donors and one hundred local employees. Per capita income in the area was $80; well over half the work force was unemployed or significantly underemployed; and the poorest took advantage of the opportunity to sell their plasma, receiving $3.50 for a liter donation. Thanks to the plasmapheresis process, which separated out the plasma to be frozen and flown to the United States and returned the red blood cells to the body, some donors could sell their plasma weekly, thus earning $182 a year.

Responding to the criticism, United Blood explained that most Americans were too affluent to be motivated to contribute blood. Furthermore, a company spokesman said, drug addicts, alcoholics, and prisoners were active blood donors in the United States and accounted for much of the hepatitis-tainted blood which resulted in thousands of deaths annually of patients receiving transfusions. Although the Central American country had high rates of tuberculosis, gastrointestinal disease, and malnutrition, its caloric intake being one of the lowest in Latin America, it had no drug problem, and there was no need to depend on alcoholics and prisoners. About 4 percent of the volunteers were rejected because of weakness or low hemoglobin count. United Blood claimed to employ inspection procedures and testing safeguards equal or superior to those in the United States, and outside observers confirmed this claim. United Blood's profit was a matter of controversy. Critics said the company netted $4.50 per liter, the company said $2.50.

Professional Trust and Patient Needs

One of the stickier but normally ignored ethical dilemmas in medicine is the problem faced by a member of the health care team who realizes that a colleague has made an obvious error in technique or ethics. From the standpoint of the observer the behavior is clearly unacceptable, but he questions his right to intervene to challenge a colleague. At the same time, he has a duty to intervene to protect the particular patient or future patients if he observes clearly unacceptable behavior. The concept of trust is crucial in resolving the dilemma.

"Trust" is an ambiguous word in medical ethics. It is touted as the moral basis of the patient-physician relationship, yet is also the foundation of the collegial relationship of one physician to another and of physicians to other members of the health care team. The Hippocratic oath is first of all an oath of secrecy and loyalty to one's medical colleagues. While the relation between the physician and the patient is one of a contract or covenant that must be based on trust, the relation to one's colleagues is also a covenantal one.

Trust between patient and physician is made even more confusing because it can be used to justify either intervention to point out a medical colleague's error or nonintervention. On the one hand, the patient's trust —in the entire health care delivery system as well as in the individual physician—can be maintained better if the patient is not informed of the error. On the other hand, the general refusal to disclose errors certainly erodes patient trust.

The dilemma of the health care team member, especially if that person is a nonphysician, is often between his duty to do what is best for the lay person, who is not necessarily his own patient, and thereby maintain the legitimate foundation of patient trust, and his need to maintain a cordial, collegial, trusting relationship with his errant colleague. The sociopsychological pressure to "be a team player" maintaining loyalty to the medical group can be great indeed.

33 THE BLUNDERED DIAGNOSIS
AND THE PHYSICIAN'S RESPONSIBILITY

William Parker, a married 57-year-old, came to the emergency room of an urban private hospital one Friday night after he had been unable to reach his private physician, who was reported by the answering service to be out of town. He gave a history of a 30-lb. weight loss over the past two months, loss of appetite, and a "lump" in his abdomen. When a physical exam revealed a melon-sized mass in the left upper quadrant of his abdomen, easily palpable, he was questioned further by the house officer, a young physician receiving hospital training, about the condition for which he was being treated by his regular physician, Dr. Gillman.

"Why, my heart condition," he answered.

"And what *is* the trouble with your heart?"

"I had a heart attack in 1968, but I've been fine since. Dr. Gillman said so."

"When did you last see Dr. Gillman?"

"Last week."

"Did you complain then about your losing weight and having lost your appetite?"

"Sure I did, and he checked me right out."

"What did he check?"

"Well, he checked my blood pressure and listened to my heart and said I was doing fine."

"Did he examine your stomach at all?"

"No. He never did that. He just checked my blood pressure, listened to my heart with his stethoscope, and told me to come back in a month. I have high blood pressure, you see."

Mr. Parker was admitted that night for a diagnostic evaluation, but since it was a weekend, no definitive studies could be done until Monday morning. Routine lab tests revealed a Hgb of 9.1, a WBC of 74,000 (70 percent lymphocytes), and a very low platelet count of 22,000. These values suggested a leukemia-like state.

Mrs. Parker confirmed that Dr. Gillman had never examined her husband's abdomen but admitted that she had not been present in the examining room. An attempt to contact Dr. Gillman was unsuccessful, his exchange stating that he was "out of town and wouldn't be back until Monday morning." He had made no arrangements with any other physicians to cover his practice for emergencies but had simply instructed his exchange to direct his patients to the hospital's emergency room. Further investigation revealed that this was a common practice of Dr. Gillman's, despite Medical Board rules requiring that staff physicians provide a back-up physician when not available themselves.

That night Mr. Parker spiked a fever to 104° F. He began to bleed from his gastrointestinal tract, and platelet transfusions were begun. Before the etiology of his fever could be determined, his blood pressure became unobtainable, he stopped breathing, and eighteen hours after admission he died. An autopsy revealed disseminated lymphosarcoma or cancer of the lymph glands, with a massively enlarged spleen weighing 200 grams and peritonitis as the cause of death.

The house officer taking care of Mr. Parker suspected that Dr. Gillman had been grossly negligent in his handling of the patient's case and probably could be found guilty of malpractice if the family filed suit. She considered making such a suggestion to the family, but was cautioned not to by her attending physician, who told a story about a doctor who was sued for libel after reporting another physician. This incident had since kept the hospital's Medical Board from taking punitive action against any doctors who failed to provide back-up coverage when not available.

The house officer was advised not to get involved and was even cautioned against writing a letter to the local medical society, with the warning that she too could be charged with libel. "After all," it was pointed out, "how do you know that Dr. Gillman didn't know that Mr. Parker had cancer but thought it would not be in Mr. Parker's best interest to tell him?"

34 THE NURSE'S RESPONSIBILITY FOR THE PHYSICIAN

A young woman came to the emergency room of a small community hospital complaining of a "sprained ankle." The nurse called the woman's private physician, and a half-hour later he arrived at the hospital and greeted the patient.

During the exam, the patient noted that the doctor appeared to be intoxicated, and she smelled a strong odor of alcohol on his breath. When the doctor left the room to examine the X-rays, the woman turned to the nurse and said half-jokingly, with a nervous laugh, "He's a little cockeyed, isn't he?" The nurse, who had also noted the doctor's apparent inebriation, did not know what to say.

CHAPTER 5

Confidentiality

"Whatever . . . I see or hear . . . which ought not to be spoken abroad, I will not divulge." So says the Hippocratic oath. Confidentiality is fundamental to interpersonal communications and is a time-honored principle of medical ethics. Yet the principle of confidence is not so simple. The ethical dilemma involves just what "ought to be spoken abroad" and how it ought to be spoken. To condemn public pronouncements on a patient's exotic illness when there are no mitigating circumstances is not hard. To scorn cocktail party gossip about the sexual behavior of the neighbor down the block is cheap ethics. Confidential treatment of patient records and disclosures is an essential for continued trust and confidence in the medical profession. It is essential to proper care of the patient. Yet the traditional codes of medical ethics always hedge on the principle of absolute confidentiality. He who says "never, ever violate any patient's confidence" probably has never been confronted with the proverbial case of the mad murderer who is passing through the physician's office for treatment so that he can return to the street for more killings. The real ethical dilemmas of medical confidentiality arise in situations that have serious extenuating circumstances, which qualify the principles in the codes.

Medical Codes on Confidentiality

The various medical codes on confidentiality are not exactly the same (see chart). In fact, the major codes of medical ethics differ remarkably

Confidentiality in Codes of Medical Ethics

Whatever, in connection with my professional practice, or not in connection with it, I see or hear, in the life of men, which ought not to be spoken abroad, I will not divulge, as reckoning that all such should be kept secret.

—Hippocratic Oath

A physician may not reveal the confidences entrusted to him in the course of medical attendance, or the deficiencies he may observe in the character of his patients, unless he is required to do so by law or unless it becomes necessary in order to protect the welfare of the individual or of the society.

—AMA Principles of Medical Ethics, 1971

It is a practitioner's obligation to observe the rule of professional secrecy by refraining from disclosing voluntarily without the consent of the patient (save with statutory sanction) to any third party information which he has learnt in his professional relationship with the patient. The complications of modern life sometimes create difficulties for the doctor in the application of this principle, and on certain occasions it may be necessary to acquiesce in some modification. Always, however, the overriding consideration must be adoption of a line of conduct that will benefit the patient, or protect his interests.

—British Medical Association, 1959

If, in the opinion of the doctor, disclosure of confidential information to a third party seems to be in the best medical interest of the patient, it is the doctor's duty to make every effort to allow the information to be given to the third party, but where the patient refuses, that refusal must be respected.

—Addition to British Medical
Association Principles, 1971

A doctor owes to his patient absolute secrecy on all which has been confided to him or which he knows because of the confidence entrusted to him.

—International Code of Medical Ethics,
World Medical Association, 1949

I will hold in confidence all that my patient confides in me.

—Declaration of Geneva, 1948

in the qualifications placed on the principle. The Hippocratic oath
specifically includes information acquired not in connection with the
professional practice. The AMA code limits the principle to confidences
disclosed "in the course of medical attendance." The oath of Hippocrates protects only that "which ought not to be spoken abroad." The
AMA code indicates three specific conditions where exceptions are made:
when required by law, when necessary to protect the welfare of the individual, and when necessary to protect the welfare of society. At the other
extreme, the International Code and the Declaration of Geneva are
blunt: "absolute secrecy on all which has been confided." This apparently places the physician beyond the requirements of the law. The BMA
code clearly allows for the statutory requirement to break confidence. In
addition, the entire principle is situationalized to allow for breaking
confidence "on certain occasions" to benefit the patient or to protect his
interests. The 1971 addition in effect nullifies this exception, providing
that the physician must try to obtain the permission of the patient to
violate the confidence when it appears to be in the patient's interest, and
that if the patient refuses, the refusal must be respected. There is no
mention in the BMA principle of violations to protect society, as there is
in the AMA position. With all of this ambiguity in the codes, the individual physician is hard pressed to sort out their implications and decide
what to do.

Breaking Confidence as Required by Law

35 THE REQUIRED STATE PSYCHIATRIC
DIAGNOSIS RECORD

For Andrew Gorly it was the second admission to the Brooklyn Psychiatric Clinic. The patient had been subdued on the corner of Rose and
Belmont Streets. He claimed that the Nazis were infiltrating the Political
Science Department of the university where he was a graduate student.
The patient had, that afternoon, assaulted three innocent passersby,
whom he accused of being part of the conspiracy. Mr. Gorly was scheduled to take his doctoral examination the coming Tuesday. He had been
up for three consecutive nights reading modern European political history, cramming for one of his exams. After completing the exams and
writing his dissertation, the patient was planning on a career in the foreign service. His professors had always thought of him as a bit strange
but considered him one of the bright young scholars in the department.
They had tried to persuade him to go into teaching, but he was an activist;
he still had faith that hard-working, intelligent foreign service officers
could do something to change American foreign policy.

His parents brought him to the Brooklyn Psychiatric Clinic late that evening. The diagnosis was an acute paranoid schizophrenic break. Dr. Lyons understood the extreme pressure of the exams. He confided to the parents that he thought the prognosis was good. Hopefully, a short stay as an inpatient would get their son through the crisis.

The doctor made appropriate notations on the chart. The patient, who was still present, insisted on knowing what was being written. Dr. Lyons explained. The doctor then picked up the Admission Form. Mr. Gorly insisted on seeing the form, and Dr. Lyons obligingly gave him a blank copy. It was a standardized, computerized form giving the patient's name, address, social security number, occupation, and psychiatric history. It also included religion, education, weekly family income, a "problem appraisal," and most significantly, the psychiatric diagnosis written as the code number based on American Psychiatric Association Manual II, 1968.

"You mean you are going to fill out this entire form so my whole life can be fed into a computer?" the patient asked. "Where does the carbon copy go?" he demanded.

"To the Department of Mental Hygiene in the state capital," was the reply.

"Do you realize what this does to my foreign service career when this reaches the government computer?"

Dr. Lyons said he was sure that the records were treated with strict confidence. The records were needed for statistical purposes only. Certainly they would not be turned over to the foreign service.

"And why do my name, address, and social security number go on the form if it is only for statistical purposes?" the patient asked. "You can't just send my name in. It violates my right to confidentiality."

"The law says I have to send in the form. It is part of a multistate information system for psychiatric patients," was the reply.

It is unlikely that Mr. Gorly will benefit in any direct sense from the reporting of his diagnosis to the state mental hygiene department. It is of course possible that, through the accumulation of statistics on acute paranoid schizophrenic breaks, treatment or preventive measures might be developed which would benefit the patient, but almost certainly this is not the justification of the reporting, and such a rationalization is best left out of the argument. Or society might possibly benefit from the reporting by accumulating masses of statistics which could contribute to the knowledge of mental illness. Whether society would benefit by having direct knowledge of Mr. Gorly's psychiatric condition, however, is questionable. One might argue that society would benefit by keeping him out of a sensitive foreign service assignment, but the connection is tenuous. If such an argument is made, it must also weigh the harm done by creating a surveillance system which infringes on personal freedom and probably prevents many persons from making constructive contributions to society.

The extent to which the medical condition of the patient is directly a threat to society may be one of the ethically significant factors in deciding whether or not a confidence should be broken. In Mr. Gorly's case the medical condition is a threat in only an indirect and tenuous way at best. In another type of case the patient's medical condition is of direct concern to society. For example, the physician's obligation is to report a patient with a contagious disease, venereal disease, or clearly present homicidal psychiatric illness. In still another type of case the medical condition itself of the patient is clearly not a threat, but he poses other threats to society.

36 REPORTING THE EPILEPTIC MOTORIST

A young man was brought into a private hospital emergency room, where the following record was kept on him over the next four days:

> 3/22/71   9:47 A.M. Admitted to seizure clinic from ER. Reported seizure while walking to work . . . Patient reports one previous seizure "just like this one" approximately four years ago . . .
> R_x diphenylhydantoin 0.1Gm.
> No.21
> sig: i tid
> 3/24/71   EEG confirms suspicion of grand mal. Patient pleads not to report case to Motor Vehicle Department. Says he only drives 2 times a month—to care for mother who lives alone on the family farm. Says distance is "about 10 miles." Will consult hospital attorney, but consider primary responsibility is to patient and patient's mother.
> 3/25/71   Attorney says law in California requires report of all seizure diagnoses. But does this conflict with medical ethics?

1. The excerpt from the record does not indicate the physician's professional relationship with the epileptic patient's mother. Suppose that he is in fact the family physician and has cared for the mother as well as the son for many years. Is this ethically relevant? Does the physician then have a special moral obligation to see that the mother is cared for, or is the situation the same ethically if the physician has never seen the mother before?

2. If the same case arises in a hospital in another city where there is no law requiring the reporting of epileptic diagnoses to the Department of

Motor Vehicles, how does this change the physician's ethical obligations?

3. How does the physician's obligation to report a diagnosis differ ethically if he is treating a patient with a venereal disease, botulism, or a gunshot wound?

37 MEDICINE IN THE SERVICE OF THE FBI

The following notice appeared in the section titled "News and Notes" in the February 1972 issue of the *Archives of Dermatology,* a publication of the AMA. It is an exact reproduction of an FBI poster:

Wanted by the FBI
On June 2, 1971, a Federal Grand Jury at Tucson, Ariz., indicted _____ for conspiring with another individual in an act which involved the interstate transportation and unregistered possession of 120 sticks of dynamite, 30 electric blasting caps, 20 fuse caps, and 50 feet of fuse. The alleged conspiracy violation occurred prior to May 2, 1970, at which time one _____ using the name William Allen Friedman, allegedly drove from Venice, Calif., to Tucson, Ariz., purchased the explosives and fuse, and returned to Venice, Calif.

CAUTION: _____ HAS BEEN KNOWN TO ASSOCIATE WITH INDIVIDUALS WHO ADVOCATE THE USE OF EXPLOSIVES AND SHE HERSELF HAS ACQUIRED EXPLOSIVES IN THE PAST. SHE REPORTEDLY MAY HAVE ACQUIRED FIREARMS AND SHOULD BE CONSIDERED DANGEROUS.

_____ is known to be afflicted with a skin condition known as acne vulgaris, which has been described as being acute and recurrent. The recurrent aspect of this skin condition could necessitate treatment by a dermatologist.

_____ is also known to frequently wear prescription eyeglasses or contact lenses, which are required for her to operate an automobile.

Notify the FBI
Any person having information which may assist in locating this fugitive is requested to immediately notify the nearest FBI field office, the telephone number of which appears on the first page of most local telephone directories.

The notice produced a major dispute about the possible necessity for the physician who sees this notice and then is asked to care for the patient to violate the assumed confidential relationship. Dr. Willard Gaylin, president of the Institute of Society, Ethics and the Life Sciences, questioned the ethical legitimacy of publishing such a poster in a professional medical journal. In an article titled "What's an FBI Poster Doing in a

Nice Journal Like That?'' he emphasized that the primary obligation of the physician is to health, specifically to the health of his patient, and that the obligations to society must be subordinated when these conflict with the right of the patient to health care:

> It seems ironic that the AMA, which has consistently opposed government intrusion into medical matters even where a legitimate public interest has been proved, should now have volunteered the services of organized medicine into a government function—and in an area so alien from the traditional medical mission as tracking down criminals. Of course, the thought occurs that it might not have been voluntary. The line between freedom and coercion is not so clearly drawn when the "petitioner" has the power of the Department of Justice. This thought, however, is only the first in the series of ethical and value questions inevitably raised by this eccentric utilization of a medical journal . . . Risks, complications, ethical dilemmas, divided loyalties, and confusing priorities crowd each other in demanding consideration —and one wonders how they were weighed, and by whom, before this decision was cast.
>
> Before even the ethical questions, what is the legal responsibility of the physician reading this? Consultation with a professor of criminal law revealed that there were indeed open questions about liability and responsibility. If he had doubts—what of the average dermatologist?
>
> The implications to the wanted person—who may or may not be a criminal—will also transcend ethical nicety. In this instance, a fatal disease is not present—although it well might be in future cases, and it has been indicated that were the condition heart disease, diabetes, glaucoma, acute depression—the wanted notices would be referred to the appropriate journal. They would make it difficult, if not impossible, to get the necessary treatment.
>
> The major question, however, seems to be whether medicine should be encouraged, or even allowed, to be an extension of the police functions of the society. There is no question that if this is seen as a legitimate function of medicine, it would represent a powerful and immense new ally for the police. In the files of physicians across the country are massive case records which would make an invaluable data bank (ready for computerization) of inestimable service in any police tracking function: the drugs one chronically uses, a tendency toward alcoholism, a hidden homosexual activity, proclivity for flirtations or other sexual idiosyncrasies, prescription glasses, specific allergies, dietary requirements, etc.
>
> There is no question that all of this information would facilitate the police functions of the state. But is that the function of medicine? And in facilitating this other function *what would it do to the primary concern of medicine, which is relief of suffering, the treatment of illness, and the saving of life?* What happens to the tradition of confidentiality —so zealously protected over hundreds of years precisely because it has been seen as fundamental to the effective function of medicine?

Such use of the profession by the police would represent the final destruction of the privacy, intimacy, and trust of a therapeutic relationship already seriously eroded. (Medicare and Medicaid, for example, now demand the right to examine *all* medical records of recipients of their beneficence.)

It is conceivable that *in extremis* an institution must abandon its traditional role. The organized church has often supported the mass killing of war when it seemed essential for the survival of the state. Perhaps medicine should be prepared to abandon certain principles, and compromise our medical goals to serve state needs. Russian psychiatry seems to be assuming just such responsiblity now.

How are we to decide, however, *when* to violate our usual primary devotion and allegiance to the private person and his well-being, for the public purpose? How are we physicians to differentiate quantitatively amongst the various crimes and conditions of criminality in which we have no training? Are we prepared to assay indictment versus conviction, versus material witness, versus "wanted for questioning"? What are the relevant weights to be placed on conspiracy to blow up a heating system of the Pentagon, versus armed robbery of a bank, versus possession of marijuana, versus massive embezzlement? How do we weigh these public dangers against the health or survival of a patient? Ought we be making these decisions—or should they be left to public decision-making via the normal legislative process which, for example, now dictates that gunshot wounds demand violation of confidentiality, but by implication of exclusion allows a host of other material the protection of confidentiality.

That prudence which is a traditional part of medical education would seem to dictate staying out of a decision-making area for which we are untrained.

Which raises the question of how such significant decisions should be made. How, for example, are the power and responsibility which influence the whole balance of medicine and government distributed by a major organization such as the American Medical Association?

The Association is formed of elected delegates. These delegates, in turn, as an organization, elect a board. There is an executive secretary who administers the organization. There is a Judicial Council with its own legal counsel that acts as an ethical watchdog. At what area of this complex apparatus was the decision discussed, debated, considered, and finally decided? A call to the Editor of the *Archives of Dermatology* indicated that he had authority and responsibility only over the scientific articles, and no responsibility for this particular poster. A call to the Corresponding Editor for the *Archives of Dermatology* confirmed that the editors of the specialty journal controlled only that localized aspect. The Chairman of the Judicial Council said the matter had never been brought to the Council, and, indeed, he was unaware of the publication of the posters when first consulted. He then suggested consulting the legal counsel of his committee who has had a long history of dealing with ethical issues and publication. *He* was unaware of the appearance of this FBI poster in the two publications [the poster also appeared in the *Archives of Internal Medicine*] until he was advised of the fact and, further, he could not recall its ever having been done before. He volunteered that when consulted in the past by various state journals, he had cautioned great prudence in publishing such material. Further calls to various anonymous sources in the American Medical Association (who must remain anonymous) indicate that it was "done somewhat experimentally" and spoke vaguely of "a great deal of pressure" having been exerted.

The interesting aspect to an outsider was the evident absence of an apparatus for consideration of new or major policy.

It was finally established that a request had been made in writing by the FBI to the Chief of the Division of Scientific Publication of the AMA, and that he made the decision, seeing no need to consult the Judicial Council, the representatives of the Board of the American Medical Association, or the Executive Secretary of the American Medical Association and his full-time professional staff. He indicated that in his mind, it was an "editorial decision" of no great moment and implied that it was a part of an ongoing tradition that preceded his assumption of office three years ago. But Dr. John Talbott, who formerly held that post for ten years, insisted that never under his tenure was an FBI poster or its equivalent published in either the *Journal of the American Medical Association* or any of its specialty journals.

Equally interesting was the gradual shift of the attitude of the staff of the Association when inquiries continued to indicate outside consideration. When they were first notified of the appearance of these pages, all seemed genuinely surprised, felt that the implications were of some moment, and suggested that, in the precedent-breaking move such as this, it seemed unlikely that one man, prudent though he be, would have initiated the action without extensive consultation.

But, by the time this initial investigation was concluded, a new official profile was emerging, minimizing the innovation, suggesting it was a routine editorial-type decision, and denying even the presence of a problem. The man who made the decision stated that he would have no hesitation printing more such posters in the future, without advice or consultation, in whatever medical journals the AMA published when there was a specific medical potential for assisting the FBI, because *"no questions of medical ethics are involved."*

The assumption that there are "no ethical issues involved" seems at this time to be the collective stance of the AMA. A formal statement read over the phone by the secretary of the AMA Judicial Council also starts with the statement that no issue of ethics is here involved. This may represent the most distressing aspect of this entire episode. Whether the publication of such material by an official medical journal is "ethical" or "unethical" may be debatable (and should be debated). That major ethical issues are raised, however, is indisputable. It involves such basic traditional questions as confidentiality and trust, private needs versus public rights, professional values versus personal ethics, the special role of the healer and saver of life, and the power of the state.

For an individual to want to avoid recognition of error is understandable. For a group to underestimate the implications of any ethical question is certainly no crime. If, however, an entire organization such as the AMA proves so insensitive to questions of ethics, as to deny their existence here—it could be disastrous.[1]

The publication of the poster by the AMA could be defended, however, by arguing that the physician may determine that he has a duty to society as a citizen which precludes maintaining confidential the fact that the fugitive-patient was in his office. If one generalized to other situations where wanted criminals could be apprehended by alerting members of a professional group who might be especially likely to come into contact with them, one might make a case that general duties as a citizen to report such criminals may take precedence over special duties believed by the professional group to apply to their profession. A journalist might believe he has a duty to report a criminal even if it means violating a duty generally recognized by his profession to maintain confidentiality. If one perceives such a general duty to report wanted persons, then the only way of not reporting this particular wanted person would be a situational analysis of the particular political charges against her. That defense would rest upon whether it is ever justifiable to violate a general principle that wanted persons should be reported to the FBI because in a particular case the individual who might do the reporting does not believe the person really committed a serious offense or any offense at all.

The physician who identifies this person in the course of medical treatment may not even have a conflict between his general duty to report and his special medical duty as a physician to keep confidences. The AMA's Principles of Ethics state that "a physician may not reveal the confidences entrusted in him in the course of medical attendance, or the deficiencies he may observe in the character of his patients, unless he is required to do so by law or unless it becomes necessary in order to protect the welfare of the individual or society." In this case, however, a physician may well interpret the case as one where it is in the interests of society to break the confidence. He may also believe it is required by law. He may even believe it is in the interests of his patient—if he fears that her continued fugitive status puts her in physical or psychological jeopardy. The AMA's code seems to leave a great deal of room for individual physicians to decide to violate confidences in just about any case where it would be plausible to do so. The physician seeing the poster may have substantial grounds for not only seeing but acting on the poster if the AMA's principles are the basis of his ethics. Whether that principle or some other one, such as the Declaration of Geneva or a more general public social ethic, ought to be the basis of his decision-making is open to question.

A physician who believes that professional ethics do not require disclosure of the knowledge of his patient, a disclosure which quite possibly is "required by law" in his state, may have a false sense of security if he believes that he has either the obligation or the right to withhold the knowledge of the whereabouts of a fugitive. In fact, the medical confidentiality laws vary greatly from state to state, and many states have no statutory professional privilege at all. Even if professional confidentiality could be invoked, it would be ironic to be more against government involvement than is organized medicine itself.

If the placement of the notice is wrong, an argument based on more general ethical and public policy grounds would seem stronger. Neither government nor society should ever be placed in the position of endorsing, defending, or enforcing the particular ethical norms of a private group, whether it be the medical profession or a religious body. Even if reporting the patient and violating confidentiality were a violation of the profession's ethics, that is no basis for societal judgments about the ethics of placing the notice.

This case poses the more general problem of wide-scale government intrusion into personal relationships. Individual freedom of communication is threatened by the "big brother" activities of the government. This threat is intensified when special groups of people are notified, whether they be journalists who obtain information in confidence, clergymen who see a person wanted for a political crime, or draft counselors who encounter a fleeing draft dodger. Each of these individuals has a legal professional service to offer, and the FBI notification would hinder the provision of that service, doing harm to the individual as well as infringing upon his freedom. Society suffers as well from a pervasive "police state" atmosphere. In the long run, freedom of communication and freedom to seek professional counsel are in the public interest. All of these considerations make it an ethically risky business to notify selective professional or social groups about fugitives, which would have a chilling effect on free speech similar to that caused by indiscriminate wiretapping, illegal search and seizure, or government surveillance of political activities. This argument makes the case against publishing the notice a broader issue of civil liberties than the seemingly simple appeal to professional ethics and reinforces the claim that a serious ethical dilemma exists.

The three previous cases are alike in one regard: violating confidentiality is, or may be, required by law. Of the three possible exceptions to the principle of confidentiality, the case where breaking a confidence is ordered by a duly constituted legal authority is the most persuasive. The physician, after all, is a citizen of the land and subject to the laws of the land. To decide to break the law, even when it appears justified by a professional code of ethics with a principle as well established as that of confidentiality, is no trivial decision; it is civil disobedience.

The principle of confidentiality can lead the physician to two kinds of action when confronted by an unjustified requirement of disclosure. First, he may appeal to the importance of confidentiality in arguing for the repeal of the legal requirement. Dr. Lyons may cite Hippocrates and the World Medical Association when going to court to block the state's required reporting of diagnoses. The San Francisco physician with the epileptic patient may do the same in fighting the law that requires reporting of epileptics. But the physician may feel morally bound to go beyond this, to refuse to file the diagnosis form or to report the epileptic. If he does so, however, he is engaged in simple civil disobedience and should recognize it as such.

Most humans recognize the need, in certain conditions, to turn to a "higher law," to appeal with Antigone to "unwritten laws, eternal in the heavens." But to reject legal authority routinely and without due thought is anarchistic. No society could survive the indiscriminate personal acceptance or rejection of law. If the physician is to avoid considering himself different from other citizens, he must treat civil disobedience with appropriate seriousness.

Breaking Confidence in the Interest of Society

In certain cases there may be no formal expression by society through its laws that disclosure is in its interest, but the physician, based on his own judgment, may believe that the welfare of the community necessitates breaking confidentiality. The physician might feel either that the general welfare of society is threatened or that specific individuals have a strong enough interest in the patient's condition to necessitate disclosure.

38 CONFIDENTIALITY, COMPUTER BANKS, AND SOCIAL WELFARE

Dr. John Webber was the director of Health Services for Space Technology Industries, a subsidiary of General Consolidated Industries and a major producer of experimental aircraft and hardware for the satellite program. He was in charge of the infirmary for the company and was thus responsible for routine medical examinations of all new employees.

A memo from the front office arrived just ahead of Thomas Carter, an astrophysicist who was joining the executive staff. The memo, addressed to Dr. Webber from the company vice-president, requested that Mr. Carter's medical processing be expedited because he was needed for new work on the JX-118 program. It was apparent that Mr. Carter, at age 30, was being groomed for an executive management position in the company.

The purpose of medically examining new employees was to screen potential employees for contagious disease and also to serve as the routine physical for the company group health plan. During the course of the examination, Mr. Carter revealed that although he felt perfectly healthy at the time, his father had died some twenty years previously of Huntington's chorea.

Suddenly Dr. Webber realized his dilemma. Huntington's chorea is an autosomal or single-gene dominant genetic disease which is distinguished by its late onset. Symptoms usually begin with personality changes, quickness of temper, moodiness, and diminished memory and judgment, evolving to involuntary and uncoordinated movements, dementia, and finally complete loss of physical control leading to death within ten to fifteen years. The onset is typically between the ages of thirty and forty.

Dr. Webber knew that his examination records would be submitted to the insurance company over his signature and that, in turn, the insurance company would make use of the centralized computer data bank of medical records now shared by the insurance industry. Some 85 percent of all insurance medical records are currently included in that data bank. If Dr. Webber reported the presence of Huntington's chorea in the family history, it would jeopardize Mr. Carter's ability to get any insurance. Mr. Carter would be excluded from the company's group health plan, which is possible under the "prior conditions exclusion clause" of the contract. His family, including his two children, would be unprotected. Dr. Webber realized that it was important to the company to have Mr. Carter on the research team, but he also realized that he had special responsibility for the medical aspects of the company, particularly for its insurance program. Failure to include the family history might increase the risk in the company insurance pool and be a disservice to the other employees insured by the company. Yet it could not be denied that Mr. Carter would be a valuable asset to the company, and Dr. Webber felt deeply that his primary moral obligation was to the individual patient.

Dr. Webber's problem was what to do with the gratuitous discovery of Mr. Carter's family history. He could attempt a tentative confirmatory test with the administration of L-dopa which is now being tested experimentally. He could report the discovery to the insurance company, which would then report it to the data bank. He could inform the business office of the company, so that it could recalculate the economic risks against the company's benefits from Mr. Carter's services.

1. Is there any sense in which Mr. Carter consented to the reporting of his medical history to the insurance company? Physical examination forms for use by insurance companies often contain a blanket permission to report the findings to the company. What would be the significance of such a blanket permission in this case if it were signed?
2. What are the implications of this case for the private practitioner who conducts physical examinations for insurance companies?
3. What are the implications for a patient submitting himself for a routine physical examination?
4. What obligations are placed on those who are responsible for data banks of medical records? To whom should data be released—insurance companies, prospective employers, or government agencies?
5. Is potential gain for the company a legitimate reason for disclosure by a physician employed by industry?
6. What are the obligations of a physician employed directly by an insurance company for the purpose of doing physical examinations? Do these differ from those of the private practitioner?

39 GENETIC COUNSELING OF RELATIVES

Mr. and Mrs. Edwall heard about the Tay-Sachs screening program at their local synagogue. The Genetics Unit at the city's teaching hospital had organized the city's Jewish religious and civic groups in an effort to identify carriers of the gene responsible for the disease. The couple's rabbi was fully behind the program. In an evening educational session at the synagogue they were told that Tay-Sachs is a genetic disease leading to a progressive mental and physical deterioration. Over a period of months, the Tay-Sachs baby develops blindness, motor paralysis, spasticity, and finally decerebrate rigidity, a rigidity of the muscles when the higher brain is not functioning. Death occurs before the third year of life. The disease is untreatable, but carriers of the recessive gene can be detected by a reduced amount of hexosaminidase in a blood analysis. When both husband and wife are carriers so that they are at risk of having an affected child, prenatal diagnosis of the disease can be carried out during the middle trimester of pregnancy, in time to give the parents the option of an abortion.

Mr. and Mrs. Edwall were confident that they were not carriers. They were both in good health. Mr. Edwall was a construction worker who had not missed a day on the job in his life. As far as they knew, there was no history of Tay-Sachs on either side of their family. The incidence of the gene in the non-Jewish population is only 1 in 300, but among Ashkenazi Jews, the group from which the Edwalls came and which makes up about 90 percent of the American Jewish population, the incidence is about 1 in 30. This is the reason for conducting a screening program through local Jewish organizations. Mr. and Mrs. Edwall were planning to start their family within the next year, so they thought they should have the test made "just to be sure."

A week after the tests, the Genetics Unit physician called to ask them to come to the hospital for consultation. He told them, "Don't worry about anything. You will never have a Tay-Sachs baby." That was reassuring, but the couple were worried. They knew the Genetics Unit did not call in everyone who was screened for a special consultation. There must be something unusual.

The chief counselor for the unit asked them into her office. After emphasizing very clearly that they could never have a Tay-Sachs baby, she disclosed to them that Mr. Edwall had a recessive Tay-Sachs gene. The counselor was most tactful, making every effort to explain to Mr. Edwall that the gene would in no way affect his health. Mr. Edwall indicated he understood, but he seemed disturbed.

Then the counselor asked about Mr. Edwall's family. He had two younger brothers, both married. The counselor advised that the other members of his family should be screened, especially since his brothers would be likely to have children soon. She suggested that the brothers be tested soon and that Mr. Edwall's parents be screened to see which side of the family carried the gene. Screening could then be carried out on those who were at especially high risk. The Genetics Unit had a carefully worded letter which could be sent by a patient to relatives informing them of the importance of the test.

Mr. Edwall was dumbfounded. He understood that the gene really would not affect his health, yet he felt that there was something wrong. Every cell in his body was marked with that "terrible disease." The counselor explained to him that everyone has some genes which could cause a genetic disease, that Mr. Edwall was just like everyone else except that, in his case, they were fortunate in being able to detect one of his genes. Mr. Edwall was not convinced. He had seen the horrible pictures of the dying Tay-Sachs babies. Somehow he was "not quite a man" if half of his children would have that same "sickness in their cells." He refused to inform his family because of the shame.

The counselor was angered. Here was a man who had two brothers who were about to start families. The brothers had a 50 percent chance of carrying the recessive gene, which meant that, with a 1-in-30 chance of the spouses having the gene, there was a 1-in-60 chance of each of the couples being able to produce a baby with Tay-Sachs disease. "It seems as if it is my duty to those relatives and to the future babies to be born to tell them of the risk they are running," the counselor argued to herself. She tried in every way possible to persuade Mr. Edwall to tell the brothers about the need for the test. Mr. Edwall struggled with his conscience, thinking that maybe he was being foolish, but he told the counselor he just could not bring himself to tell his brothers.

That afternoon, the counselor took her pen and wrote two very cautiously worded letters to the two brothers.

---

1. Is this a situation where, in the words of the AMA Principles of Medical Ethics, the "welfare of the community" requires revealing the medical knowledge, or should the more inclusive principle of the World Medical Association apply, to the effect that a "doctor owes to his patient absolute secrecy on all which has been confided to him"?
2. The counselor, according to the case record, never asked Mr. Edwall for permission to contact his brothers. Thus she was not directly violating the patient's judgment. Does the disclosure in these circumstances differ ethically from a case where there is a direct refusal of permission on the part of the patient? Should the counselor have asked for permission first?
3. What will be the long-term effect on the Genetics Unit of the counselor's letters?
4. If the two brothers were by chance ongoing patients of the counselor, would her ethical obligations differ?

Breaking Confidence in the Interest of the Patient

The third exception to the general principle of confidentiality as stated by the AMA Principles of Medical Ethics occurs when disclosure is seen as being in the interests of the patient. In most such cases the patient would agree that his interests require disclosure, whether in a court case where insanity is the patient's defense or in an insurance case where the patient wishes to collect benefits. But if the patient believes that disclosure is not in his interest and the physician disagrees, the situation poses an ethical issue.

40 WARNING: PREMARITAL SEX MAY BE DANGEROUS TO YOUR HEALTH

The British General Medical Council's Disciplinary Committee was charged in 1971 with the task of deciding whether or not a physician was guilty of "serious professional misconduct," whereupon it made the following report:

> The Committee next inquired into the charge against Dr. Robert John Denis Browne of Birmingham, that he had disclosed to the father of a Miss X that an oral contraceptive had been prescribed for her by the

Birmingham Brook Advisory Centre, notwithstanding that he had been given the information in confidence by the centre and that he had neither sought nor received her permission to make the disclosure.

The complainant was the Birmingham Brook Advisory Centre which was represented by Mr. G. S. Jonas, Solicitor . . .

Mr. Jonas said that it was only after the most anxious thought and deliberation, including meetings with Dr. Browne, that the matter had been brought before the Disciplinary Committee. Dr. Browne had practiced in Birmingham since 1941 and was highly regarded by his patients. Mr. Jonas alleged that in his capacity as a doctor he had received confidential information about one of his patients and quite deliberately and for no valid medical reason had betrayed that confidence by telling the patient's father what he had been told . . .

At the time Miss X called at the centre she was just over 16, a highly intelligent, attractive, and mature young woman. Mr. Jonas told the Committee that when an oral contraceptive was prescribed it was the practice of the clinic to inform the family doctor unless the patient specifically forbade it. In this instance Miss X agreed to her doctor being informed. Dr. Browne had informed the girl's father that she was on the pill. No effort had been made by Dr. Browne to discuss the matter with his patient, and the patient's consent to this disclosure was neither sought nor obtained . . .

Dr. Browne had said he would have to do the same again in every case that came to his notice, and the only situation he could see was that the centre should never again inform him if one of his patients came to see them. He had said it was all very well the clinic prescribing the pill but if anything went wrong he would have to deal with the problem. The burden of the complaint was that the doctor let his views interfere with the objectivity demanded of a professional man.

The press had said the issue was important for doctors, and also to patients, but in Mr. Jonas's submission it was primarily important to patients, whose confidence must be kept. The confidence was always with the patient, it was never that of the doctor.

[A clinic physician testified that he] felt it important that the general practitioner should be informed so that if there were any side effect the doctor would have knowledge that the girl was taking oral contraceptives . . .

Mr. R. Alexander, Counsel . . . for Dr. Browne submitted that this was not in any sense a test case. The sole issue was whether this respected doctor had been guilty of the offence of serious professional misconduct. There were three issues: firstly, could one doctor unilaterally impose a confidence upon another, and by unilaterally he meant could he do so without seeking the consent of the other doctor; secondly, what was the position with regard to the duty or right of a doctor to tell the parents of a child who had not reached the age of majority of the medical treatment that child was receiving; and the third issue was that medical confidence existed for the benefit of the patient. If the doctor believed it to be in the interests of the patient to reveal the confidence to a third party then he was entitled to do so . . .

Dr. Browne, in evidence, said that he was 63 years of age and was married with three children, including a girl of 18. He had qualified in 1941 and had been in practice in Birmingham for about 30 years. The parents of the girl had been his patients for many years and he had been their doctor at the time of her birth. She had been his patient all her life. She still was his patient, and he had seen her professionally quite recently.

When he had received the letter from the Brook Centre it sounded an alarm bell in his mind. He was concerned that a girl only just 16 had been placed on a contraceptive pill without prior knowledge or consultation with the family doctor. It was a stable family with the daughter living at home. He had discussed the matter, which gave him great anxiety, with professional colleagues. He tried to get an estimate of the situation without mentioning anyone's name, and considered the problem carefully.

The girl's father happened to come to the surgery shortly after this, and he asked him if his daughter was getting married. The father said that she was not, but that she had a steady boy friend and was still at school. Dr. Browne said he thought hard and then made up his mind—bearing in mind the girl's best interests, and for that reason solely—and handed the father a copy of the letter from the centre and explained what it meant . . .

Dr. Browne said that he had had two motives in informing the parents. One was the physical hazards of the pill, and the second was the moral and psychological hazards. He was not standing in judgment, but with his knowledge of the home background, and knowing the parents were sympathetic and kindly and could handle the situation with care and tact, he considered they were the best people to counsel her in their own way. He also saw psychological hazards, for if she were keeping a secret she might have a sense of guilt, which could have a harmful effect on her emotionally. He pointed out that it would have been difficult for him to contact the girl without arousing parental suspicion. The episode did not appear to have impaired his relationship with Miss X.

In reply to cross-examination by Mr. Jonas, Dr. Browne said that his interests were primarily for the patient and for her alone. He had no other interest except what was best for her. His patient was being placed on a dangerous drug without his prior knowledge or consent with all the hazards that might involve—and steroid drugs were a particular hazard . . .

Dr. Walter Woolley, ex-Chairman of the Central Ethical Committee of the British Medical Association, told the Committee he had been a family doctor since 1933. In his view a third party could not fetter the right of the doctor—for instance, by a letter such as the one from the Brook Centre—to exercise his own judgment.

Dame Annis Gillie said that she had had 38 years' experience in general practice, and in her view professional secrecy existed in the interest of the patient. She considered that there could be situations in which the benefit of the patient meant that a confidence must be disclosed. Every case should be judged on its own merits by the practitioner involved . . .

The final witness was Dr. J. C. Cameron, Chairman of the General Medical Services Committee of the British Medical Association. He had been in general practice for many years, and considered that a longstanding knowledge of a patient was of great advantage in forming an assessment of a situation. He would have preferred that, if possible, the girl's consent should have been sought prior to the disclosure to her parents, but there might be circumstances in which this was impracticable . . .

After consideration in camera the President said: "The Committee has found proved that the information you received from the Birmingham Brook Advisory Centre was in confidence, and that you had neither sought nor received the patient's permission to make the disclosure; but in the particular circumstances of this case . . . the Committee do not regard your action in disclosing the information referred to in the charge as improper. The Committee therefore has not found that the whole of the facts alleged in the charge, including the word 'improperly,' have been proved. It has accordingly recorded a finding that you are not guilty of serious professional misconduct."[2]

The BMA principle of confidentiality as adopted by the Representative Body in 1959 was in effect at the time of the Browne case. It stated clearly that "the overriding consideration must be adoption of a line of conduct that will benefit the patient, or protect his interests." Dr. Browne was claiming that his patient's interests required the disclosure to her parents. Furthermore, he was arguing from what is normally considered to be an enlightened broad conception of health which includes social and psychological considerations. Sex for the single girl, according to his considered "medical" judgment, was unhealthy, which he felt obliged him to disclose the information.

In light of the Browne case, the BMA in 1971 adopted an amendment to its principle of confidentiality, which in effect rejects the "patient's interest" grounds for violating confidentiality. The physician, according to the revised principle, cannot ethically second-guess the patient's judgment of his or her own best interest and must respect the patient's refusal to allow information to be given to a third party.

The Second National House Staff Conference Delegates meeting in Atlanta in 1972 went even further. Recognizing the psychological power of the physician to persuade some patients, they stated simply, "When the physician believes that confidence should be violated for the patient's own interest, he must abide by the patient's own decision.''

In contrast to the House Staff Conference, the AMA code indicates that confidences may have to be broken to protect the welfare of the individual patient. The physician thus has a problem deciding what to do. Even if he accepts the professional codes of medical ethics as normative, he must resolve the conflicts among the codes.

CHAPTER 6

Truth-Telling

Probably no subject generates more heated controversy when physician and nonphysician meet to discuss the ethics of medical practice than the apparently simple yet subtly complex question of what the patient should be told. In spite of the fact that these discussions tend to produce more heat than light, the issue of truth-telling lends itself more directly than most other problems in the medical context to formal ethical analysis of the norms or principles on which decisions are based. One aspect of the problem is to determine what in fact is the "truth" of a situation. Conflicts can then arise between a duty to withhold information because of anticipated consequences, and to disclose information because of its possible meaning, use, or interest to the patient. Special problems are raised by the placebo, the patient's or family's request that information be withheld, and the disclosure of staff negligence. Another aspect of the question concerns the patient's right to his own medical records.

The Condition of Doubt

Frequently the problem of what to tell a patient arises when those who are in a position to know cannot be sure of the accuracy of information or of its meaning. Were the prognosis of a terminally ill patient certain, there would still be controversy over what that patient should be told. In reality, however, the prognosis is never known for sure, or at least the medical professional cannot put an exact time on the remaining length of life to come. The already difficult problem of what to tell is compounded by doubt about the prognosis. What to do in this "condition of doubt" depends on the stance one takes regarding basic ethical issues and value orientations.

41   THE UNEXPECTED CHROMOSOME

Martha Lawrence was tense and nervous when she came to the Human Genetics Unit on December 12, 1971. She had been referred by her own physician because, unexpectedly pregnant at the age of 41, she was considered at risk for the birth of a Mongoloid child. She was eighteen weeks pregnant, which would not leave much time for a potential abortion.

Down's syndrome or Mongoloid babies are twenty times as likely to be born to women over 40 as to women under 25. About 50 percent of all such babies are born to mothers over 35, and 25 percent to mothers over 50.

Mrs. Lawrence's first two pregnancies had been uncomplicated, and her two sons, ages 16 and 13, were both in good health. The genetic counselor, Dr. Brenda Gould, recommended amniocentesis, the withdrawal of a sample of the amniotic fluid surrounding the fetus, drawn from the abdomen with a needle. The fluid contains enough fetal cells for biochemical or chromosomal analysis.

The sample showed that the fetus had no extra twenty-first chromosome and thus was free of translocational Mongolism. But the sex chromosomes, rather than being XX for female or XY for male, showed the abnormal XYY composition. Some research suggests that XYY males might be "supermales," inclined to violent acts, including sexual offenses, while other recent studies do not confirm this finding. Considering the inconclusive nature of such research, the possible danger to society and the Lawrence family, and the impact of the information on the way the Lawrences might treat the child, Dr. Gould faced a dilemma: what to tell Mrs. Lawrence.

Dr. Gould's dilemma should dispel the common but naive assumption that the medical practitioner's role, even as a genetic counselor, is simply to provide "the facts" to the patient. Dr. Gould has to decide not only which facts to communicate, but what the facts actually are. She must determine which facts fulfill her responsibilities as a counselor, and which fulfill her moral obligation to the couple who have sought her advice.

One clear fact, however, is that Dr. Gould has to act; she has to decide something. There is no way out. It is the type of dilemma which is becoming more common in the medical-scientific professions: a very human problem arises for which there is only a little bit of scientific evidence, a promising theory, or perhaps only a wild hypothesis. Some day there may be more evidence, but the decision is demanded today. The professional is thus in what might be called a condition of doubt.

Whether patients who seek the professional's knowledge will get it depends in part on the physician's views about what to do when there is serious doubt. On the one hand, the cautious person may say, "When there is real doubt, wait!" She feels a moral imperative to wait until more evidence is in before acting positively. This cautious, evidence-demanding view is firmly rooted in the Western scientific tradition, but clearly it is not itself based on scientific evidence. It is an expression of a judgment about the nature of the world.

At the other extreme is the position that when there is serious doubt, "proceed unless there is good reason not to." It makes sense to demand scientific evidence for confirming scientific propositions, for establishing facts, as required by the Western scientific tradition, but deciding whether to act positively in a practical setting such as clinical medicine or counseling is a very different world. Some decision is demanded.

In this case Dr. Gould could take the more cautious view. She could reason that there is no clear evidence of the correlation between the XYY chromosome pattern and antisocial behavior. Since it is not yet a proved relationship nothing need be said about it. In fact, she might conclude that nothing ought to be said. She could give as reasons for this decision the potentially harmful consequences of telling the parent of the possibility that her child will be aggressive or violent, or she might reach the decision on the ethically different grounds that her contract with her patient does not call for disclosure of this finding but only a diagnosis of Mongolism. She might conclude, however, that she ought not to tell simply because the information is very uncertain. If her reason for nondisclosure were the nature of her limited contract, clarification of the relationship between XYY and antisocial behavior would not make any difference in the decision. If it were the potential bad consequences of a prediction that might be self-fulfilling, establishment of a positive correlation should logically make her even less inclined to disclose the finding. If, however, her decision is based on the uncertainty of the accuracy of the correlation and she takes a cautious, evidence-demanding view, she will be opposed to disclosure only as long as the evidence is so uncertain.

If, on the contrary, Dr. Gould takes a different value stance, she might emphasize the difference between deciding the correlation is proved, which is a scientific question, and deciding that the available information, uncertain as it is, should be disclosed to her patient. She could hold that it is not irrational to base the clinical decision on the available information. She might then give the patient the option of working with the uncertain information. The decision-makers can act as if the preliminary findings showing the correlation are correct, just as they can act presuming the contrary findings are. Since a decision must be made before the definitive findings are available, Dr. Gould might decide for disclosure in the condition of doubt just as she might decide against it.

42 SICKLE CELL CARRIER PARENTS

Jean Dunbar, a black 22-year-old, was a volunteer worker in the New York Sickle Cell Counseling Service. She was engaged to a black community organizer in the city's Youth Job Corps. During the week she worked as a secretary, but three evenings a week she came to the clinic to process the long line of people who queued up for their tests for sickle cell carrier status. She was not responsible for counseling, which was handled by trained counselors, but she filled out initial records and guided patients to the counselors prior to their testing.

Her fiancé became interested in the program and came for testing. To his amazement he was identified as a carrier. Having had a basic genetics course while in college, he had some understanding of what it meant to be a carrier. The counseling that followed the positive test for carrier status further clarified the implications. Since he had only one of the genes and two are necessary to produce the disease, he himself would never be affected. If, however, he married and his spouse were also a carrier of one of the genes, their offspring would each have one chance in four of having sickle cell disease. Furthermore, there would be two chances in four that each offspring would be carriers of the disease but would, like the parents, be themselves unaffected.

Only at this point did Ms. Dunbar appreciate the fact that, although working in the program, she had never bothered to have herself tested. No one in her family had ever been affected with sickle cell disease. After the test, her finding of a positive carrier status was a shock.

The couple, who were planning to marry within three months, entered a counseling program. In a session with the two of them together, the counselor became convinced that they understood their situation realistically. Probing seemed to uncover little or no confusion about the fact that the odds of sickle cell disease would apply to every child they had.

The couple now began to ask about sickle cell disease in more precise terms. After questions about its effect on the baby and chances of survival, the question of possible treatment came up. The counselor had to ask himself whether to tell the couple about potential treatments under study with urea and cyanate ion. Although the couple did not ask, the counselor also pondered revealing to them that research was currently under way on prenatal diagnosis using a fetal blood sample. The first prenatal blood test for sickle cell had just been reported in tests on aborted fetuses. It would be several years, however, before the technique would be available for general use. To disclose these facts might build false hopes for the couple that sickle cell disease could be either treated or prevented by possible prenatal diagnosis and abortion. To fail to reveal these facts could seriously affect the couple's planning of their family. They were clearly unsettled at the thought of bringing a sickle cell baby into the world if it might mean he would suffer in any serious way. They wanted to have children, but expressed a willingness to consider the alternatives of adoption or a childless marriage. They also discussed artificial insemination briefly, but ruled it out as unacceptable for them.

The same condition of doubt problem that arose in the XYY chromosome case arises here. However, in this case the nature of the ''disease'' is not in doubt. The nature of sickle cell disease is well known. Further, the psychological impact of revealing the diagnosis to the couple is not of overriding concern, although this cannot be overlooked and must be treated delicately. Basically, the doubt exists over the status of the treatment and prenatal diagnosis. It simply is not known at the time of this case whether either treatment or prenatal diagnosis will be developed in time for the couple to make effective use of them during the period when they are raising a family.

There are those who argue that the counselor's task is simply to reveal what is known at this point in time. Scientists know what sickle cell disease is, they understand the genetic transmission, and they can predict the odds of a couple, both of whom are carriers, having a child with either carrier status or the disease itself. The counselor's job is simply to explain this information in a way that the couple can understand and not to get involved in a scientific review of the state of research. Yet the same counselors, both physician and nonphysician, who might be inclined to withhold information from the couple about possible scientific breakthroughs, probably would not want to dash the hopes of the terminal cancer patient who can be buoyed by pointing out that research is going on at a tremendous pace, including some research that might have an effect on his particular malignancy.

The ''we don't know for sure'' argument is often used by physicians to justify the failure to disclose information. It is clearly wrong to tell a patient that there is a certainty he will be dead within six months when the fact is that no prognoses are ever so accurate and miracles do happen. Although this is a sound reason for not telling the patient that he has a fixed period left to live, it is not a valid reason for failing to tell him what is known according to the best medical knowledge available. It may be wrong to tell the patient, even in a gentle and kind way, that he for sure has less than one chance in a hundred to live more than six months, but the "we'll never know for sure" argument cannot justify failure to disclose that the best estimate of survival is less than one in a hundred. If that information is not to be transmitted, the concealment has to be justified on some other basis.

The same condition of doubt exists regarding sickle cell treatment and cure. It is illogical to justify the failure to disclose the fact that research is going on in these areas by arguing that the answers are not in yet. The information that research is taking place can reasonably be expected to be useful to the couple, either in planning their family or in deciding when and if to have children. The counselor may be of the view that only scientifically supported clinical information about what can be done at present should be transmtted to the counselees, but that choice cannot be based on the fact that all the answers are not yet available.

How the counselor behaves in such a situation will depend on a basic philosophical value orientation. When there is doubt in the clinical setting, he can take the optimistic, interventionist position on the assumption that when in doubt, one should give things a try, or he can take the more conservative position that trying new alternatives is generally or frequently counterproductive. The choice between the two is not based on the amount of scientific evidence available. All would agree that the situation could be evaluated more accurately if there were more data. The problem is that there are no more data at this moment and some decision must be made. It must rest upon one's philosophical biases about the nature of good and evil in the world.

Duties and Consequences in Truth-Telling

The condition of doubt is a special circumstance in the general problem of what the patient should be told. The more ordinary situation is for the facts of the case to be relatively straightforward but the evaluation of the consequences and moral implications not to be.

43   THE DYING CANCER PATIENT

This was the first hospitalization for the 54-year-old patient. She was born in Puerto Rico but had lived in the States for the last ten years. She had come to the emergency room two weeks before with a severe pain and a mass in the right lower quadrant. The previous December the patient had had a severe attack in the same area. Her history revealed that she was past menopause. She had worked in a nursing home and so was familiar with medical procedure. A third-year medical student obtained the pertinent material in her medical history and engaged in a brief conversation with her. The patient explained that she was afraid she had cancer. The student assured her that she would have a complete work-up. She replied in a sad manner that she knew, "If it was cancer, you doctors wouldn't tell me." The student did not comment on the patient's statement but said that the lab test and examinations would tell them much more about the possible causes of the trouble.

Two days later, after the patient had been examined by the medical students, the resident, the chief resident, and the attending physician, the diagnosis was made of a degenerating fibroid. This would explain the severe pain and the mass, although it was pointed out that after menopause the most common cause of painful mass is cancer.

The patient went to surgery Wednesday morning. The medical student spoke to the resident the same day. He reported that she had stage IV cancer of the cervix, the most advanced stage. They had cleaned out all the tumor they could see, but since the tumor had spread to the pelvic wall, all they could now do was to try chemotherapy and radiation. The five-year survival rate of stage IV cancer is 0 to 20 percent.

When the patient awoke from surgery, the medical student's first reaction was to go to her and explain the findings. He felt that he should speak frankly with her, attempt to share the grief, and be there for support. However, since he had not had much experience with cancer and this was the first patient of his "who had been given a death notice," he decided to speak first to the chief resident about how best to approach telling this woman.

The chief resident was sitting in the lounge. The medical student explained that he wanted to tell the patient she had cancer, and that he felt close enough to her to share some of the process. The chief resident's reaction was agitated. "Never use the word 'cancer' with a patient," he said, "because then they give up hope." He suggested using other words or medical jargon.

The student's mind was in a turmoil. He felt that it was important to convey to the patient what he knew himself. According to their best medical understanding of her condition, she had a limited time to live. New biomedical technology and medical discoveries had resulted in several possible treatments, and these would be tried. New discoveries were also being made which might help. But somehow he wanted to convey to her that, knowing what they did, the chances were not good that she would live out her normal life span. In fact, the chances were that she would not survive more than a few years.

The discussion got more heated. The resident angrily asked, "I'd like to know how you'll feel when the patient jumps out the window?" The student's response was that he felt he had to evaluate the patient's desire to know and that this woman had given a clear message that she wished to know.

The resident told the young student a story about the senior attending physician on their service, an internist and an internationally known author of a major medical textbook, who on rounds one day had asked if there was anyone present who would tell the patient they had just seen that he had cancer. When one medical student raised his hand, the internist, who was the awesome patriarch of the medical school, said, "You march down to the Dean's office and tell him that I said you are to be kicked out of medical school." Since an authoritarian and often hostile relation between master and student is not unusual in the clinical teaching setting, the student took him very seriously and turned toward the door. At that point the internist said, "Now you know what it's like to be told you have cancer. Tell a patient that, and it will destroy the last years of his life."

The student left the meeting with the chief resident wondering what should be told to the patient and who should do the telling. He had a good idea what would be said by the senior attending, by the resident, and by himself.[1]

This case raises all of the classical issues in the morality of what the patient should be told. The issues divide into three separate problems of ethics: whether the consequences have been accurately determined (value theory); whether consequences are definitive or moral principles indicate right and wrong in a particular situation independent of consequences (normative ethics); and whether situations should be evaluated individually or general moral rules should apply.

The physician chooses in this case to withhold the terminal cancer diagnosis from the patient because of what he thinks would be the consequences of telling it. Cost-benefit analysis is one of the classical methods for resolving ethical dilemmas and is particularly favored by the physician. The Hippocratic oath pledges the physician to do that which, according to his judgment and ability, will benefit the patient and protect him from harm. In this case the costs and benefits are clearly not thought of primarily in economic terms. The focus is on the psychological impact of the disclosure of the ultimate bad news. Concern is expressed over the possibility of suicide following the disclosure and more generally over the needless suffering, anxiety, and depression upon learning of her fate.

Yet there are dangers in leaping quickly to the conclusion that these possible consequences imply that the patient should not be told of the diagnosis or even that they create a predisposition not to tell. In ethical theory the position that rightness or wrongness of an action is determined by the consequences, called utilitarianism or consequentialism, is hotly debated, but even if consequences are accepted as the determinant, there are reasons to argue for telling the patient of her cancer diagnosis.

Some of those consequences are apparent to the medical student and probably even to the chief resident who is so vehemently opposed to the disclosure. The uncertainty of not knowing can produce anxiety. With knowledge, financial budgeting can take place more accurately. Two other problems derive from depending on the medical professional's calculation of the consequences. First, he may not have included some values that are important to the patient. This woman may have grand-children in Puerto Rico whom she would want to see more than anything in the world before she dies. She may value conversation with her priest or the Catholic last rite. Some patients may value human freedom and self-determination very highly. The consequences to the patient of being told or not being told can be accurately determined only if the proper values are included in the calculation and if they are given the proper weighting.

The second problem is that even if the proper values have been included, there may be differences between the physician and the patient which lead to serious errors in calculating the consequences. Suppose both patient and physician agree that psychological consequences are crucial and that serious anxiety and mental suffering are to be avoided. Suppose also, however, that the thought of death produces high anxiety in the mind of the physician, whereas the patient can handle the thought with comparatively little psychological trauma. Some patients reportedly are able to adjust to the thought of their own death because of particular religious convictions, because they have worked through their feelings, or because they can come to grips with the psychological impact rapidly once given the news. In fact, one psychological study of physicians suggests they have a uniquely high anxiety when confronted with the subject of death.[2] If this is so, then one can anticipate systematic errors in estimating the psychological harm done by telling the patient of a fatal diagnosis. The same would be true in the opposite case, if the physician is eager to tell while the patient shows a uniquely high anxiety on the subject of death.

Even if the physician uses the same values as the patient, weighs them properly, and quantifies the benefit or harm in the correct way, there still are moral problems in deciding whether to tell something to the patient on the basis of estimating the consequences. The patient may make moral judgments using considerations other than consequences.

Many systems of ethical reasoning emphasize factors other than the consequences in deciding which actions are right and which are wrong. In fact, the utilitarian or consequentialist position has been treated rather harshly in discussions of normative philosophical theory.[3] Those who are not satisfied with the utilitarian position claim that there are right-making characteristics inherent in actions independent of their con-sequences. Holders of this position, called the formalist or deontological position, claim that the utilitarians cannot adequately account for intuitive moral judgments and that honesty, promise-keeping, justice, and similar characteristics are important even if they do not necessarily lead to the best consequences. One need not be personally convinced of the formalist position to recognize the problems it raises for the decision about whether to tell the dying cancer patient of the diagnosis. One need only recognize the undisputable fact that some patients do hold such a position. Certain sophisticated forms of the formalist position do not deny the importance of consequences but claim that there are other important considerations as well.

Kant was a representative of the formalist tradition. On the subject of truth-telling he argued:

> The duty of being truthful . . . is unconditional . . . Although in telling a certain lie I do not actually do anyone a wrong, I formally but not materially violate the principle of right . . . To be truthful (honest) in all declarations, therefore, is a sacred and absolutely commanding decree of reason, limited by no expediency.
>
> Thus, the definition of a lie as merely an intentional untruthful declaration to another person does not require the additional condition that it must harm another . . . For a lie always harms another; if not some other particular man, still it harms mankind generally, for it vitiates the source of law itself.[4]

Kant may have stated the matter more strongly than the typical twentieth-century patient, but it seems clear that some of those patients give importance to truth-telling independent of or in addition to the consequences. For those patients, the argument that the deception is justified by the harmful consequences of the disclosure is not necessarily sufficient.

Some who feel that withholding of information is the right course may reply that withholding the information is not the same as lying. They grant the duty to tell the truth, but not the duty to tell the whole truth. The distinction is between actions and omissions, and it is one that troubles medical ethics at many points, not only in comparing lying with withholding information but also in comparing the killing of a dying patient with not starting a respirator or abandoning a patient with failing to take him on in the first place.

Whether the distinction is valid is debatable. But even if one concludes that it is valid, the issue is not resolved. The question is still open whether inherently it is morally acceptable to withhold information which is potentially meaningful to a patient even if that action is different from lying. The formalist may well take the position that in addition to the moral duty to avoid lying, there is another moral duty to disclose information which is potentially meaningful when one is in a position to do so conveniently.

The duty to disclose information that is potentially meaningful is not the only formalist or nonconsequentialist factor in deciding whether the woman should be told about her diagnosis. Some would hold that the patient has the right and the duty to give informed consent for medical treatment, and that right and duty exist independent of the consequences of giving that consent. Not only may failure to disclose the diagnosis make it difficult to get patient cooperation in therapy, but continued treatment of the patient may also violate the requirements of reasonably informed consent and thus be assault and battery.

The conclusion seems clear, that one reason the issue of what to tell a dying patient is so controversial is that different people in the debate have widely differing ethical norms which they bring to bear on the decision. If one person has the objective of doing what will have the best consequences and another has the objective of disclosing potentially meaningful information or of obtaining informed consent or of protecting patient dignity, the moral conclusions may be quite different, even if the two can agree on what values are important and what the consequences will be.

The third major issue in ethics raised by this case is the conflict between those who insist that moral rules must be followed in specific cases and those who argue that each situation, each case, is unique and must be evaluated anew. The formalists are often accused of being legalistic, of insisting on the rules of truth-telling or promise-keeping or consent-getting. But the rules-situation debate is really independent of the utilitarian-formalist debate. It is quite possible to argue that a rule to tell the truth should be followed even if in a particular case it appears that the consequences would be better if the rule were not followed, and to argue this on the grounds that following the rule will produce the best consequences in the long run. It is also possible, even for the formalist, to argue that on the question of what to tell the patient every case must be treated as a unique entity in which no general rules can be followed. In every case the situation would therefore have to be examined to determine what formal right-making characteristics are present and how they can be balanced, independent of the consequences or with the consequences being only one consideration.

The case of the woman who has cancer and does not yet know it is a good case to test the value of the rule. The evidence from surveys indicates that the overwhelming percentage of physicians would tend not to tell patients of a cancer diagnosis. According to Donald Oken, the figure is 88 percent.[5] In contrast, an overwhelming percentage of lay people, between 82 and 98 percent, say they would like to be told of such a diagnosis.[6] Of course, some might argue that they say they want to be told when they really do not want to, but such a judgment requires a paternalistic second-guessing of the lay person's judgment, which has moral implications of its own. In any case it would appear that the gap in judgment between the professional and the lay person is extremely great. If every physician considered each case as a special situation and did what he thought best, then it seems very likely that in many cases he would make a judgment in which the lay person would not concur. He may do so because he is a consequentialist while his patient is a formalist; he may do so because he is considering some consequences while his patient would have considered others; or he may do so because he evaluates some consequences, such as anxiety in the face of death, as much more serious than his patient would. There are good and predictable reasons why the problem of the medical student and his mentors about what to tell the woman with cancer creates heated ethical disputes in the hospital as well as in the classroom.

One kind of difference in the consequences considered is between those that are long-range and those that are short-range. When the woman with cancer says, "if it was cancer, you doctors wouldn't tell me," she is making a statement based on prior experience or beliefs. If many years ago her dying mother was not told of a cancer, she may have learned that in some cases the physician will not disclose the true diagnosis and prognosis to the patient. It is unlikely that the physician caring for her mother would have included in his calculation of consequences the impact on this patient who is now in the miserable condition of not being able to depend on the word of the medical profession. It may be that some people, including physicians, are uniquely committed to considering short-range consequences. If the physician's duty is to his patient and not to others, it might even be considered immoral to include such consequences. On the contrary, the classical utilitarian may well be very interested in such long-term consequences.

44   THE STUDENT DOCTOR: TRAINING IN DECEPTION

Mary Rogers was expecting a baby. Her husband was a student at State University so she was entitled to care in the school's medical center prenatal clinic. She made her first visit when two months pregnant, having reservations about not getting a private obstetrician, but confident that she would have available the best obstetrical care in the state if not the entire Northeast. She argued with herself, "If the baby is normal, then a midwife could handle the delivery, but if something goes wrong, they can call on the whole medical school faculty." Mr. and Mrs. Rogers were also happy that the clinic fee was only $400 compared to a total fee of about $1000 which they would have to pay for hospital and obstetrician fees if Mrs. Rogers were a private patient.

She was now attending the clinic monthly but would soon change to visits every two weeks. She was a bit disturbed by having to see a differ-ent physician on each visit, but the procedures were simple, and she recognized that it was more efficient. She was also struck by how young some of the doctors were. She remarked to her husband that the one she had seen this week could barely be out of medical school.

Howard Colvin was that young "doctor." He was indeed hardly out of medical school. In fact, he was a third-year medical student on his clinical rotation through the Obstetrics and Gynecology Department. It was a six-week rotation: three weeks on obstetrics and three on gynecol-ogy. He was now in his second week. He had begun caring for patients last year, taking histories and doing physical examinations in the "Intro-duction to the Patient" course. He had been very uncomfortable in his role at first, not knowing how to introduce himself to the patients he saw. The medical school issued a white jacket to him with "Dr. H. Colvin" printed on it. None of the students brought the matter up with the pre-ceptors, the physicians who worked with the students in the course. They did talk about it among themselves, though. An informal poll among the students in the second-year class had revealed that only about a third introduced themselves to the patients as "Dr. _____." A few introduced themselves as "student doctor" or "Dr. _____, a student doctor." Two said they were medical students. Another group introduced themselves simply by their names and let the white coat with stethoscope dangling from the pocket create an impression.

Now, as third-year students, virtually the entire class were introducing themselves as doctors. Several reasons were given by those who had thought about it. The most common was that the patient would be dis-tressed if she knew the "doctor" examining her was a student. By acci-dent, as Howard Colvin was wrestling with the problem, he encountered a letter in the *New England Journal of Medicine* in which Lewis Glick-man, a physician at Downstate Medical Center in Brooklyn, was re-sponding to an earlier letter advocating that attending physicians begin introducing their students as students and asking for permission from the patient to let the student gain experience. Dr. Glickman, in opposing this proposal, argued:

> The anxiety that students manifest when they begin to see patients is a result of the start of their transformation from student to physician. This change cannot be achieved, nor can the students learn the skills of obtaining information from and reassuring frightened people, unless they are involved in a doctor-patient relation. To this end, they must identify themselves to the patients and think of themselves as function-ing as physicians not students.
>
> If patients are interviewed or examined by students who have no responsibility for their care they are annoyed at being involved in a situation that they see as irrelevant. They will also reveal less, for they are no longer motivated to reveal anxiety-laden information . . .

One solution to the difficulty is having the students in history taking and physical diagnosis attached to the wards as part of the ward staff, as are the clinical clerks, interns and residents . . . Another is for the students to have the responsibility of communicating their findings to those who are responsible for the patients' care. If students had this responsibility there would be no question of "exploitative role playing" or "fraud." If students are addressed as "Doctor" it would be because they would be assuming one of the essential functions of a physician.[7]

Howard Colvin was not worried that Mrs. Rogers would get inferior care. He had confidence in what he was doing, and his work was supposed to be checked by the resident on duty in the clinic. He was concerned, however, that he was somehow being dishonest.

---

1. Is the medical student learning that he can deceive patients when it may be for their benefit, or even for his own benefit? How should he resolve the problem?
2. If the medical student or his supervising physician is convinced that the patient is getting high-quality medical care and would only be unnecessarily bothered by being told Howard Colvin is a medical student, is that sufficient to justify not telling Mrs. Rogers?
3. The student had one of his clinical rotations at Jefferson Hospital, a private general hospital caring primarily for chronic diseases, where he was issued an identification badge saying simply "Howard Colvin." How does that change the case?
4. If a student is justified in using the title "doctor" because he is adequately assuming one of the essential functions of a physician, is Rosalie Morse, RN, the nursing supervisor of the intensive care unit for the past twenty-two years, also entitled to identify herself as a doctor for the same reason?
5. If Howard Colvin were an intern or a resident—a recent medical school graduate getting supervised practice in a hospital for one to five years—would he have any obligation to tell Mrs. Rogers of his status?
6. What actions should Mrs. Rogers take? Would her situation change vis-à-vis being informed she is cared for by a student if she were a private patient rather than a clinic patient?

45 THIS WON'T HURT A BIT

Clara Glover brought Tommy and Michael, her two sons ages four and two, to Dr. Stephen Huntington, the family pediatrician, for routine examinations. Michael, the older boy, was getting ready to enter kindergarten, so he needed a medical form filled out for school. Dr. Huntington had a reputation for being kind and gentle with children, always willing to take a worried mother's call. He had been practicing pediatrics for twenty-seven years and had learned many tricks of the trade.

He began Michael's examination by looking at his throat, ears, and eyes. When he got to the examination of the fundus of the eye, he made use of a clever idea he had learned from a tip in *Medical Economics*, a widely read magazine distributed to physicians free of charge for the advertising. He showed Michael his ophthalmoscope and asked, "Would you rather see a doggie, a kitten, or a butterfly?" Michael replied, "A doggie." Lawrence Garner, who sent in the tip to *Medical Economics*, remarked that the child will usually pick the first. Dr. Huntington, following the advice from the magazine, told Michael he was going to shine the light into his eye. Michael should look into it to see if he could see the doggie. Michael did not seem to see anything and began to get restless, so Dr. Huntington said, "The doggie is a little afraid, but I'll get him to come out for you. I see him, do you? He has one black eye and one white eye." Michael did not appear convinced but looked into the ophthalmoscope a bit longer. Dr. Huntington, having completed his examination of the right eye, now told Michael he thought the doggie had jumped into the other eye. The examination of the fundus was completed.

Examination of the heart and lungs and a blood pressure reading followed, building up to what they all knew was the climax. Michael was required by state law to have a rubella immunization. The nurse had been preparing the syringe carefully outside the vision of Michael and his mother. Dr. Huntington opened a drawer and took out a wrapped piece of hard candy. He handed it to Michael's left hand while simultaneously reaching for the vaccine-filled syringe. He took hold of Michael's right arm, inviting Michael to unwrap the candy with his left hand and teeth. As Michael glanced over to the syringe, Dr. Huntington said, "This won't hurt a bit." Michael winced slightly as the needle went in. His mother left the office marveling at what a wonderful doctor Dr. Huntington was.

———————————

1. Is there any possible relation between the attitude of the dying cancer patient in case 43 and Dr. Huntington's behavior?
2. Dr. Huntington's techniques please Michael's mother at least as much as Michael. Should this be a relevant factor in the decision to use such techniques?
3. In a case where there are both short- and long-range consequences of an action, how are they to be compared?
4. Suppose Dr. Huntington reflects upon the long-range impact on Michael of the petty deceptions he uses and decides that, on balance, the short-range benefits, including the establishment of a cordial

relation between Michael and the medical community, outweighs any long-range harm done to Michael, but he also decides that if all physicians used these techniques for all their patients, it would contribute to a general mistrust of the medical profession. How should the good, on balance, in the single isolated case be related to the conclusion that if the general practice is established in all patient-physician relationships, the total consequences are judged bad on balance?

Complications in Truth-Telling

The reasons, or principles, for deciding either to tell a patient about a potentially relevant piece of information or not to disclose it can be applied to a special group of problems of truth-telling that arise routinely in the medical setting. One such problem involves the use of the placebo in therapy. It can be viewed either as a benevolent deception because the clinician believes that, all things considered, it will benefit the patient, or as no benefit at all because of the long-term consequences. The defense of the placebo derives from the principle that the physician's duty is to do what he thinks will benefit the patient, but other principles, such as the duty to tell the truth or to keep the patient/physician contract, would lead to a very different evaluation of the placebo.

Another special problem involves waiving the right to know. One issue is whether the family ought to be able to waive the right to know for a competent patient on the ground that it is for the patient's own good that information be withheld. Another issue is whether the patient himself ought to be able to waive the right to know. A question concerns the duty of auxiliary medical personnel to disclose important information.

46 THE POTENT PLACEBO

Dorothy Abraham had been bedridden for the last twelve of her 72 years. Cancer of the colon had been treated through three operations and chemotherapy. During the active therapeutic intervention, a period of about three years, Mrs. Abraham was in severe pain, for which she received meperidine, a narcotic analgesic. She also had a great deal of difficulty sleeping, for which her physician, Dr. Martha Little, gave her secobarbital, 1/2 gr., a fast-acting barbiturate. Eventually Mrs. Abraham was able to decrease the dose of the analgesic and had not taken any for several years. As tolerance for the secobarbital developed, however, Dr. Little had increased the dose to 1-1/2 grains. Although she could find nothing organic to account for the insomnia, the patient still was unable to sleep without the barbiturate. Mrs. Abraham continued taking the

1-1/2-gr. secobarbital for about two more years, when Dr. Little became convinced that she had a barbiturate addict on her hands. She did not object to sick patients getting the medication they needed even if it meant addiction, but she saw no reason to support Mrs. Abraham's habit, even if it had begun in the most innocent manner.

Through the local drugstore, which delivered all of Mrs. Abraham's medical supplies, Dr. Little arranged to prescribe a specially formulated secobarbital with an increasing amount of lactose, the pharmacologically inert milk sugar, and a correspondingly decreasing amount of the barbiturate. The pharmacist began replacing 10 percent of the active drug with lactose. After a month the formula was changed to 20 percent lactose. Special arrangement was made with the manufacturer of the drug to obtain the distinctive red, bullet-shaped capsules so that they looked exactly like the full-strength barbiturate.

Over a period of about a year the lactose proportion was gradually increased. For the last several years, once a month, Mrs. Abraham had had delivered to her apartment a prescription for thirty 1-1/2-gr. capsules of placebo. The pharmacist currently charged $4 a month, the same price he would have charged for the real barbiturate, despite the fact that his labor cost for hand-filling the capsules with lactose was much higher than would be the cost of the active drug. He had known Mrs. Abraham for many years and was aware that she and her husband lived on a modest Social Security check, so he felt he should give her the specially low price.

Dr. Little continued to see Mrs. Abraham and to write the monthly prescriptions for the pharmacist's files. She had reduced her charge for the prescription to one dollar a month out of a similar respect for the Abrahams' modest means. To give the prescriptions without charge, she feared, would run the risk of losing the therapeutic effect of the placebo.

A new pharmacist had just been hired to work evenings in the local drugstore to relieve the overworked owner. He had been asked to fill the placebo prescription for the thirty tablets. He was disturbed. The owner explained to him the long history of the case—the cancer, the barbiturate addiction, the gradual withdrawal several years ago. He ended with a plea that it would be cruel to Mrs. Abraham ever to suggest that she was not getting the real drug. The new pharmacist was still perplexed. He recognized how disturbing it would be to be told of the placebo. Mrs. Abraham would not only run the risk of insomnia and even real addiction but also might lose confidence in her physician of many years. But he was also concerned about the expense to her—$60 a year for nothing more than milk sugar. More than that, he was vaguely disturbed that he was becoming part of a conspiracy to deceive a patient, to trick her into thinking she was getting real pharmacological help. He found the whole enterprise demeaning, an insult to this patient and to patients in general, yet he conceded that Mrs. Abraham might be better off spending her last years happily thinking she was getting the potent drug.

---

1. Is giving a placebo a deception of the patient? If so, can it be justified?
2. Assuming that Dr. Little is committed to the principle that she should do what she thinks is for the benefit of her patient, that she believes it is wrong for her to be addicted to secobarbital, and that she thinks she can relieve her of her addiction, what ought she to do?
3. On what possible grounds could the new pharmacist or anyone else oppose the use of the placebo in this manner?
4. Does the pharmacist have any responsibility for the ethical judgment in the use of these placebos?
5. If the placebo were supplied to Mrs. Abraham free of cost to her, how would that change the ethical implications of the case?
6. How does the use of the placebo for therapy compare ethically to the use of the placebo for double-blind paired-comparison of an experimental drug? Is there any way in which the subject for a drug experiment can consent to the use of the placebo? Is there any way Mrs. Abraham could?

47   WHEN THE FAMILY SAYS NOT TO TELL

Recently Thomas Dundee, an athletic man and writer in his early forties, had a stroke and was admitted to Putnam Institute, the neurological center of a major teaching hospital. For some months before the stroke he had been bothered by headaches and nausea, and his wife had complained that he was listless and moody, but until that time he had been in generally good health. After a neurological work-up Mr. Dundee was prepared for immediate surgery. Finding a glioblastoma multiforma, a cerebral tumor that is a particularly malignant form of glioma, depressed Dr. Miles Foreman, the neurosurgeon with the responsibility of communicating with Mr. Dundee and his wife.

He approached Mrs. Dundee, a firm, heavy-set woman of 46 who had been responsible for getting her husband transferred from the community hospital to Putnam and for bringing Dr. Foreman into the case. Mr. Dundee was not yet sufficiently recovered from the surgery to be able to communicate. Dr. Foreman explained to Mrs. Dundee that her husband was in a critical position. He probably had five months, at best. Dr. Foreman found these conversations after the surgery the most difficult part of his task. "Give me the operating room," he would sputter, "where I am in control and the patient is unconscious." The emotional strain of communicating with the patient and family members, particularly when the news was this bad, ripped at his feelings. He felt particularly helpless when the patient or the family member would lose control and burst into tears.

Mrs. Dundee was not going to lose control, however, at least not in Dr. Foreman's presence. She was stunned, but seemed to take charge quickly. She told the physician that her husband ought not to be told anything about the tumor. "Tell him he is going to need more treatments for the stroke," she said, "but he couldn't handle anything that sounds like cancer. It wouldn't be fair to him to make his last days so miserable." She pointed out that her husband had always handled things in the past by denying reality.

Dr. Foreman explained to her that her husband was going to need radiation treatments and it would probably be impossible to keep him completely unaware that there was a tumor, but he might well not comprehend the malignancy of it. Like most physicians, he handled the problem of what to tell his patients on a "situational" or case-by-case basis. He was discouraged by this case, but he recalled the closing sentences of one of his medical texts. After discussing the pathology of brain tumors, it suggested that although the results of therapy are usually disappointing, the occasional dramatic recoveries always give great hope for the next case. Dr. Foreman wanted his patient sufficiently aware of his condition so that he would cooperate fully in treatment, but he did not want to disturb him. The firm instructions from Mr. Dundee's wife added another dimension to his decision as to what to tell the patient.

---

1. Can one assume that the next of kin is the presumed guardian for a patient when he is incompetent?
2. Is the disclosure of the patient's condition to the presumed guardian an appropriate conversation or is it a violation of confidentiality to which the physician is pledged?
3. If Dr. Foreman is thoroughly convinced that it is in Mr. Dundee's interest to have the diagnosis disclosed to him, because he thinks it will facilitate helpful treatment, what ought he to do?
4. What will be the proper course if both Mrs. Dundee and Dr. Foreman agree that the patient should not be told? Does the patient still have any right to know? If so, how should the decision be made?
5. Could any arrangements have been made before surgery to avoid the dilemma posed by this case?

48   WHEN THE PATIENT SAYS NOT TO TELL

Wesley Crossman was a 43-year-old real estate broker who had just been hospitalized for persistent pain in the bone of his hips. At first he thought he must have pulled a muscle, but the pain gradually became more severe. About six months ago, after he had had the pain for almost a month, he went to his family physician, who made a tentative diagnosis of arthritis. After several months of treatment with indomethacin, an antiarthritic drug, during which time the pain became unbearable, referral was made to an orthopedic specialist for further tests.

Mr. Crossman was the proprietor of a small agency in a suburb of Phoenix, Arizona, in the path of urban growth. Although only marginally successful, he earned enough to support his wife and three children who were now 18, 14, and 12. The rapid development of the area gave him new hope for a financial bonanza. With one child in college and two more on the way, he could use the money. He had recently sold a tract of land to a local group, including a physician and two lawyers, who were planning to build a shopping center. After overcoming his wife's reservations ("She's always too hesitant to take a chance"), he invested $20,000 from their savings account in the project. It would take a few years to pay off, but he was tired of making fortunes on land for everyone else while he and his family put their savings into a bank which added only a dribble of interest twice a year.

Mr. Crossman felt tense when he went to the appointment with Dr. Marvin Greenblatt, the orthopedic specialist. He had not said anything explicit to his wife, but they were both thinking about the neighbor who had succumbed to bone cancer. During the examination, Mr. Crossman remarked that he was a busy man who did not have time for a lot of conversation. "Doctor, you do what you have to do to get rid of this pain," he said. "Put me in the hospital if you have to, but don't trouble me with all the details. Do what you think is best. Even if it's awful, I'd just as soon not know." Both Mr. Crossman and Dr. Greenblatt knew that "cancer" was the word they would not or could not say.

Dr. Greenblatt had seen patients like Mr. Crossman before. Some patients give signals, just as clear as can be, that a diagnosis of a terminal illness would be more than they could handle psychologically. Dr. Greenblatt asked himself, however, "Does he have a right not to know the truth?"

This case leads to conclusions that are atypical of most truth-telling cases. Whereas in most cases the principle of patient self-determination would lead to a decision to disclose a diagnosis or prognosis, and the consideration of consequences for the patient would support nondisclosure, at least from some points of view, in this case these arguments seem to lead to the reverse conclusions. If patient freedom and self-determination are dominant, then the clearly expressed wishes of the patient not to be bothered with the details certainly support nondisclosure, even if the physician feels Mr. Crossman would be better off knowing. On the contrary , if Dr. Greenblatt considers the consequences, he might conclude that Mr. Crossman ought to be told. If he limits the relevant consequences to those related to the patient, he might consider the better therapy as well as psychological adjustment that can be made over the next few months if the patient knows his condition. These consequences alone, however, probably will not be decisive in a decision to disclose because of the consequences. If, however, Dr. Greenblatt considers the consequences for Mr. Crossman's three teenage children of having a father speculate with the family's modest savings in a venture that will not pay off for several years, he might well conclude that the total consequences will be better if he tells Mr. Crossman of his condition. Even if he limits his concern only to patient-related consequences, this might be relevant. If Mr. Crossman will later be disturbed at the realization that he has squandered the resources his children need, then the consequences for Mr. Crossman himself might more decisively justify the disclosure.

The case can be approached from another perspective. Instead of asking what Dr. Greenblatt ought to do, one can ask what Mr. Crossman ought to have done. While the principle of patient self-determination might well justify the physician's agreement with the request of the patient not to disclose, it is irrelevant to the patient-centered question. Assuming that Mr. Crossman has the freedom to request nondisclosure, ought he to do so? While the consequences for the family must be excluded from the physician's judgment if he follows the principle of doing what he thinks will benefit his patient, those familial consequences certainly are not irrelevant to Mr. Crossman's own moral decision-making. He has an obligation to provide for his family and presumably an interest in their welfare as well. From the standpoint of consequences it seems that he has a strong obligation to have the important information about his future.

What, however, if there were no family members in the picture? Would there then be any reason for Mr. Crossman to accept the information if he would rather not be troubled with it? While the freedom of choice of the competent patient might justify his right to refuse the information, some would nevertheless hold that such refusal is still not ethically the best course. According to this view, a mature adult has an obligation as well as a right to make decisions about his own medical care. The fact that to avoid unpleasant information makes life more comfortable would not necessarily make it right. Some would make the case that Mr. Crossman ought not to have requested the nondisclosure even if the interests of his children were excluded from the case.

49 AUXILIARY PERSONNEL AND MEDICAL NEGLIGENCE

Henry Arnold, a 44-year-old electrician, was married and had four children. At age 14 he had had rheumatic fever, and shortly thereafter a heart murmur was noted during a routine physical examination. He was without symptoms until five years prior to admission when he began to notice fatigue and shortness of breath with only slight exertion. He was referred by his family doctor to a cardiologist, who diagnosed rheumatic heart disease with a damaged heart valve. His symptoms became progressively more serious as he developed severe congestive heart failure. The decision was made to replace the damaged valve with an artificial prosthetic valve.

A week later he underwent open-heart surgery on cardiopulmonary bypass or artificial heart-lung pump and a mitral valve prosthesis was implanted. Early in the procedure, one of the pump technicians noted that there was a large pool of blood on the floor of the operating room; the tubing connecting the pump to the patient had either failed to be connected or had been insecurely fastened at the locking connector. Judging from the volume of blood on the floor and the rate of flow of the pump, the technician estimated the length of time Mr. Arnold's brain was without blood and therefore without oxygen as being six minutes. Four minutes of cerebral anoxia is sufficient to produce irreversible brain damage. The surgeon decided to reconnect the pump, complete the operation, and "hope for the best" since the actual time of cerebral anoxia was unknown.

Postoperatively, Mr. Arnold was transferred to the intensive care unit, which was routine procedure for post-open-heart surgery patients. The rumor of the "accident" in the operating room spread quickly through the nursing and professional staff of the intensive care unit and soon after through the rest of the hospital. Mr. Arnold never regained consciousness, although his surgery was successful and his cardiac function improved remarkably. He made random spontaneous movements of his left arm, smacked his lips, and occasionally furrowed his brow. His family had been prepared before the surgery for the possibility of death or disablement as a result of the "unavoidable consequences of high-risk surgery" and never thought to question what had gone wrong.

The staff taking care of Mr. Arnold in the intensive care unit wanted to tell his wife but, since they had not been present in the operating room, felt that they might "just be passing on a rumor." The surgeons never made any mention about what had happened. At two weeks postoperatively, Mr. Arnold was transferred to an extended care facility, where he died nine months later from pneumonia.

Mrs. Arnold received a bill from her insurance company for $5500, the portion of her bill not covered by her husband's health insurance, plus the portion of the nursing home bill exceeding the allowable ninety days coverage provided in his policy.

The Right to Medical Records

The consumer protection movement has made a cause of obtaining the right to see financial records that may include adverse information used to block an individual's credit. The advent of the computer means that medical records can be stored, displayed at remote terminals, and read by anyone with access to the computerized data, including insurance and government agents. Yet, except where state laws take precedence, access to medical information is limited. It is excluded from the list of information that must be disclosed according to the 1971 federal Fair Credit Reporting Act.

The arguments about access to medical records are structured similarly to other arguments about what the patient should be told. According to some views, the patient may benefit from having the information withheld, but according to other views, civil liberties as well as the dignity of the individual patient and his right to self-determination may require disclosure to the patient himself of some of the same information that the patient can already authorize to be disclosed to others.

50   THE CANCER DIAGNOSIS RECORD

The patient, a 72-year-old man, had had a small abdominal growth discovered one year previously during a routine physical examination. The rapid expansion of the growth during the year led to a further examination and exploratory surgery. The surgeon reported a tumor, which the patient understood to be malignant, but he was assured by the surgeon that they had "gotten it all out." No radiation or chemotherapy was prescribed. The large tumor (22 x 8 cm) was described as being in the connective tissue of the abdomen and near the right kidney and small intestine.

The patient was naturally disturbed at the cancer diagnosis and anxious about the future. He was in the process of purchasing a retirement home and wanted to make plans for his retirement with his wife, who was younger and in good health.

Four months after the operation he complained to his family physician during the course of a checkup that he was having continual trouble with loose bowel movements. The physician remarked that this was normal for a man who had lost several feet of his small intestine and a third of his large intestine. This was the first knowledge that the patient had of the removal of the intestine. He sought access to his medical record to no avail. He has been preparing for his funeral since that time.

51 THE CHILD'S IQ

Marilyn Johnson, the middle-class wife of a graduate student, enrolled in a prenatal clinic for families of students in an Eastern school. She was asked, and with her husband consented, to participate in a longitudinal study of the relationship between prenatal factors and child health and development. She and the baby boy were examined at various times throughout the next seven years. On the occasion of the seven-year examination, the parents were concerned that a great deal of psychological and neurological data were being gathered about their apparently normal child. They indicated that they would continue to participate in the study only if they could examine the records up to that point. Their request was originally denied by Dr. Shirley Long, the head of the study. At one point the explanation was given that the study was funded by the government, and that although provision had been made for sending the results of the exam to the child's pediatrician, no budget provision was made for the xeroxing expense to give the record to the parents.

Upon hearing that the government was funding the study, the parents asked if the government received copies of the results. They were informed for the first time that it did, although the form of the government record file was never made clear. This aroused the parents further, who envisaged a full psychological history of their child on store in government files.

The thorough examination by this major medical research center was considered to be of great value to the parents, who did not have access to comparably thorough examinations for the child elsewhere. Thus they had an interest in having the exam done if they could satisfy themselves that the records were not damaging or in error. An agreement was made that the child would be examined and the mother could examine some of the previous records. It was stipulated that no IQ scores could be examined. The parents agreed and examined some records from the previous years, but to date had not seen the records of the seven-year exam or any indication of what was submitted to the government.

52 THE COMPUTERIZED INSURANCE EXAM

A middle-aged man with a history of inactive diabetes was employed by a small new company which was beginning a group medical insurance policy. Because of his diabetes, he was excluded from his company's medical insurance coverage. Out of concern for him, his fellow employees agreed to change insurance companies if another would agree to include him. They found such a company and made the switch.

The man was informed by the insurance agent that he should be quiet about the diabetes since the centralized computer used by the insurance industry for storage of patient medical records did not yet have the information. According to one report, this computer has stored medical records of 12,500,000 persons. It is a strict policy of insurance companies that access to these computer records be available only to their medical departments, never the agents. The man, alarmed as well as concerned as to the type of data that might be stored on him, sought to find out more about the computer. He confirmed its existence but was able to discover very little more.

Earlier in life he had had two medical examinations prior to obtaining life insurance. He would now like to see if those records were in the computer. He had been told that this information was privileged but that upon his written authorization the insurance company would send a letter to his personal physician summarizing the relevant information.

The man, however, did not have a close relationship with a physician. He had seen one about once a year for the past four years, but he did not want to have the information summarized by the insurance company and reinterpreted by a physician whom he did not know well. He wanted to have an actual copy of the insurance company's computer record in his hands for his own examination.

In all three cases there are reasons for not disclosing the information to the patient. In the case of the 72-year-old man with cancer, there had been a breakdown in communication and trust between the physician and the patient as well as a lack of communication between surgeon and family physician. Perhaps the patient has not made clear to the surgeon or his family physician how disturbed he is by not knowing. Perhaps he can sue to get the information. But this will force the case to a legalistic resolution. The moral problem is whether, on balance, it is right to withhold these records, which is somewhat different from whether it is legally required. As with the other cases involving what the patient should be told, there are questions of which kinds of benefits should be counted, how much they should be weighed, and how much benefit and harm will come from alternative courses; there are questions of whether the consequences necessarily dictate the course of action preferred or whether other considerations, such as patient self-determination, are also significant; there are questions of whether in the long run decision-makers would more often be right by following a rule to disclose or not disclose, because of the gradual buildup of mistrust and the possibility of error, even when someone believes that in an individual case more good might come from another course.

The commonest argument for withholding the records from the patient is that the records are complex and might be confusing to the patient. He might suffer needlessly from a fear produced by a misunderstanding. This is the thrust of the position of Dr. Paul Entmacher, medical director of Metropolitan Life:

> Insurance companies are happy to release the medical information that they have in their files, but this is done through the applicants' or policyholders' personal physicians for several reasons. Primarily there is concern that the applicant or policyholder will be given medical information that he or she will not be able to interpret or that the physician feels should not be made known to the patient. When a medical report is obtained, it is obtained with the understanding that the contents of the report will remain confidential and will not be divulged to the patient or to any other person not directly involved in evaluating the insurance risk. The reports, therefore, contain detailed medical information that a lay person may misinterpret and become unduly alarmed by what appear to be serious abnormalities which are, in reality, inconsequential. On the other hand, the person may become aware of very serious abnormalities, knowledge of which the physician has withheld, feeling that the patient may be unable to cope with the problem. For example, an electrocardiogram may reveal changes which are significant, and yet no specific therapy may be necessary. Or a patient may have been operated on for a malignant tumor and not be told the exact diagnosis because the physician and the patient's family feel he or she should not be made aware of the diagnosis. Under these circumstances it would be harmful and not in the patient's best interest for an insurance company to discuss the medical diagnoses and finding directly with the patient.[8]

Clearly a physician employee of a commercial company has obligations to that company which raise problems worthy of consideration, but the main thrust of this defense is in terms of the principle of protection of the patient himself, the Hippocratic principle that focuses on patient-centered consequences.

A second, less patient-centered defense of withholding patients' records appeared in a New York law suit. Edward and Dorothy Siemer sued the executor of the estate of their physician, Dr. Harold Culbertson, to obtain a copy of their medical records.[9] Dr. Culbertson had directed in his will that his executor burn and destroy all office records without opening or examining them. The court ruled that the "records taken by a doctor in the examination and treatment of a patient become property belonging to the doctor." In reaching this decision, they appealed to five excerpts from the Principles of Professional Conduct of the American

Medical Association. Those principles include the position that whether or not the records are given to the patient "rests with the decision of the doctor who knows all the circumstances involved in the situation."

The court ruled, however, that the records would unquestionably be of extreme value to a subsequent examining physician and that their destruction could have grave consequences. It therefore ordered that they be turned over not to the patient but to the succeeding physician. This ruling suggests that while the court recognized a principle of ownership resting with the physician which overrides the patient's wishes, the principle of patient benefit found in the professional ethics literature of the AMA is still an important factor. The court decision seems most implausible in its reliance on the AMA as the determiner of both legal principle and patient benefit. It seems unlikely that Dr. Culbertson had this particular couple's interests in mind when he ordered his records burned. Even if he did, however, the question remains open whether the physician is indeed the best person to determine the patient's best interests. The question also remains open whether the court is justified in appealing to the AMA's principles for determining the proper course. Nevertheless, the court appears to have held that the records are the physician's and not the patient's.

This conclusion is now being questioned in other cases and in certain state laws.[10] Massachusetts currently has a statute specifying that patients have a legal right to access to their records and to copies for a reasonable fee. The moral case in favor of the right of patients to their own medical records can be made in terms of either the consequences or the fundamental rights or civil liberties independent of the consequences. In the three preceding cases it seems reasonable that good consequences can be anticipated from accepting the patient's right to see his records. In the case of the cancer patient, anxiety will be reduced; in the case of the child in the neurological study, possibly dangerous and inaccurate information will be kept out of government files. The goods in the insurance industry computer case are less obvious, but general experience with computerized records justifies the fear that there may be errors. The insured patient will certainly benefit from correcting any errors that exist. In general, the poor communication among physicians and hospitals might make it worthwhile for patients routinely to be the custodians of a copy of their own records.

A more plausible case for the patient's right of access is independent of the consequences. Jeremiah Gutman, a lawyer with experience in the civil liberties field, has argued with regard to the insurance indistry computer case that, especially in the commercial use of medical records, the insurance industry owes the insured "the right to verify the accuracy of the entries made with respect to him; assurance that it does maintain the information under strict standards of confidentiality; and notification of each request for access to data concerning him so that he can withhold or grant consent as he deems best.''[11]

Underlying these rights is a more fundamental moral principle, one which is basic to human relations, including the medical relation. Treatment of the individual with dignity and respect requires a positive response to a request for information, or so the holders of this position argue. They agree that medical information about one's own person is an extension of the self. For the physician to deny this information when obtained in a patient-physician relationship with at least the implied consent of the patient is to destroy the basis of that relationship of mutual respect and confidence. A resolution of the question of the right to medical records will depend not only upon the fundamental questions of ethics, such as the evaluation of consequences and the comparison of consequences with inherent moral obligations, but also upon an understanding of the relation between the patient and the physician. The issue of access to medical records may take on a symbolic meaning signifying how that relationship is to be understood.

PART THREE

SPECIAL
PROBLEM AREAS

7

Abortion,
Sterilization,
and Contraception

Sometimes medical ethics is approached by focusing on special issue areas, such as abortion, human experimentation, or death and dying, rather than on basic themes, such as the individual and society, justice and health care delivery, confidentiality, or truth-telling. There is in fact an overlap between the theme and issue orientations. One special group of problems arises in the area of obstetrics and gynecology. It includes cases on abortion, sterilization, and contraception, as well as on genetics and the new methods of conceiving and bearing children resulting from what might be called the biological revolution. Other issues of current debate in medical ethics are transplantation, hemodialysis, and the allocation of scarce resources; psychiatry and the control of human behavior; and experimentation on human beings. Consent and the right to refuse treatment is another issue, relevant to virtually all the cases in this volume. Finally, a unique problem is raised by death and dying.

Abortion, sterilization, and contraception have been dominant among the issues of medical ethics for many years. Though the specific problems have changed as a result of new laws, court decisions, and attitudes, these remain central ethical problems.

Abortion

The one issue in medical ethics that has generated the most heat and the least light is the problem of abortion. For some, abortion is a simple matter: the right of a human being to life. For others, it is equally simple:

the right of a woman to control her own body. Yet even after the Supreme Court decision of 1973 to the effect that with certain limitations a woman has a right to an abortion, it remains one of the most controversial and complex issues of social policy and personal moral responsibility.

One reason is that the stakes are so high. If advocates of the right and responsibility to have an abortion are correct, the woman who is required to bear a child against her will is having forced upon her an enormous economic and psychological burden. If those who see abortion as a moral outrage are correct, the act is among the worst forms of the taking of human life—the willful destruction of an innocent, helpless person.

Another reason for the clamor of the abortion debate is that in reality many different issues are buried in what appears to be a simple argument. First, there is a radical difference between arguing that abortion should be legal and arguing that it is moral in a particular case. The question for medical ethics is not what abortions are legal, a subject for legal medicine, but rather what abortions, if any, are moral. The two cannot be entirely separated, however, because to many persons the willful violation of the law takes on a moral character of its own.

A second issue in the abortion debate is that of who ought to decide when an abortion is acceptable, whether legally or ethically. Possible decision-makers are the pregnant woman, the father, the physician, and a hospital committee. Conflicts can arise between any or all of these elements.

A third issue in the abortion debate is summarized in the slogans of the different factions: the right to life, the right to control one's own body, or in the case of the physician, the right to practice medicine as one sees fit. All these slogans claim certain rights. A right, as used in ethics and public policy, is something to which one is thought to have a morally justified claim. There are two significant characteristics of the language of rights, which contrast with both the language of moral duties and the language of ethical principles. First, rights contrast with duties in being summary statements of freedoms to which one is thought to be entitled. Duties may be implied in rights. The right to health care, for example, may imply someone's duty to provide health care; the right to practice family planning may imply the duty of the government to provide contraceptives. Even so, the duty is not normally specified. It is unclear what duties are generated by the claim of the right to an abortion. This right probably does not mean that a certain physician has a duty to perform the abortion. It may or may not mean that the hospital has a duty to make facilities available or that medical insurance has a duty to pay for the procedure. To claim a right is to claim a freedom, but freedom may be either positive or negative. A negative freedom is merely the right to act without being restrained. A positive freedom requires much more: the facilitation of the act by providing the resources and means necessary to carry it out.

The second main characteristic of rights which differs from ethical principles is that they are normally more specific. They are summary statements of a specific freedom to which one is thought to be entitled. In this sense they are analogous to "summary rules," which state that a specific behavior is required, such as the rule that signed consent must be obtained before a human is used as an experimental subject. Rights state a specific behavior that one is free to perform. In both cases the behavior is limited: getting consent for an experiment, obtaining medical treatment, or procuring an abortion. These behaviors contrast with the more general values and obligations that are summarized in ethical principles, such as freedom, justice, or the duty to avoid harm.

The problem with specific summary statements of duties and rights is that the moral conflict becomes interesting only when those rights and duties conflict with other equally impressive rights and duties, and it is at this point that the summary statements are of no help whatsoever. Thus, although a woman should have the right to control her own body, many would deny that the woman's right to control her body is the only right at stake in an abortion. Many would accept, in the abstract, that physicians have the right to practice medicine as they see fit, but would also insist that competent patients have the right to refuse any medical treatments they choose. The dilemma occurs when a woman wants to control her own body by having an abortion and her physician decides that performing one would not be practicing medicine as he sees fit. All recognize that at some point a right to life exists in the specific sense that a minimal moral and legal right exists requiring society to protect that life with constitutional guarantees. Yet controversy remains over what the beginning and ending points of that protection ought to be. The right to have one's life protected may be in direct conflict with the rights of others who wish to control their bodies or to practice medicine as they see fit. When a woman wants to control her own body by destroying an eight-and-a-half-month-old fetus which she calls a "uterine tumor," she is deciding that the point at which life ought to be protected has not yet arrived and therefore only her own rights are at stake. When the opponent of such action claims that the eight-and-a-half-month-old fetus has a right to life, the opponent is making a different evaluation of the moral status of that fetus.

What is significant is that both positions rest on a moral evaluation of the claims. In all likelihood the most critical variable in such disputes is the moral status of the fetus. That moral status is clearly linked to a series of biological processes, but the crux of the issue is that no matter what evaluation is made at any point in fetal development, it is always an evaluation, a process of making moral and other value choices. It is logically impossible to offer a strictly biological argument for the status of the fetus, although it may be possible to claim that some biological event, such as conception, implantation, or the beginning of breathing, is the factor that ought to be given moral significance. The many possible events during the development of the fetus which have been considered significant include the following:

Fertilization
Fixation of the genetic code (soon after fertilization)
Implantation (about one week)
Last chance for change in the genetic code (two to four weeks)[1]
Central nervous system activity (detectable electroencephalogram at about eight weeks)
Spontaneous movement (ten weeks)
Brain structure complete (twelve weeks)
Cardiac system activity (electrocardiogram at twelve weeks)
Quickening (thirteen to sixteen weeks)
Viability at present point in technology (normally twenty-four to twenty-eight weeks; occasionally as early as twenty weeks)
Integrated functioning of the nervous system
Birth
Breathing
Consciousness
Social interaction
Acceptance by other people
Development of language
Development of nervous system complete

The choice among these various candidates for the point at which the fetus is considered to have moral claims depends on a fundamentally philosophical or ethical decision about what it is that gives significance to human life and must therefore be provided moral and legal protection. The choices fall into three broad groups. One group focuses on bio-physical developments: fertilization, implantation, spontaneous move-ment, cardiac system activity, birth, and breathing. Those who hold that these biological or physical events are of utmost value—or are "sacred," to use the religious language—see man's nature as essentially biological. Man is close to his animal forerunners. Little significance is attributed to the mere presence of respiratory activity and motion per se in human cells, since neither human sperm nor unfertilized eggs nor still respiring hair and blood cells are given any status. Yet according to one view of man's nature, he is first of all a biological creature and at least some biological events have great moral significance. The biological events tend to take place early in fetal development, but they can occur later or even, as in the case of first breathing, after the time of birth.

A second group of choices about what is morally significant in human life is avowedly sociocultural. Quickening (as opposed to the first spontaneous movement), social interaction, acceptance by other people, and the development of language all require a social context and the response of other human beings to the fetus or baby. They reflect a belief that the human person is more than a biological organism. Human personhood, according to this perspective, is a social phenomenon. Man is a social rather than a biological animal. His significance lies in his relation with his fellow man.

One argument against such a completely sociocultural view is that it makes human significance depend on the sensitivity and goodwill of other people. The young child totally rejected by its parents and isolated from other human contact would, according to this view, not be worthy of legal and moral protections. This sociocultural stance also has the unattractive feature of making the point at which protection is warranted extremely variable. If acceptance by other people is taken as the crucial element, for instance, some will accept a fetus as a human person worthy of protection from the earliest stages of development, while others will not. Such a policy could require the protection of a fetus it it were accepted by anyone, including a stranger, even if it were rejected by the pregnant woman, while at the same time a fetus would not be given protection even at eight-and-a-half months if no one were available to accept it as a person. This sociocultural conception of what is significant in man's nature tends to initiate protection at a much later point in the development of the fetus/baby than the biological perspective does, although such events as quickening or acceptance by others may take place at a very early embryological stage.

A third group of choices combine both biological and sociocultural elements. The appearance of activity in the central nervous system, completion of the brain structure, viability, integrated functioning of the nervous system, consciousness, and completion of neurological development are all biological events. Yet they have a special sociocultural significance. The development of the central nervous system and its capacity to function is the basis of the human characteristics of emotion, intellect, responsivity, and awareness. Viability is the initial point of the capacity for social independence and is also dependent upon the social phenomenon of the state of technology. The choice of these events, which range from as early as the eighth week to well after birth, combines an understanding of man as both a biological and a social creature. It avoids making moral and legal rights wholly dependent either on the whims of others or on biology. It has the added advantage of being compatible with more recent developments in understanding the meaning of death, of what is so significant in human life that a person can be called dead or alive.

Proponents of both the biological and the sociocultural choices have objections to this understanding of man's nature. Those who defend the early biological choices—fertilization and implantation—argue that the potential for all of these developments arises in the genetic events and that it is potential rather than actual capacity which is so significant as to introduce legal and moral rights. The last chance for modifying the embryo's genetic endowment is seen as the establishment of the unique potential of a human individual. Advocates of this position also use a "wedge" argument. They point out that there is a continuum of development up to and even after birth and since it is difficult to choose among the fine gradations of change in such development, the only way to avoid a position that would justify infanticide is to take a firm stand at the first potentially significant event. The proponents of the later points, which usually emphasize the sociocultural dimension, reject the wedge argument. They directly challenge the significance of the events of nervous system development or viability, arguing that man is much more a social animal than the others are willing to grant.

The abortion cases require a choice about what it is in human life which is its essence, what it is which is so significant that it introduces moral and legal rights. The first problem is to determine who ought to decide about an abortion, especially when there is disagreement. There are several possible candidates besides the parents, who themselves may disagree. One is a hospital abortion committee. The contemporary abortion debate also focuses on the role of the state and the church.

Even after the problem of who ought to decide is resolved, the fundamental moral question remains of deciding when abortion is morally acceptable. During the 1960s the American Law Institute Model Penal Code became the standard for abortion law reform. It permitted abortion in the "hard cases," that is, on grounds of the life and health of the woman, rape, incest, or the substantial possibility that the child would be born with a grave physical or mental defect. Each of these cases requires a somewhat different moral justification. Abortion in the case of grave defects in the unborn is often defended on the basis that the future child itself would be better off not being born. It is also sometimes justified on the theory that the future child's impact on other family members, children as well as parents, would be too much to demand. The cases of rape and incest involving underage children hinge on a different argument that it is morally acceptable to interrupt a pregnancy if the pregnant woman in no way consented to it. Abortions justified because the life or health of the woman is jeopardized are often thought to involve a tragic conflict between two moral claims. Especially when the life of the woman is at stake, the conflict is seen as a forced choice between two competing claims. If abortion is accepted, it may be as the lesser of two evils.

Justifying abortion in the hard cases, however, requires a judgment that the fetus' life can be morally compromised. Thus, the laws patterned after the model code of the American Law Institute open the way for a wider acceptance of abortion for social and economic reasons. Once one accepts that the moral claims of the fetus, at least prior to a certain stage of development, are not the same as those of a postnatal human, abortions need not be justified only for rape, incest, and medical or genetic reasons. Certainly the medical needs of a woman might be less serious than the social or economic needs of that woman or her family. The resolution of the abortion debate will depend upon defining the moral status of the fetus.

Finally, the most dramatic ethical problem related to abortion arises after the decision to abort has been made, whether morally correct or not. It is the tragic problem of how to care for the unexpectedly viable abortus.

53 ABORTION CONFLICT BETWEEN SPOUSES

John and Evelyn O'Brien had enjoyed a happy, religiously mixed marriage for twelve years. Although John had been raised as a Catholic, he had not been particularly active in the church since their marriage. They were a typical middle class family, living comfortably, if modestly, in a Long Island suburb of New York City. They had planned their family well, first using a diaphragm and then birth control pills when they became available. They now had a boy, aged ten, and a girl of eight. Evelyn had been working for the last six years as a teacher in the local high school. John commuted to Manhattan where he was a teller at a bank. Even before the publicity about women's liberation, they had shared equally in the household responsibilities and the care of the children. John agreed that, as long as Evelyn wanted to continue her career, it was only fair that he should play an equal part in the domestic responsibilities.

Then the crisis came. At first, when Evelyn's period did not start on schedule, they treated it as a private joke. About a week later they began to get worried. Five weeks after the missed period, the pregnancy test confirmed what they had feared.

"Finances will be tight, but we can't let it upset us," John commented, mumbling about the gynecologist who had said the pills were "virtually one hundred percent sure." He was shocked when Evelyn told him she had decided there would have to be an abortion. In New York State any woman may obtain a legal abortion upon request up until the twenty-fourth week of pregnancy. "Every woman shall have the right to control her own body" is the slogan that cleared the way for the law change. Now it was a question not only of Evelyn's body but of her career, her peace of mind, even the welfare of their children. John assured her that in any event he would continue to carry his share of the household responsibilities, but that the thought of aborting a child of his was abhorrent. They just could not in cold blood decide to extinguish a life they had created. After all, he suggested, if the husband is equally responsible for child care, the responsibility should surely begin with this decision.

Like it or not, they agreed that the law was clear. If Evelyn went to the hospital and demanded the abortion, she would get it. But their marriage was too strong for a legalistic solution. This was something they would have to work out together for themselves. Simply because the abortion would be legal did not necessarily mean to them it was right.

54   ABORTION FOR PSYCHIATRIC REASONS

On June 7, 1970, a 38-year-old woman with five children received confirmation that she was pregnant. She had become very distraught as soon as her period was overdue, fearing that she already had as many children as she could adequately handle, both emotionally and financially. She had always thought that abortion was wrong, but now she felt quite desperate because she did not want another child.

She was using a diaphragm as a contraceptive, having quit birth control pills for fear of their ill effects. She had talked to her husband about abortion, and he had told her he would go along with whatever she decided.

The woman came to her physician to see if she could get a recommendation for an abortion. She admitted to having thoughts of suicide, but added that she did not think she would do it. She was also concerned that no one should find out about the pregnancy, because she suspected that her friends and family would not accept the idea of an abortion.

---

1. This case arose prior to the United States Supreme Court decisions on abortion in a state where the authorization of a physician for an abortion based on psychiatric reasons was required. What is the logical and ethical foundation of the physician's authorization under such a system?
2. Should a physician in such a situation dishonestly certify that the woman is suicidal if such is necessary to obtain an abortion to which the physician thinks she is entitled?
3. Suppose that the case had occurred after the Supreme Court decision, when the woman could have obtained an abortion without a physician's authorization of medical or psychiatric need. What should the woman do in a circumstance where bearing another child will be a serious psychological burden, but not such a burden that suicide is contemplated?

4. Why are the psychiatric effects on the mother, as opposed to the social and economic effects on her and her family often emphasized in the abortion debate? Are medical, including psychiatric, effects more weighty in considering an abortion?
5. Should the husband have given some other answer when discussing the abortion with his wife?

55   ABORTION FOR TEENAGE PREGNANCY

An 18-year-old single girl was three months pregnant. She had been in psychotherapy because of feelings of inadequacy. In her relationships with men she had frequently been exploited, but she repeatedly engaged in such relationships because sexual intercourse gave her a feeling of acceptance and seemed to prove to her that she possessed adequacy as a woman. She did not use birth control pills because she never expected to have intercourse.

She was undecided about marrying the father of the child because she was not sure she loved him. He had offered to marry her, but his interest appeared to be mainly one of duty. She also was undecided about whether or not to have the child. She had spoken to friends, some of whom advised one course of action and others advised the opposite.

She was mildly depressed about her state and felt that this was just another in a lifelong series of mistakes. She wanted advice on what to do.

56   ABORTION FOR POSSIBLE HEMOPHILIAC SON

Ruth Mason's sister had just had a boy. Within hours it was clear that the child had classic hemophilia. Among the children of Mrs. Mason's sisters he was the second son to be born with hemophilia. Because hemophilia of this kind, type A, is caused by a gene on the X chromosome which is passed from mother to daughter, Mrs. Mason had a one in two chance of being a carrier herself. If she were a carrier, approximately half of her male offspring would receive the X chromosome with the hemophilia gene and half of her daughters would be carriers like herself; the other half would be normal. She had been planning to have a child and now wanted desperately to know what she could do in these circumstances.

Her obstetrician told her about a new test which she could take before becoming pregnant to determine if she were a carrier of hemophilia. He emphasized that if the test were positive, it would definitely mean that she had the gene, but that it picks up only 80-95 percent of the women who are carriers. Should she become pregnant, the obstetrician informed her, a prenatal test called amniocentesis could be done around the sixteenth week of pregnancy, which would tell her within days whether or not she was carrying a male fetus. In the current state of medical technology, however, he pointed out that there is virtually no way to ascertain whether the fetus is normal or destined to be a hemophiliac. The doctor told Mrs. Mason that she could then choose an abortion in the latter half of the second trimester of her pregnancy. She realized that if she were positively identified as a carrier, she would then be faced with the prospect of an abortion in which there would be a fifty-fifty chance of aborting a hemophiliac male—or a normal son. And if she were negative, she still could not be sure of not having a hemophiliac because the carrier detection test misses almost one in every five who have the hemophilia gene.

Mrs. Mason decided to find out more about the disease and called the National Hemophilia Foundation, which told her of new developments in the care and treatment of hemophiliac boys. There was a new means of preparing the anticlotting factor cryoprecipitate, and home therapy programs could greatly reduce the cost of home treatment to approximately $6000 per year. She also learned that a prophylactic schedule of treatments, administered once every other day, greatly reduces the insidious bleeding which in the past caused much of the disability experienced by hemophiliacs in their joints. She returned to the obstetrician, troubled and confused. She was uncertain whether to go ahead and take the test to determine if she were a carrier. Even then she would not know how to decide whether or not to become pregnant and possibly have to abort.

Abortion is the first, but only the first, moral problem posed by recent developments in genetics and in prenatal diagnosis of genetic conditions, which also raise other ethical issues. At this point in the development of technologies, however, often the only intervention available is to determine the presence of risk of a genetic condition and then to abort. Thus, the ethics of abortion has become directly linked to the ethics of genetics. Put most bluntly, the problem is how serious a genetic condition must be and how great the risk of that condition must be before an abortion is justified.

Mrs. Mason has an opportunity to learn with great probability if she is a carrier of the sex-linked disease of hemophilia. Sissela Bok, a philosopher who teaches medical ethics at the Harvard Medical School, has reviewed Mrs. Mason's alternatives, arguing that an abortion should be averted, if possible, by foregoing pregnancy, but also that hemophilia is so serious that prenatal detection of the sex of the fetus and then abortion if it is a male—despite the fact that it has a 50 percent chance of being a normal male—is preferable to the substantial risk of bringing the hemophiliac fetus to term:

Ruth Mason must first decide whether to attempt to learn if she is a carrier of hemophilia. In the past, before such knowledge was possible, there could be no parental responsibility for any suffering on the part of afflicted children. But to avoid seeking information *now* is to shirk such a responsibility, and severe recriminations within the family might well ensue. Consider the analogy of a mother planning a trip with a child into a region where the air in some states affects 25 percent of all children with permanent symptoms resembling those of hemophilia. If the information concerning the state where she wishes to go is easily available, what would we say about the mother's decision to refuse to find out whether there are such risks for her child?

As a first step, then, Ruth Mason should find out whether she is likely to be a carrier. If she is, agonizing questions will arise testing her very sense of herself as a woman and as a mother, and her deepest beliefs concerning responsibility for unborn children. How can she feel in advance the suffering to which she might expose a child, or measure her own ability to deal with it? How can she evaluate the help from community and federal programs, and gauge their continued availability in a world of rapid shifts of policy and growing scarcity of resources? How can she weigh the very natural urge to be the biological mother of her children against that, equally natural, of wishing to give her children the healthiest possible start in life?

If Ruth Mason learns that she is a carrier while she is still *not pregnant,* she has three different kinds of options:

1. The first is to forgo pregnancy, either through contraception or through voluntary sterilization. It does not present the ethical problems of the latter two. She can then either remain childless (as more and more women are choosing to do) or seek to adopt children. She will thus avoid the dilemma of whether to consider aborting male fetuses and won't expose daughters to being carriers in turn.

2. The second choice is to become pregnant with the intention of undergoing amniocentesis and aborting the fetus if it should be male. I would find a planned policy of this kind, continued until the desired family size is reached, more difficult to justify ethically. This is because abortion is not a last resort here (even for those who want to bring up children), since the alternative of adoption does exist. In addition, since abortion after amniocentesis takes place later in the pregnancy than most (in the latter half of the second trimester), the procedure is more problematic for both the mother and the physician. And the fact that there is a 50 percent possibility that the abortus will be free from hemophilia should cause hesitation. If, on the other hand, a technique is developed whereby *affected* male fetuses can be detected early in pregnancy, these last two difficulties would vanish.

3. The third alternative which is, in my opinion, the least defensible, is to decide in favor of becoming pregnant and giving birth, thus exposing one's baby to a substantial risk of suffering from hemophilia for life. If reluctance to have an abortion is thought of as a reason for such a choice, it must be remembered that adoption likewise avoids

abortion, without therefore exposing children to risks of this magnitude.

I find the first alternative preferable. If, however, Ruth Mason does not learn that she is a carrier until *after she is already pregnant,* her choices are more restricted. There is now no longer a chance of avoiding a risk to the fetus—a 25 percent risk of hemophilia, a 50 percent risk of abortion. The religious views of some parents may lead them to reject amniocentesis followed by abortion of a male fetus, even under these conditions. I would be inclined to make the choice to have the amniocentesis and possible abortion out of a concern not to bring into the world a child afflicted for life.

Whatever choice parents make, it is crucial that they not be subjected to coercion in this matter, either to abort or to carry the baby to birth.[2]

Marc Lappé, program director of the Research Group on Ethical, Social and Legal Issues in Genetic Counseling and Genetic Engineering at the Institute of Society, Ethics and the Life Sciences, takes a very different stand, emphasizing the qualities needed in parents of a hemophiliac but concluding that, if the parents could provide necessary support of the child, a 50 percent risk of hemophilia would not justify the abortion:

Societal "cost-estimates" for many genetic diseases, where the affected individual's potential as a human being is essentially unimpaired, are inherently suspect. There are statistically calculable "costs" for every prospective person, irrespective of what is known about his or her genotype. While it might be morally wrong to knowingly bring a truly defective child into the world—where the parents cannot afford to give it the amenities of human existence unaided by society—in a pregnancy at risk for hemophilia one can neither "know" with certainty that the male fetus is hemophilic, nor know the true "cost" of dealing with the defect. Moreover, hemophilia is a highly heterogeneous disease. Only slightly more than half of all hemophiliacs require the constant (i.e., once every other day) and expensive prophylactic treatment to avoid spontaneous bleeding episodes. With new technologies, hemophilic boys could likely be given the promise of avoiding the joint disabilities which previously made hemophilia crippling.

Because the currently available tests for detection of carrier females and affected fetuses allow only a statistical estimate of the chance that a fetus is a prospective hemophiliac, Ruth Mason could only avoid all risk of having a child with hemophilia by deciding to abort all male fetuses—*irrespective* of the test's outcome. (Recall that the test may miss one in five carriers.) Here there is an extra moral weight to the decision to abort, since on the average, one or more normal male fetuses would have to be sacrificed to avoid the *prospect* of the birth of one with hemophilia. Nevertheless, the Masons might justify the decision to avoid the birth of hemophilic children by citing the psychological burden to themselves, and the possibility of bringing into the world a life whose existence would be fraught with suffering. But like some moral reasoning, these arguments are weakened by the inherent uncertainty of future events.

The truly difficult question is if the Masons could morally proceed with a pregnancy where there *was* a chance of having a hemophilic child. I think they could. Indeed, were she to believe that the possible ambiguities of a carrier test would aggravate the psychological burden of the pregnancy, Ruth Mason might justifiably even refuse the carrier test. To refuse, she should be able to justify her presumptive right to conceive a child where there was a substantial risk of having an infant who would require special and perhaps expensive care on a lifetime basis.

To do this, I believe that Ruth Mason would need to examine some or all of the following factors: 1) her valuation of human life; 2) her psychological ability to nurture a child who will necessarily experience *some* suffering, both physical and psychological; 3) her family's resources—emotional, psychological, and monetary—to care for this child; 4) the possibility that her own or her husband's expectations in having male children are incompatible with the life style dictated by hemophilia; 5) her recognition that such a child may himself have deep psychological problems from overprotection afforded by well-meaning others.

To my mind, a final test for this couple is whether or not they can give the prospective hemophilic child an assurance of independent existence, even where risks of his safety are still apparent. If they cannot, then perhaps they ought to consider those options which avoid his birth. They might well decide that sterilization is the only moral course open to them. Or, wishing to avoid the anxiety, costs and possible guilt of an "at-risk" pregnancy, they could adopt a child, especially if they consider abortion morally unacceptable.

But assuming they have weighed all the factors, and could accept the risk of a "worst" outcome, I think the Masons could go ahead and have a child. I know I would.[3]

57   ATTEMPTED ABORTION RESULTING IN LIVE BIRTH

Janice Ralston, a 24-year-old unmarried woman who worked as a maid for a large business office, came to the hospital clinic in labor. She reported that the previous day an abortion had been induced at a hospital in another part of the city. When she had become pregnant, she at first delayed and then went to a private physician who had been recommended by a friend. He was unable to see her for twelve days, and then three weeks passed before pregnancy tests were reported to the woman at her next office visit. At that time she brought up the possibility of an abortion. He was not in favor but referred her to a clinic where she could receive obstetrical care at a cost she could afford.

Delays caused by the woman's fear of offending her employer by missing work and crowded clinic schedules consumed several more weeks. She finally became convinced that she would not be able to obtain an abortion at the clinic and, through another friend, went to the hospital where the abortion was induced. A check of the records in that hospital showed that the abortion had been induced by the withdrawal of 1800 cc's of amniotic fluid and its replacement by an equal volume of saline solution. The hospital records also showed that, based on the report of the patient, pregnancy had been estimated as of twenty-two weeks' duration.

While the patient lay unattended in bed in the second hospital, she delivered. A heartbeat was discovered in the newborn baby. Over a period of approximately two hours the staff were uncertain about the proper course of action. No resuscitation was attempted. At the end of this time there were no vital signs. It was reported that during the labor process the woman had showed no interest in the birth and had given no indication of a willingness to keep the child once it was born alive. By visual examination, the attending physician estimated the weight of the newborn to be 1700 grams; it was eventually weighed, revealing a weight of approximately 2000 grams. The policy in the Obstetrics Department of the hospital was normally to attempt resuscitation for any newborn in the 500-1000 gram range.

---

1. Under what conditions, if any, is it morally acceptable knowingly to induce an abortion in a viable fetus?
2. Assuming that a competent physician should be able to discern that a fetus is really about thirty-two rather than twenty-two weeks old, what is the moral and legal status of the physician who induces the abortion? Under what conditions, if any, is a physician morally justified in violating the law? Do arguments for civil disobedience apply in this case?
3. Suppose that Ms. Ralston decided to carry the child to term, placing it up for adoption, and then delivered the fetus/baby prematurely at thirty-two weeks? Should the physician's response be the same? What morally significant differences exist in the two situations?
4. In a saline-induced abortion the fetus may be affected by the saline, producing some risk of damage to the central nervous system. How should this fact affect the decision about resuscitation? How should it affect the decision to use saline in late abortions if the only alternative is a hysterotomy, which has a higher risk to the woman?
5. What steps should be taken to avoid the confusion of not knowing what to do during the two hours after delivery of an unexpectedly viable fetus? What should be done by the woman, by the delivering physician, and by the hospital?

Sterilization

Ethical conflict over sterilization has long divided theologians and policy-makers, physicians and their patients. Sterilization provokes dispute because it touches on many basic value orientations of the human species. Procreation itself is fundamental to the species, and sacred traditions have naturally grown up around it. Man's relationship to nature and to the "natural" body processes is crucial in determining attitudes about medical interventions. Sterilization is only a particularly dramatic example.

Pope Pius XI's encyclical on marriage summarizes the objections to sterilization according to one tradition: "Private individuals have no other power over the members of their bodies than that which pertains to their natural ends. They are not free to destroy or to mutilate their members or in any other way render themselves unfit for their natural functions, except where no other provision can be made for the good of the whole body."[4]

Orthodox Judaism also vigorously opposes sterilization, often referring to it as "mutilation of the reproductive organs."[5] The Protestant tradition is more ambiguous. A pluralistic tradition, it has at various times and in various forms argued that sterilization is morally outrageous or perfectly acceptable. The objections tend to be based less on the natural functions of the body and more on practical considerations like the importance of the family, the need to preserve the option to have more children, and even the fear of promiscuity.

Physicians, as members of a wide variety of social and religious groups, share in this diversity of judgment about the ethics of sterilization. One interpretation of the Hippocratic oath sees it as opposing sterilization when it forbids "cutting for the stone."[6] There is a fascinating controversy over whether this prohibition means that sterilization is wrong per se, that such surgery is acceptable so long as it is not performed by Hippocratic physicians, or that, as Ludwig Edelstein argues, the oath's provision does not apply to sterilization at all, but to the less provocative procedure of cutting the bladder to remove stones.

Whether or not the ancient physician opposed sterilization, there is disagreement among contemporary physicians. The disagreement has to do more with the physicians' general attitude about intervention in the body processes and preservation of procreative options than with specific prohibitions in the tradition of physician ethics. In a national survey physicians were asked whether they agreed with the statement: "The forces of nature are awe-inspiring. The physician best serves his function if he has respect for the complexity of the human body and counts on nature to do its own healing." In that study 45 percent agreed.[7] Their anti-interventionistic perspective might make them very skeptical about significant interventions like sterilization.

Even the conservative traditions that generally prohibit sterilization make exceptions in the case where life is at stake—where it is "for the good of the whole body," to use the Pope's phrase. Some, however, would argue that many or all sterilizations are for the good of the whole body.

58 SELLING STERILIZATION

Dolores Johnson was a 24-year-old black patient being seen by gynecologist Dr. Benjamin Clarke. Dr. Clarke was deeply troubled. Mrs. Johnson had delivered a baby girl six months ago and had almost died in the process. She had hemoglobin HbSS, or sickle cell anemia. Dr. Clarke wondered why he could not convince the patient of the seriousness of her case. Recently her sickle cell crises had not been severe. The pain could be controlled by narcotic analgesics. She had been hospitalized four times in the past five years, substantially less often than she had been earlier in life.

"It's foolish for her to run the risk of pregnancy again," Dr. Clarke said to himself as he looked at her chart. Not only was the risk to the baby great—over 50 percent of pregnancies end in spontaneous abortion, stillbirth, or neonatal death in women with the full sickle cell anemia. Dr. Clarke was especially concerned about what he considered to be an incredibly high mortality risk for Mrs. Johnson herself.

Dr. Clarke had recently read an article by Fort et al. in the *American Journal of Obstetrics and Gynecology,* which painted a horrendous picture of the dangers of pregnancy for women with sickle cell disease. In monitoring 97 pregnancies in 35 homozygous sickle women, the authors had found six deaths associated with pregnancy. Furthermore, some of the women had demonstrated that they were unusually low-risk because they were multiparous, having between five and eleven pregnancies each. If they were eliminated from the group, the risk of maternal mortality rose to 10 percent for each pregnancy. The authors also questioned the mothers' long-term capacity to rear their offspring, pointing out that severe and chronic anemia interferes with all body functions, making it difficult to nurse, train, or support a child. Life expectancy is shorter than normal. The article concluded with a strong recommendation to the obstetrician/gynecologists reading the journal: "We advocate primary sterilization, abortion if conception occurs, and sterilization for those that have completed pregnancies. Patients with sickle cell disease should be unhesitatingly thus counseled."[8]

Dr. Clarke was torn. He had gone over many times with Mrs. Johnson the dangers of pregnancy, although he had tried to do so in a neutral, nonthreatening way. Now one of his patients was behaving in what he thought was a foolish manner. "No rational person would knowingly take that risk," he thought. He was sure he could persuade the patient to be sterilized if he were dramatic enough. Especially an appeal to the interests of the existing child would convince her she had no business having any more children.

Although there is said to be a specific medical indication for the sterilization in this case, the value framework dictates the position of both patient and physician. It is not clear whether Dr. Clarke perceives sterilization advocacy as the value-laden issue it is or whether he sees it merely as a "medical fact" that she ought to be sterilized. Certainly a 10 percent death risk does seem high, even for the presumed good of having a desired child. A value premise is hidden in Dr. Clarke's position. If one holds that a 10 percent risk of death is not worth it (value language), even for a desired pregnancy, then the fact of the 10 percent risk of death is critical. It leads to the conclusion that one ought (value terms again) not become pregnant and probably also to the derivative conclusion that one ought to take the steps necessary to best insure against pregnancy—in this case possibly sterilization.

All that is needed, however, to challenge this conclusion is to question the value premise that the 10 percent death risk is not worth it. This leads to the question of why Mrs. Johnson might want to bear another child. Undoubtedly this question introduces psychological as well as value issues. A line of analysis might lead to a psychological explanation of her desire for a child—her need to fulfill a mothering role, her need to satisfy her husband, or her husband's need to demonstrate his sexuality.

There is something offensive, however, about the psychological rationalization of patient behavior, particularly when it is used to imply that the patient is not really responsible for her behavior. There might also be sound reasons for Mrs. Johnson's desire to become pregnant again, reasons rooted in her system of values. Although desire for anything is presumably rooted in one's psychological history, that fact alone cannot make desires irrational or even nonrational. Mrs. Johnson may be committed to the widely held view that siblings are important for a child; that is, she may be acting out of a commitment to her present child. She may hold that family interactions are important or that there are genocidal implications in the pressures on blacks to be sterilized. The first critical issue in this case is the realization that the behavior of both physician and patient is rooted in a system of values. It is not clear that Mrs. Johnson is behaving as she is merely because she does not grasp the medical facts or because she is psychologically forced into the child-bearing role.

The question of psychological coercion raises a second question. Dr.

Clarke is in a position of substantial power over Mrs. Johnson. His presentation of the facts and the value implications of those facts could well influence her behavior. While this is not a blatant case of compulsory sterilization, it raises similar problems in a provocative way.

Compulsory sterilization statutes were enacted several decades ago, leading to the famous Supreme Court decision of 1927 in *Buck* v. *Bell*. The Court found that Carrie Buck, who was allegedly mentally retarded and promiscuous, was "the probable potential parent of socially inadequate offspring, likewise afflicted, that she may be sexually sterilized without detriment to her general health and that her welfare and that of society will be promoted by her sterilization."[9]

The grounds justifying the coercion were both the welfare of the individual *and* the welfare of society. Dr. Clarke could make a similar argument on the first ground with regard to Mrs. Johnson, for he seems convinced that her welfare is at stake, and he might well argue that the welfare of her present child is as well. But there is no evidence that he bases his concern on the welfare of society, though others might introduce that argument. Both the cost of future care and the original eugenic concern—the protection of the gene pool—might be cited. Some are convinced that these considerations alone justify the infringement on personal procreative freedom.

Not only does Dr. Clarke fail to base his concern on the interests of society, either economic or genetic, but he does not even think of his persuasive argument to Mrs. Johnson as coercive. Rather, he sees himself as acting in a traditional Hippocratic fashion to pursue what he thinks to be in the interests of the patient, making use of the right to voluntary sterilization in the process. Even voluntary sterilization, however, has recently been criticized. A newspaper story began, "Doctors in some cities are 'cavalierly' subjecting women, most of them poor and black, to surgical sterilization without explaining either potential hazards or alternate methods of birth control, the Health Research Group charged in a study released today."[10]

The public outcry began with the report that two black girls, ages 12 and 14, had been sterilized in 1973 in Alabama at the Montgomery Family Planning Clinic, a federally funded social agency. Reportedly the 12-year-old was mentally retarded and the 14-year-old was either a fourth or sixth grade student. The mother signed the consent form with an "X," later claiming she had thought she was signing a permission slip for vaccinations. The hospital director claimed that a notary public quizzed the mother about her awareness of what she had signed before he stamped the document.

This and similar cases gave rise to new regulations from the Department of Health, Education, and Welfare. Competent adults can now be sterilized only after giving their written informed consent, indicating that they are aware both of the costs and benefits of the sterilization and of the fact that they can decline the procedure without losing federal benefits. For minors or incompetent adults, not only is written consent of the minor or incompetent required, but a special review committee has to determine whether the sterilization is in the best interests of the person. The expected mental and physical effects of pregnancy and motherhood or fatherhood and the expected immediate and long-term mental and physical results of the sterilization must be considered.

In 1974 the case of the two Alabama girls reached federal Judge Gerhard Gesell. He was even more concerned than the authors of the HEW guidelines about the risk of coercion in procuring consent for sterilization. He strengthened the requirement that for competent adults it must be made clear that no federal benefits can be withdrawn because of failure to accept sterilization. For minors and incompetent adults he prohibited sterilization even with consent and committee review, maintaining that they cannot volunteer such consent and that the consent of others should not be accepted on a procedure as significant and irreversible as sterilization. Apparently he was not persuaded by arguments that the sterilization was for the individual's own good rather than for the good of others.[11]

Although Mrs. Johnson had the capacity to consent, Judge Gesell's concern over the risks of coercion are important for her case as well. While the old compulsory eugenic sterilization laws at least had the advantage of some semblance of due process, for court hearings were required, the apparently voluntary sterilization of the competent adult poses a moral dilemma. The risk of quasi-coercive pressures by the physician, sometimes in medical language that makes the case appear to be one of medical facts alone, leads to objections to easy volunteering. The suggestion, however, that the patient is not able to withstand the coercive forces of the physician, is not able to judge for himself or herself what is in his or her interests, smacks of condescension, of an indignity to the patient. Dr. Clarke has to walk the line between these two dangers.

59 FOOD INCENTIVES FOR STERILIZATION

The population of a very poor country in Asia was doubling every twenty-one years. This growth had negated economic gains and hindered meaningful economic development.

The country's Family Planning Council, after a massive study, concluded that continued rapid population growth jeopardized the health and welfare of its citizens as well as the very existence of the country. The council recommended drastic action: that every citizen who voluntarily agreed to accept sterilization be given coupons redeemable for one hundred kadis (U.S. $20) worth of food. Any individual who voluntarily requested sterilization after no more than two children would get another hundred-kadi coupon. To increase recruiting, a similar coupon would be provided for persons bringing to a government clinic anyone who subsequently accepted sterilization.

In defense of this proposal, the council argued: "No one will be penalized for having children; no one will be forced to refrain from having children; no one will suffer. In accord with the U.N. Declaration of Human Rights, every citizen should have available those means of controlling family size which are consistent with his own values and religious beliefs."

The traditional religious beliefs of the country apparently offered some resistance to limitation of family size on the grounds that such matters should be in the hands of God. However, studies of past population programs in the country suggested that in practice, the religious objection was limited to a very small minority of the population.

This case raises the problem of pressure or inducement for sterilization in quite a different way from the coercing physician. Here the problem is in part society's, or whether society should make use of inducements to motivate sterilization. It is also in part the problem of the physician's or medical professional's participation in national programs such as government sterilization incentive plans.

Two divergent views have been expressed on the subject. Edward Pohlman, professor of counseling psychology at the University of the Pacific and the author of *Incentives and Compensations in Birth Planning,* makes a case for the legitimacy of the sterilization incentive scheme:

> The father of two children can either get sterilized and get 200 kadis, or not; under the status quo he does not have these options. Not to offer the scheme might restrict freedom. Rapid increases in population growth will probably result in many restrictions on true freedom. Freedom may be like seed: giving up a little for a population limitation scheme may produce a harvest of freedoms later—and avoid increasing regimentation.
>
> In this Asian country most citizens are desperately poor peasants with limited education and few genuine options. They must be farmers, marry young, follow prescribed life styles. They enjoy "freedom" as an abstract concept. Genuine freedoms—education with its broadened vision, nutrition and medical care that produce the vitality and intellectual alertness to make choices, options in jobs and life styles— would be encouraged by sharp increases in per capita income. *If* population limitation produces such increases, and *if* incentive

schemes produce population limitation (both big "if's"), then the schemes may advance freedom.

Incentives like these might limit population, boost the economy of an entire nation, and make national per capita income spurt forward. If so, even families with many children, no sterilization, and no kadis would be better off financially than without the scheme.

This scheme is a way for government to manipulate individual behavior for group goals; government already does this; it discourages murder, theft, driving through stop lights, dumping garbage in rivers and streets, shooting pheasants out of season, etc. Family size may seem more "intimate" than these things; but laws forbid incest, bigamy, homosexuality and adultery, also "private" matters. There is no evidence that any of these hurts society more than continued population growth will. If the law can discourage two wives, why not five children? The supposed "right" to have all the children one wants may conflict with the right to education, food, medical care, pure water and air. The "right" to live seems sacred, yet the death penalty and compulsory military service remove it.

Incentives seem "artificial"; so are irrigation systems, duties and customs on imports, compulsory school attendance and social security schemes, and taxes. Economists abandoned "laissez-faire" long ago, yet it is worshipped as an ideal in family size. Each child born in California costs taxpayers many thousands of dollars through hidden public welfare, education, etc. The state is massively subsidizing child-production; "laissez-faire" is an illusion. In Bombay it is more expensive to rear children than in the village, and so city dwellers may want and have fewer children. Ethically pure family planners may welcome this urban-rural difference because it results from "natural" economic factors. These "natural" factors actually result from a myriad of man-made changes.

Thus incentive schemes may be condemned because they deliberately plan to rig economic influences to make families smaller, whereas we welcome haphazard, unplanned economic changes that accidentally have the same effect as a spin-off. The spectre of "Big Brother" manipulating society so frightens many citizens that they prefer stumbling backwards blindly into the future because that is "natural"— meaning not rationally planned.

In my view society has a right to manipulate family size if (and only if) anticipated rates of population growth are judged to be severely harmful to the well-being of present and future members of the society as a whole. Knowing when this point is reached is difficult; in practice it is a political decision. At the more abstract level, we stoutly deny that the burden of proof lies solely with those who would change the status quo and introduce more extreme measures of population limitation such as this incentive scheme. The effects of rapid population growth, effects on resources, pollution, environment, present and future generations, cannot always be predicted with certainty. To require absolute proof from the innovators and let the defenders of the status quo preserve it without proof is to weigh the balances for conservatism, and for sins of commission. It is the easy path, politically and ethically, but doing nothing may harm the future by default. Probability rather than certainties are the name of the game; we must gamble either way; and the stakes are the total lives of our children and grandchildren and their planet home.[12]

Daniel Callahan, a philosopher and director of the Institute of Society, Ethics and the Life Sciences, argues a rather different point of view:

The assumption behind any incentive program is that it is possible to induce, bribe or otherwise manipulate people into doing that which someone else wants them to do. Incentives would not be necessary if people were prepared, on the basis of their own motivations, to take the steps desired (by someone else). When they are not so prepared, then bait must be put before them.

In this instance the bait is food, no doubt chosen because in a poor country, with pockets of malnutrition, the procurement of food is an endless and pressing concern, particularly for those with families.

But note a significant lack of symmetry in the proposal. The benefit of a food bonus is temporary, good this year but gone next year. By contrast, sterilization is for all practical purposes irreversible. Thus the government gets a permanent benefit in return for taking a temporary step. On the face of it, this strikes me as unjust, a one-sided bargain. Had the proposal called for a food bonus in return for the use of contraceptives—a temporary benefit for a temporary avoidance of children—the transaction would be more just.

The point of asking for a symmetrical plan is not only to serve higher forms of justice. In a poor country, children are social and old-age security. In poverty-stricken agricultural areas, children are necessary in order that sufficient food may be raised. In the absence of pension and old-age security systems (virtually unknown in poor countries), one's children are the only source of support in old age. High infant mortality rates (another characteristic of the kind of country described) require that a large number of children be born in order that a small number will survive to adulthood. In that kind of setting, the permanent foregoing of further children is something more than the sacrifice of whatever satisfaction there may be in having children as such. It may seriously, permanently and irreversibly threaten the future welfare of those sterilized.

Note that my objection to the proposed plan is not an objection to incentive plans as such; it is to the details and conditions of the incentive plan described. But are there not more serious and fundamental objections to the plan? Of course there are. The Council argues that "no one will be penalized for having children." The deprivation of needed food, for failure to meet a governmental requirement, would strike me as a serious penalty. It also argues that "no one will be forced to refrain from having children." In the context of poverty and malnutrition, the choice between no food or no children could surely be defined as a forced choice. Finally, the government contends that "no one will suffer." Are we really to believe that parents of under-nourished children, who might otherwise want more children, would undergo no suffering in having to make the choice between food and sterilization?

Those are all very serious objections. The very nature of incentive programs in poor countries is to trade upon the needs of the poor, pushing them to make choices they would not otherwise make.

Moreover, it has to be assumed that the government can at least afford to make some food or money available, otherwise it could not initiate the program at all. But then, one must ask, is an incentive plan for sterilization the most equitable way of making available surplus food (or the funds to buy food)? Why do those willing to be sterilized "deserve" the food more than others, e.g., more than the old, past childbearing age, or more than the very young?

The only possible rationale for this kind of selectivity is that population growth is the single most important problem facing a nation, sufficient to justify the making of benefits available to one group (albeit at a price) which will not be made available to another. If that proposition can really be proved, then incentive plans might be in order. But it is by no means easy, with any nation, to prove that population growth is the "single most important problem," a very different matter from proving it is *a* serious problem. But assuming someone (somehow) could prove such a proposition, then incentive plans could be made ethically viable. The one condition I would stipulate is that the bargain struck be fair to both sides: permanent sterilization requires a permanent bonus or benefit.[13]

Contraception

Another of the classical moral problems in medicine is contraception. Although the use of contraceptives within marriage is now widely accepted, moral problems remain. The traditional Roman Catholic objections to any form of "unnatural" intervention in the process of conception are well known. Not so well known are the nuances of that tradition and the ambivalence of the attitude of other Western traditions.

The main strand of Catholic thought remains opposed to all forms of contraception, with the grudging concession that rhythm is tolerable.[14] The argument is that depriving the sexual act of its procreative potential divorces it from the end of marriage which legitimates the act in the first place. Pius XI articulated the position definitively in the encyclical *Casti connubii,* referred to in English as "On Christian Marriage," when he said: "the Catholic Church, to whom God has entrusted the defense of the integrity and purity of morals, standing erect in the midst of the moral ruin which surrounds her, in order that she may preserve the chastity of the nuptial union from being defiled by this foul stain, raises her voice in token of Divine ambassadorship and through Our mouth proclaims anew: Any use whatsoever of matrimony exercised in such a way that the act is deliberately frustrated in its natural power to generate life is an offense against the law of God and of nature, and those who indulge in such are branded with the guilt of a grave sin."[15]

By the 1960s the debate among Catholic theologians and lay people had reached the point where John XXIII appointed a special papal commission to deal with the problem of contraception. The commission was so deeply split that two reports were issued. The majority, however, emphasized the notion that the obligation of marriage includes education as well as procreation. They concluded: "The regulation of conception appears necessary for many couples who wish to achieve a responsible, open and reasonable parenthood in today's circumstances. If they are to observe and cultivate all the essential values of marriage, married people need decent and human means for the regulation of conception."[16] Pope Paul VI then put an end to speculation about possible change in the position of the Catholic Church in 1968 when, in the encyclical "On Human Life," he condemned all "artificial" methods of birth control.[17]

Other major Western traditions have not escaped an ambivalence on birth control. Malthus, an Anglican clergyman, was pessimistic about population growth, in large part because he could not conceive of birth control within marriage. Protestants well into the twentieth century had serious reservations about birth control, although often for different reasons than Catholics. Readily accessible birth control would lead to promiscuity, they feared. It was not until 1930 that the Anglicans cautiously approved of contraception while maintaining that "the primary and obvious method is complete abstinence from intercourse . . . in a life of discipline and self-control lived in the power of the Holy Spirit."

Although Jews in practice vary widely in their views of contraception, Orthodox Jews have traditionally opposed all methods of birth control where no medical or psychiatric threat to the mother or child is indicated. The argument against birth control is two-dimensional, involving both the positive commandment to procreate and the prohibition against improper emission of seed. While the procreative duty is not absolute or limitless, the prohibition against the improper emission of seed acts as a general deterrent against the use of any contraceptive device.

In cases of medical hazard, the situation is more ambiguous, and concessions have been made by the rabbis. The use of the condom or coitus interruptus are in all cases considered unacceptable because they allow the unnatural and purposeless emission of seed. Furthermore, abstinence is in most cases not regarded as an appropriate alternative.

This has led to a search for the "least objectionable method of birth control," that is, the method that least interferes with the natural sex act and with the full mobility of the sperm and its natural course, to be used when pregnancy poses dangers and when rabbinic sanction for the use of birth control has been obtained. Within this context, modern halakic opinion tolerates contraceptive methods such as the diaphragm, cervical caps, or sterilization where pregnancy may prove hazardous to the life of the mother. Rabbinic opinion, however, favors oral contraception by pill as the "least objectionable method" and sanctions its use for lesser medical considerations that do not involve a threat to the life of the pregnant woman or her children, such as to space one's family for medical, though not for economic, reasons.[18]

Muslims have never formally opposed contraception. Medieval texts in fact approve it. But the folk belief in the power of Allah often gives rise to a norm of leaving conception in His hands.

This mixture of moral arguments against contraception—involving the duty to procreate, the violation of natural processes, the fear of promiscuity, and the objection to tampering with the spontaneous—still gives rise to moral problems related to contraception. The problem is especially severe with respect to provision of contraceptive medical services to young, unmarried, but sexually active patients.

60 CONTRACEPTION FOR THE UNWED TEENAGER

A 12-year-old girl came with her parents on a return visit to the County Hospital pediatric emergency clinic for a follow-up report on a pregnancy test, VDRL, and gonorrhea culture smear taken earlier. Her initial complaint had been irregular menses and amenorrhea for two months, and during the original interview with her alone she had indicated a very active sexual history for her age. All test results were negative, however, showing that she was neither pregnant nor infected. The irregularity of her menses was considered normal for her age. Because of the onset of another menses since her previous visit, she did not require the induction of menses medically.

The resident physician who talked to her had resolved the problem and was ready for the next case. However, the medical student who had been observing the interview stopped him in the hallway outside the patient's room. She asked: "What if she does get pregnant? She's not married, quite naive, but certainly sexually active. Should we instruct her now on birth control methods and, in fact, initiate oral contraceptives?"

The resident seemed surprised, because he had not thought of the possibility. He said, "She's so young . . . You're right, though, she's sexually active . . . Birth control at her age? Her parents don't even know why she is here. I don't see how I could recommend the pill to her.''

——————

1. Assuming the resident physician finds sexual activity for this unwed teenager morally objectionable, what ought he to do?
2. Assuming the medical student finds sexual activity for this unwed teenager moral or at least tolerable and also feels the obligation to make sure she has potentially useful medical information about contraception, what ought she to do?
3. In the state this case took place, there was no law explicitly permitting medical services for sexually active teenagers without parental consent. How does that affect the case? How would circumstances change if there were such a law?
4. Which of the following moral objections to contraception, if any, are defensible?
    a. It is an infringement on the natural functions of the body.
    b. It makes sexual promiscuity more widespread.
    c. In the case of oral contraceptives, it exposes the user to intolerable and unknown medical risks.
    d. While generally acceptable, in certain situations it interferes with the growth of an ethnic, racial, or social group, such as the Jews in Israel, the blacks in the United States, or persons with high IQ's.
5. The medical student apparently feels that it is in this patient's interest to have knowledge of contraception to protect her health and welfare. Should a physician initiate conversation about contraception with a 26-year-old unmarried woman for similar reasons? Or would this be condescending on the party of the physician?
6. Might it be acceptable for a physician to initiate discussion of contraception with a patient for any of the following reasons:
    a. Recognition that the patient is from a low-income group
    b. Knowledge that the couple already have many children
    c. Concern about world population growth
Or should a physician never suggest that contraception might be appropriate for a patient?

CHAPTER 8

Genetics, Birth, and the Biological Revolution

But the God in fashioning those of you who are fitted to hold rule
mingled gold in their generation, for which reason they are the most
precious—but in the helpers silver, and iron and brass in the farmers
and other craftsmen. And as you are all akin, though for the most
part you will breed after your kinds, it may sometimes happen that
a golden father would beget a silver son and that a golden offspring
would come from a silver sire and that the rest would in like manner be born of one another. (Plato, *The Republic,* Book III, lines
415 ab)

The flow of gold, silver, iron, and brass from parent to child has, in
the twentieth century, become a major fascination. Since W. Johannsen
gave the name "gene" to the basic unit of heredity in 1909, it has been
possible to speak more precisely of this transmission from parent to
child. There has also been a basis for understanding the occasional
alchemical wonder of changing iron to gold or the more common bun-
gling of the alchemist when the gold of the parents produces the tragedy
of a child of baser metal. Perhaps nowhere else in creation has so much
mystery and so much controversy been packed into such a small space as
in what has come to be called the gene—unless it be in the atom itself.
Much of the mystery as well as the controversy, however, is already in
that Platonic view of the world: the genetic determinism, the value loading of varying genetic potentials, and the linking of social position to
genetic endowment.

The excitement and controversy of genetics and human intervention in the process of procreation and birth has mushroomed in recent decades. The social and ethical dilemmas have grown in proportion. Some of the controversies are not really new. They are the same problems that arise whenever man intervenes medically in the human process. Other problems, however, are quite new, or at least are posed in new and dramatic ways.[1]

In identifying the values in these cases, eight questions ought to be asked. First, what is meant by genetic health? Deciding that one has a medical problem requires, by definition, the superimposing of a set of values on a medical condition. It is impossible either to call something a problem without drawing on values or to make a medical choice among alternative treatment possibilities without evaluating those alternatives. Health itself is a value-laden concept.

This is clearly the case when speaking of genetic health, although only recently has its value loading begun to be realized.[2] In some cases, as in retinoblastoma, there is consensus that a condition is unhealthy, but in others the label is more problematic. Is the mother who may be carrying a gene for muscular dystrophy diseased, or are only those who actually have the disease? Would the mother be in a healthier state if a test determined that she was clearly a carrier, eliminating the psychic trauma of uncertainty, or would she be less healthy? Deciding that a condition is unhealthy often legitimates medical intervention. In many of the cases of prenatal genetic experimentation the value judgments necessary to consider the person in need of medical help are particularly apparent. Infertility can give rise to a proposal for medical artificial insemination; the infertile person's medical condition is judged sufficient to warrant the intervention. But infertility can also lead to an attempt to produce a baby by extracorporeal means, that is, a test-tube baby, or to reproduce a genetic copy of another person. In all such cases it is essential to identify the values used to justify the medical intervention.

The second key question for determining values is who should decide about genetic intervention? In genetic counseling the problem of separating the roles of physician, patient, relatives, and society is controversial. Ought the genetic counselor to be a counselor in the sense of advising the patient/client about the best course of action? Ought he to recommend an abortion, urge it, insist on it, or only pose it for consideration? Or ought he never to mention the possibility unless it is brought up by the patient?

Directive counseling, in which the counselor actively recommends a course of action, began with the more obvious genetic conditions, such as Down's syndrome or Tay-Sachs disease, where there is no real doubt about whether the condition is a problem. Directive counseling, however, thrusts the genetic counselor into the role of moral counselor. Abortion is obviously a value-laden issue, but so is the decision to institutionalize a child or to treat a child with a serious illness.

The problems associated with directive counseling, especially the necessity of the counselor to incorporate his personal values and impose them on his clients, have given rise to the advocacy of value-free or nondirective counseling. The counselor's role, according to this view, is to give the patient the facts about the genetic condition—to explain the nature of the disease, the risk, the possible treatments, and the possible ways of avoiding the risk. It is then the patient's job to make the critical decision. This approach avoids the unfortunate priestly quality of directive counseling, but it has its own problems. For one thing, no counselor can in practice be really value-free. All human beings have value perspectives, which creep into communication no matter how hard they guard against them. Simple shifts, such as the difference between saying that a woman has a 50 percent chance of having a diseased baby or a 50 percent chance of having a normal baby, convey value perspectives. Painting a horrible picture of institutionalized care at its worst or an optimistic picture of loving parental care also communicates values. In fact, it is logically impossible to be a value-free counselor because one must select the facts thought to be significant for discussion, and choosing what is significant requires evaluation. Different cases may require different resolutions of this paradox. Deciding roles in the decision-making is particularly crucial in genetics cases.

Third, how should conflict between the interests of the patient and society be resolved? The classical principle of medical ethics—that the physician should do what he thinks will benefit his patient—presents serious problems in many cases, but in genetics cases the problems are especially acute. For example, it is not always clear who the patient is. Is it the woman who comes for genetic counseling? Is it the couple? Is it the fetus? Or is it even possible that a yet-to-be conceived child could be thought of as the patient? If so, how ought the counselor to handle a case where the potential child's interests— if that has any meaning—conflict with the parent's? The current proposals for mass genetic screening force the issue of conflict between the individual and society. Should screening be compulsory? If so, why? To protect the fetus, to protect the economic interests of society, or simply to give potential parents the option of free and informed choice?

Fourth, is the most beneficial course always the right or just course? The conflict between the individual and society is closely related to the conflict between right and good. For example, producing the most social benefit in health care delivery may conflict with promoting justice, as in the case of money spent on a particular institution, which might not produce the greatest good for the greatest number (the classical utilitarian good-maximizing formula), but still might help a small group who have suffered greatly. According to one major tradition in ethics, the course that does the most good, all things considered, may still not be the one that is right. There may be inherent characteristics in alternative courses, such as justice, which make them right even though they do not maximize the benefits. In fact, whenever a physician says he has a duty to do what he thinks will benefit his patient, he is probably saying that there is something more important than worrying about the total good which might come from his actions, namely, doing the best he can for the individual patient.

Fifth, must genetic and other prenatal interventions be kept confidential? Another principle besides justice determining whether actions are right, independent of whether they do the most good, is the principle of confidentiality. This is really a medical application of the principle of promise-keeping or contract-keeping, in which there is an implied promise to keep medical information confidential. Genetic information is among the most fascinating of all types of medical information and among the most significant, especially for relatives who may be genetically at risk. At issue is the extent of the duty to tell relatives of a potentially important piece of genetic information.

Sixth, does the genetic counselor have a duty always to tell the truth, or only if it will be beneficial? Still another principle which some hold to make an action inherently right is that of honesty or truth-telling. The question arises frequently in the context of genetics. The techniques available to monitor and control genetic and other prenatal development are great. Speculation about future capacities to intervene in order to control or treat genetic conditions might provide valuable information, but it might also prove disturbing. It might, for instance, condition a parent to believe that a child is in some way abnormal.

Seventh, what is the relation of abortion to the problem presented? Abortion is intimately connected to the ethical evaluation of many genetics cases, at least in this day when one of the primary methods of intervention is prenatal diagnosis and abortion. This is the alternative faced, for example, by the woman who discovers that she may be carrying a child with hemophilia or muscular dystrophy.

The ethics of abortion is logically separate from the ethics of genetics. At the same time, it would be dangerous to assume that abortion is always morally acceptable simply because the fetus will be genetically abnormal. In the end the resolution of the moral dilemma of abortion will influence the answers reached in cases involving genetics and birth.

And eighth, what is the nature of man and how should man use medical technology to change that nature? This is a fundamental question in all of medical ethics, but it is posed most dramatically by genetics, particularly by the new techniques of genetic manipulation and fetal research. Answers to the problems posed by these techniques will depend heavily on one's understanding of man's nature and of whether or not man ought to use technology to change the fundamental building materials of that nature.

Genetic Counseling and Care

The problems in genetics and birth can be divided into three groups: counseling and care, mass genetic screening, and experimental interventions in the process of procreation and birth. Genetic counseling and care are now becoming routine in medical centers and physician's offices. Decisions about the funding of these services are made regularly in policy-making bodies in state and federal governments, although the services themselves are being offered more or less in the context of traditional medical services.

61 STATISTICAL MORALITY: GENETIC COUNSELING FOR MUSCULAR DYSTROPHY

Margaret Farrow, a 27-year-old in the twentieth week of her third pregnancy, requested genetic counseling and amniocentesis, a procedure permitting study of the amniotic fluid surrounding the fetus. She had been referred to the counselor by her obstetrician. She had three brothers with Duchenne muscular dystrophy, two of whom were hospitalized. The illness begins in early childhood with a pelvic girdle weakness, causing frequent falls and difficulty in rising. It progresses through childhood, and by early adolescence the patient is confined to a wheelchair, continues to deteriorate, and life expectancy for the greatest number of patients is middle life.

Mr. and Mrs. Farrow already had a 7-year-old son and a 3-year-old daughter, both in good health and born before she was aware that the new genetic tests were available. Earlier tests to determine if she were a carrier of muscular dystrophy, administered in another hospital, had been inconclusive. She stated to the physician in the initial session, "If you cannot show me that the baby is normal, I am going to have an abortion. If the baby is normal, I want it." She stressed how much strain her brothers' illnesses had put on the family.

The physician-counselor explained to her that Duchenne muscular dystrophy is a sex-linked disease. Females do not have the disease, but because it was known that her brothers had the disease, there was a 50 percent chance that she was a carrier. There was therefore a 25 percent risk that any male born to her would be affected by muscular dystrophy. The physician explained that whereas amniocentesis could assist in detecting the sex of the fetus, no technique was yet available for discerning the extent to which muscular dystrophy would be present in the child. He recommended amniocentesis coupled with other new attempts to determine whether Mrs. Farrow was a carrier. If it were determined that she was, then the risk of a male child having muscular dystrophy would increase to 50 percent.

An amniocentesis tap was performed the same day. In addition, arrangements were made for Mrs. Farrow, her mother, and her two children to obtain creatine phosphokinase studies at the National Institutes of Health. These enzyme studies could show that Mrs. Farrow was definitely a carrier, but the test is not yet sensitive enough to show that she definitely was not. If either child were shown to be a carrier, she could also conclude that she was a carrier.

The tap showed the fetus to be male. Mrs. Farrow decided that she wanted an abortion, as well as a hysterotomy for purposes of sterilization, without waiting for the results of the tests to determine if she were a carrier. She explained her decision to a pastoral counselor to whom she had turned for counsel: "I will not know any more after the tests than I know now. The test cannot tell me for sure that I am not a carrier. The tap showed that I am carrying a boy and the chance of him having muscular dystrophy is high (25 percent). I guess it boils down to a decision based on chances."

The counselor pointed out that she might know for sure after the test results were in that she was definitely a carrier. This additional knowledge, added to the result of amniocentesis, might have served as the most complete basis for a decision. She replied that if she could not be told with certainty that she was not a carrier and that the fetus was normal, she did not want to run the risk of having the child: "After growing up with it in my brothers, if there is the slightest chance, I want to avoid it."

The geneticist, in a separate discussion, agreed with her reasoning about the abortion but not about sterilization. He felt that she should retain the possibility of bearing children because, if she became pregnant again, tests could be made to determine if she were carrying a female. If she were, the child would definitely not have the disease. If it were a male, there would be the same 50 percent chance it would have muscular dystrophy. He added: "Is there an ethics for calculated gambling? There is a chance that a healthy life may be destroyed to prevent a supposed unhealthy life."[3]

62   RETINOBLASTOMA: GENETIC RESPONSIBILITY AND DOMINANT INHERITANCE

Following is an interoffice memo from Ian Ward of the Genetic Diseases Unit of the State Department of Health to Michael Hobbs, state health commissioner:

In response to your request for a memo on our need to develop a policy on limiting genetic transmission of retinoblastoma, here is the present situation together with alternative policies. I'll begin drafting legislation as soon as you give me the word.

Retinoblastoma is a rare, malignant eye tumor which occurs early in childhood. Until recently it was invariably fatal. In the 1950s about 5 in every 100,000 children were born with retinoblastoma—on the average one of them (20%) carried a dominant gene which caused the tumor. Before effective treatment was instituted some 25 years ago (the treatment includes removal of one or rarely both eyes), the one case in five was the result of a new mutation. Today, the incidence of retinoblastoma is greater than 5 per 100,000, more than one case in five has a genetic basis, and a smaller proportion of genetic (usually bilateral) cases are due to new mutations now than in the 1940s and 1950s.

This new pattern of retinoblastoma is almost certainly due to the survival and reproduction of those individuals who in previous generations would have succumbed to this fatal tumor before reproducing. (Because only 80% of the individuals receiving the gene actually develop retinoblastoma, a portion of the cases which appear to be "new" are the result of unaffected individuals also transmitting their genes. Such individuals cannot currently be detected by any genetic test, but if they have affected brothers or sisters they would be suspected as being carriers.) On the average, half of the children of a person with the genetic form of retinoblastoma will develop the condition, even though he will almost certainly be married to a "normal" individual. If they too are treated successfully and reproduce, there will be a rapid increase in the frequency of the gene responsible for retinoblastoma. (For example, the results of early diagnosis and treatment of retinoblastoma between 1930 and 1960 in the Netherlands led to a two-fold increase in the incidence of retinoblastoma.)

In the first treatment generation, the incidence of a disease previously fatal (prior to reproduction) will double, and increase incrementally proportional to the rate of mutation, so that in ten generations the gene frequency will be 0.011 percent, in thirty generations it will be 0.031 percent, and in a hundred generations 0.099 percent.

Policy Alternatives

1. Those families in which retinoblastoma can be demonstrated to have a genetic cause shall (shall not) be aggressively treated by systematic screening of eye-grounds of newborns and children.

2. Treatment of retinoblastoma shall be contingent on submission of the successfully treated individual to sterilization before marriage.

3. Treated individuals with genetic retinoblastoma will be actively encouraged to have 1/2 the prevailing average number of children.

4. Individuals with genetic retinoblastoma will be subject to mandatory genetic counseling prior to their marriage as a prerequisite to being given a marriage license.

5. Marriage licenses shall not be given to individuals proven to be carrying the gene for retinoblastoma. Reproduction without a license shall be punished as a misdemeanor.

6. Individuals with genetic retinoblastoma who submit voluntarily to sterilization will be compensated by the state.

7. Individuals with genetic retinoblastoma or their affected children

who have lost eyes as a result of treatment should be compensated by the state for this loss.

8. Genetic counseling shall be proffered on a voluntary basis to individuals with genetic retinoblastoma.

9. No restraints on childbearing shall be imposed on those having genetic retinoblastoma.

Mike, these are the options. I don't see how we can go on inflicting this kind of suffering on innocent children. If we keep going as we are there will be more and more cases. I favor at least some state restraints. I am concerned that we know that we cannot currently distinguish between genetic and non-genetic forms of the disease until we have a family history. I'm also worried about the 20 percent of individuals who carry the genes but never develop the symptoms. What do we do?

63   JUSTICE AND EFFICIENCY IN CARE FOR THE MENTALLY RETARDED

The hearings for State Bill 529 had been called to order. The bill, introduced by State Representative John Sheehan, provided for the establishment of community-based homes for the care and education of the mentally retarded. There would be one home for every fifteen of the presently institutionalized mentally retarded in the state. The estimated cost to the state for this care would be $70 million a year, in comparison with the present budget of $55.8 million for the four state institutions for the mentally retarded. These four institutions currently served 7600 people.

Representative Sheehan spoke in favor of the bill. He painted a picture of hundreds of human beings, many with no clothing, huddled in the dark, drab rooms of the present institutions. Built before the turn of the century, they remained as they were decades ago, without even the basics of furniture. Recreation and educational equipment were nonexistent; aesthetics were ignored. The institutions were terribly understaffed, and many staff members had no professional training. Representative Sheehan, who had the support of the parents' organization, the State Department of Mental Health, the local chapter of the American Civil Liberties Union, and the religious leadership, concluded his case by pleading, "Justice requires that we extend this token contribution to this group of our citizens most burdened by incredible medical expenses, by physical and psychological suffering, and by the degradation of our society's past inhumanity to its fellow humans."

Representative Janet Hudson and Dr. Robert Simmons were the primary spokespersons in opposition. Representative Hudson emphasized that she was concerned about the care of the mentally retarded but that she was also the elected representative of all the citizens of her district.

She argued that the representatives had an obligation to examine possible alternative uses of the $14.2 million in increased funds called for by the bill; not to do so would be fiscally irresponsible. She had some facts to back up her point. The $70 million needed for the new program would represent 1.5 percent of the state's annual budget, a budget raised by all its citizens. Yet the institutionalized population to be assisted by the program equaled only one-tenth of one percent of the state population. The proposed increase of $14.2 million could also buy hot lunches for all of the school children in the state or provide job training for persons to become productive members of society. The fairest thing to do, she argued, would be to spread the money more evenly and to spend it on those who would be productive. "Our task as legislators," she argued, "must be to serve the greatest good of the greatest number."

Dr. Simmons took a similar position but, as a physician, he felt the money would be used more efficiently in providing health care for three groups: normal or nearly normal children, thousands of whom could be reached for every mentally retarded child in the Sheehan bill, adults potentially engaged in productive labor, and pregnant women. He emphasized that he was concerned about the plight of the mentally retarded. He showed, however, that much mental retardation could be eliminated with prenatal diagnosis. He estimated the cost of the prenatal elimination of Down's syndrome, for example, to be $200 per case, compared to an average of $60,000 for every child institutionalized. Although acknowledging the fact that some of the institutionalized retarded might be gainfully employed if they were in high-quality, small-scale, community-based homes, he argued that the savings from spending the funds on detection rather than on more expensive forms of institutionalization would be enormous.

The legislative committee then moved into closed session to make its decision on the bill.

Genetic Screening

The increased capability to detect, control, and in some cases treat genetic conditions has given rise not only to genetic counseling and care but also to more systematic efforts to screen for those conditions. Programs to screen a population systematically for genetic traits began in 1971 in Baltimore where a voluntary, community-wide program to detect Tay-Sachs disease carriers was developed in the Jewish community, the dominant population group affected by the disease.

Mass genetic screening is more in the tradition of public health than is genetic counseling and care. It raises all of the social and ethical problems of genetic counseling plus additional ones. In public, large-scale programs the contact between genetic counselor and client is much more tenuous. Often no real counselor-client relationship exists at all. The programs may be run by community groups or others who for the most part do not have behind them a tradition of medical ethics which emphasizes such issues as confidentiality and patient, rather than social, benefits.

Some programs are government mandated. Twenty-nine states now have some kind of mass genetic screening legislation. In several cases the screening is actually compulsory. The kind of screening, the disease for which the screening is carried out, and the time of screening vary considerably. Screening programs for Tay-Sachs, sickle cell, and phenylkentonuria or PKU have received the most attention. Screening may be for carrier status, as in Tay-Sachs and sickle cell disease. In such cases the screening may take place at the time that marriage is contemplated. Some states mandate sickle cell trait screening as part of the medical exam when a child enters school. PKU screening is required at birth in some jurisdictions. Prenatal screening of fetuses using techniques such as amniocentesis or ultrasound is becoming more routine for diseases such as Tay-Sachs when both parents are identified as having the trait or for Down's syndrome in the case of the older pregnant woman. In some cases a couple can be screened for the presence of the trait, but no satisfactory test is available for detection of the disease itself in time for an abortion to be chosen. Sickle cell disease is one such case.

64   SICKLE CELL AND BLACK GENOCIDE

Wilbur Johnson and Mae Sanford, both black, had met while working on a community action project in a large Eastern city. After going together for a year, they decided to get married and have a family.

When they appeared for the premarital blood test, which their state required for venereal diseases, they discovered that the state also required black marriage license applicants to be tested for the carrier state or "trait" of sickle cell disease. The disease itself is an inherited abnormality in the structure of hemoglobin, which at a minimum almost always severely handicaps its victims, and kills half of them before the age of 20. It is an autosomal recessive; that is, both parents must be carriers (heterozygotes) before there is a risk of producing children with the disease (homozygotes). When both parents are carriers, the risk of bearing such a child is 25 percent with each pregnancy. Carriers themselves are almost symptomless and have no idea of their status unless they are screened.

Mr. Johnson's younger brother had died in adolescence from the disease, after many painful and debilitating attacks. He thus knew something about it, including the fact that there was a good possibility that he himself was a carrier. Since both his parents were carriers, there was a 50 percent chance that each of their children would be one. Mr. Johnson also knew that the trait is fairly common among black Americans, about one in twelve of them being a carrier, so that there was a good chance his fiancée was a carrier too.

There is currently no widely available, low-risk prenatal diagnosis for sickle cell disease, and although treatments are available, they are not satisfactory enough to make possible a near-normal life for most victims. Thus, two prospective parents who know they both are carriers have only three options: they can risk a 25 percent chance of having a child with the disease itself with each pregnancy, living with the attendant anxiety; they can resort to artificial insemination with a noncarrier donor; or they can forgo childbearing altogether, perhaps adopting if the short supply of adoptable babies permits.

Mr. Johnson found each of these alternatives infuriatingly unacceptable. He argued that the compulsory premarital screening of blacks for the sickle cell trait, which is not a clinical condition and about which nothing can be done, was just another government attempt to cripple black reproductive capability. In the context of black history, he viewed it as an attempt by white society to control his fecundity in the beneficent guise of providing free medical information. Since he could do nothing with the information except undergo great anxiety or refrain from fathering children, he charged that the law was simply camouflaged genocide. He was particularly annoyed that while the state rushed in to mandate compulsory screening—screening which might suggest that blacks should have no children—it paid no attention to the need for counseling connected with that screening which would help those identified as having a sickle cell trait to understand their situation and the alternatives for having children.

Ms. Sanford did not feel so strongly, but she agreed that there was a danger whenever the state singled out black citizens as targets for a compulsory medical program. She decided that she wanted to oppose the test too.

The social and ethical problems of mass genetic screening have been explored by the Genetics Research Group of the Institute of Society, Ethics and the Life Sciences, which proposes eleven principles for the design and operation of screening programs:

1. Attainable Purpose. Purposes should be articulated before the program is undertaken.
2. Community Participation. From the outset, program planners should involve the community affected by screening in the formulation, design, and objectives of the program and in its administration, actual operation, and review of results.
3. Equal Access to Facilities. Information facilities related to the program should be available to all, though priority should be

given to populations which are well defined and in which there is known to be a greater frequency of the occurrence of genetic defects.

4. Adequate Testing Procedures. Tests for autosomal recessive conditions, for example, should include tests to distinguish persons carrying the trait from those who have two of the variant genes and will thus have the disease.

5. Absence of Compulsion. The screening program should have no policies that impose constraints on childbearing or stigmatize those who still desire to have their own children. Screening programs should be conducted on a voluntary basis.

6. Informed Consent. It should be the obligation of the program director to obtain signed consent documents from those tested or from their legal representative in order to assure knowledgeable consent, to design and implement proper information procedures, and to review the consent procedures for effectiveness. The recommended guidelines for consent are suggested by the Department of Health, Education, and Welfare (HEW).

7. Protection of Subjects. Screening ought to be considered a form of human experimentation. Since it carries a risk of possible psychological or social injury, programs should follow the HEW guidelines for such studies.

8. Access to Information. Those who are to implement a program should fully and clearly disclose to the community, and to all persons being screened, the policies on informing those screened of the results of the tests performed on them.

9. Provision of Counseling. Well-trained genetic counselors should be readily available. As a general rule, counseling should be nondirective, with the emphasis on informing the client and not making decisions for him.

10. Understandable Relation to Therapy. Before the testing begins, all persons being screened should be informed about the nature and cost of the available therapies or maintenance programs and should be given a description of their benefits and risks.

11. Right of Privacy. The screening program should have a policy of informing only the person to be screened, or with his permission, a designated physician or medical facility, and records should be kept in code.[4]

These principles have been criticized from two quarters. The Subsection on Heterozygous Carriers of the Task Force on Genetics and Reproduction at Yale University disagrees with the opposition to compulsory screening. They give as an example PKU screening, in which early detection of this metabolic disease in infants permits them to be placed on a diet excluding phenylalanine, the protein constituent responsible for the mental retardation in such cases. Although this argument based on possible diet control is not directly applicable to the screening program for sickle cell in adults, it suggests a principle whereby mass genetic screening might be mandatory. If there were a safe, simple, and sure diagnosis of a genetic condition which, if identified, could be counteracted by a safe, simple, and sure treatment, it might be reasonable to make screening mandatory in cases where the potential patient is not capable of consenting or refusing consent. This is close to the condition in PKU, where the infant obviously cannot give or refuse consent. The PKU diagnosis has been known to be made in error, however, and the dietary treatment is not all that simple; at least, it is considered by many to be a very bland diet. That the Yale group would accept such reasoning is suggested by their application to screening of parents in cases where knowledge that the parents are carriers might lead to diagnosis and treatment of a pre- or postnatal infant. They argue: "As we approach a period when in utero therapy may prevent or minimize the effects of a genetic disease, we suggest that a diseased fetus has the right to optimal therapy. This will often necessitate screening of the parents." Parental screening for sickle cell can currently alert medical personnel to the need to monitor a newborn infant when both parents are carriers. Potentially, it could be useful for the in utero detection and treatment of sickle cell disease.[5]

The other criticism of the proposed principles comes from precisely the opposite direction. James E. Bowman of the University of Chicago criticizes them for failing explicitly to condemn compulsory mass genetic screening programs, including the sickle cell screening of school children in Virginia and the District of Columbia and of marriage applicants in Virginia. Bowman argues that the next step will be to legislate mandatory amniocentesis for mothers whose embryos or fetuses are at risk for sickle cell disease. He also attacks the Virginia marriage application law on grounds of cruelty, "for the decision has then already been made to marry." He maintains that social reform programs, such as reducing the high rates of maternal and infant mortality or malnutrition in ghettoes, ought to have a higher priority.[6]

Since compulsory sickle cell screening laws do not imply compulsory in utero testing, which at present is not generally feasible, and since they certainly do not imply compulsory abortion, the question remains what good is served by requiring the screening in those couples who actively resist the screening. The responsibility to make informed parental decisions does not necessarily justify a compulsory information supplying program.

Prenatal and Genetic Experimentation

The work in genetics and other prenatal manipulation that commands the biggest headlines is far more futuristic than counseling or screening.

It is the experimentation on new techniques to intervene in the process of procreation and birth. The techniques include genetic interventions, such as cloning, or creation of an exact genetic copy of a human, and efforts to change the human genetic code in order to correct for an error. They also include attempts at extracorporeal or in vitro fertilization of a human egg (the test-tube baby), research on living human fetuses, and artificial insemination. Many issues are raised by these innovations. Perhaps the most significant is how they affect the understanding of human nature and of man's capacity to manipulate human nature in order to improve on nature's lottery.

65   THE INNOCENT CASE FOR THE CLONE

Charles and Doris Schmidt were both 23 years old when they had Johnny, an adorable, healthy, apparently bright child who rapidly became the center of their joyous marriage. They had feared that they would not be able to have children of their own since Mrs. Schmidt's mother had an unusually structured uterus, an anomaly that the daughter inherited. Following her birth, her parents had been unable to have additional children of their own. They finally adopted a boy six years younger. The boy had created problems for the family, doing poorly in school and having several scrapes with the law. He had not been heard from since he left home at age fourteen.

Charles and Doris Schmidt were thus overjoyed at the birth of Johnny. Doris had feared having a girl, who might inherit the abnormal uterine structure. They now had the child they wanted. Since they were also concerned about the possible danger of a second pregnancy, Mrs. Schmidt had a tubal ligation at the time of Johnny's birth.

A year-and-a-half later tragedy struck. Johnny wandered between two parked cars and was critically injured when a neighbor backed the car into him. Rushed to the hospital, he was given only a slim chance of recovery from major head injuries. Soon it was determined through neurological consultation that there was complete and irreversible destruction of the brain measured according to the Harvard Criteria for irreversible coma. Johhny was being maintained on a respirator, which might support him, the parents were told, for several months at the most. There was no hope of recovery or even of regaining consciousness.

The Schmidts were horror-stricken. Johnny had been their greatest joy. Mrs. Schmidt was now sterilized and dreaded lest, if an effort were made surgically to reconstruct the tubes connecting the ovaries to the uterus so that she might conceive again, she would pass on the abnormal uterine structure to a girl. The bitter memories of her parents' experience with adoption led them to conclude that they would never be able to handle the adoption process. Yet they desperately wanted another child. What they really wanted was another Johnny.

That same week they read in the Sunday supplement of the newspaper that work was being done on the cloning of higher animals. Cloning is a process of asexual reproduction, in which the genetic material from one animal is transferred to another by implanting the nucleus from a cell of that animal into an egg cell whose own genetic material has been removed or destroyed. The egg cell is then implanted in a host mother for the period of fetal development. The new individual is genetically identical to the one from which the cell nucleus was taken. The Schmidts read that cloning had been accomplished in lower animals, including the frog and toad, and that scientists were speculating about the possibility of replicating the cloning procedure in humans. They realized that Mrs. Schmidt could volunteer to supply the egg cell and carry the newly created embryo to term. The Schmidts returned to their doctor to ask, "Can't we give Johnny another chance?"

66 THE TEST-TUBE BABY

John E. Del Zio and Doris Del Zio were married on December 22, 1968; it was a second marriage for each. For a number of years thereafter, they tried determinedly but without success to have a child. Physicians were consulted often and at great cost; a variety of techniques were attempted. Mrs. Del Zio's physician performed a hysterosalpingogram, revealing that her fallopian tubes were blocked, preventing pregnancy.

The couple were referred to Dr. William J. Sweeney, who proposed an in vitro fertilization procedure. Ovarian tissue and the fluid from the follicles of the woman's ovaries would be removed by a surgical procedure known as laparotomy. A sterile culture of the fluid and ovarian matter, presumably including egg cells to be fertilized, would then be combined with semen from the woman's husband and incubated. The culture was to remain for four days so that if fertilization took place, the cell divisions could occur until a blastocyst emerged, after which it would be implanted in the uterus in the hope that the pregnancy would proceed normally. Dr. Sweeney reportedly detailed the hazards and expenses of the procedure, while warning the couple that up to that date no successful human transplant was known. They accepted the risks.

The laparotomy was performed. Mrs. Del Zio returned from the operating room in good condition, and the sterile culture tube was prepared by Dr. Landrum Shettles, the physician called in to aid Dr. Sweeney in the fertilization.

On the following day, Dr. Shettles was summoned by Dr. Raymond Vande Wiele, his superior at the hospital. The tube containing the possibly fertilized in vitro culture lay on his desk; the stopper had been removed, destroying its sterile condition and rendering the entire operation useless.

Mr. and Mrs. Del Zio claimed that Dr. Vande Wiele had said he destroyed the culture in compliance with a proscription against in vitro fertilization by the National Institutes of Health. Inquiry was subsequently made of the institute, which reported that no such proscription existed, either by law or by official institute policy.[7]

67   CHANGING MAN'S GENETIC CODE

Ulrike and Marie Steinhegger, aged 5 years and 18 months respectively, suffered from hyperargininemia, a hereditary deficiency of the enzyme arginase. Arginase deficiency leads to high concentrations of arginine in the blood and cerebrospinal fluid, which in Ulrike's case was already associated with severe mental retardation, and Marie seemed to be developing the same mental retardation symptoms. These two children were apparently the first reported cases of hyperargininemia. There was thus no accepted method of treating their genetic disease.

The pediatrician in charge of caring for the girls was approached by an expert who proposed a novel treatment for their condition. He suggested trying to correct the hereditary defect at the genetic level by injecting Shope papilloma virus into the children. Earlier a scientist had discovered that the Shope papilloma virus infection of rabbit skin stimulated the synthesis of arginase, and the resulting arginase had some properties that were different from the normal enzyme of rabbit liver, suggesting it might come from a new source. When the scientist first reported these experiments in 1963, he postulated that the viral DNA carried a gene for a viral arginase different from the cellular enzyme. Since that time the scientist had observed that about 35 percent of the laboratory workers tested, who had worked with and thus been exposed to Shope papilloma virus, exhibited lower serum arginine contents than control hospital patients who had not knowingly been exposed to the virus. Thus, the scientist argued, there was some ground for believing that the inadvertent Shope papilloma virus infection of humans could lower serum arginine levels without apparent harmful effects, since the laboratory workers with the low serum arginine levels showed no overt signs of disease.

The children's pediatrician learned, however, that the interpretation that Shope papilloma virus codes for viral arginase had been seriously questioned as a result of more recent experiments by other scientists, which made it appear likely that virus infection merely stimulated the production of a cellular arginase. Whether the arginase was derived from viral or cellular genes was important to the rationale of the treatment. If virus infection induced the synthesis of cellular arginase, then infecting the girls, who were deficient in the genes responsible for production of that cellular arginase, with Shope papilloma virus might not have any possibility of correcting their condition. In addition, although Shope papilloma virus had no known harmful effects on humans, tests to establish the safety of large doses had not been carried out.

The unhappy parents of Ulrike and Marie Steinhegger were pressing the pediatrician to tell them whether anything could be done to help their children.[8]

68   THE HUMAN FETUS AS RESEARCH MATERIAL

The government's Committee on Biological Research Review examined all research proposals submitted for funding by government grants and contracts. This day's meeting was devoted to examining one specific proposal that came from the world-famous Institute of Embryology at a prestigious university teaching hospital. No one on the committee doubted the scientific merit of the proposed research or the ability of the research team that would undertake this major study. Their doubts were fundamentally ethical.

The Institute of Embryology had long been concerned with the plight of women who were prone to spontaneous abortions. They had pioneered in the development of acute care facilities for premature newborns. Now they were eager to develop techniques that would permit the salvaging of previable and marginally viable fetuses in the 300- to 1200-gram range. The research proposed for review and funding was to develop an artificial placenta. Fetuses would be obtained from pregnant women who were aborted voluntarily by hysterotomy under the country's uniform abortion statute, which permitted abortion up to the twenty-fourth week of gestation. The fetuses would then be transferred to the institute's research facilities. The technique would involve cannulation of the internal iliac vessels, that is, placing a small tube in them, permitting total perfusion of the fetus/infant.

It was recognized that success would be limited during the early stages of the research. The research team anticipated maintenance of the vital signs of the fetuses for periods of no more than a few hours. It was hoped, however, especially with fetuses in the 1000-gram range, that survival time would gradually increase as the technique was perfected. For this phase of the research it was decided that because of possible fetal damage during the critical period of transfer to the artificial placenta, no fetus would be maintained for more than a two-week period. Fetuses would be obtained from the obstetrical services of the six hospitals in the immediate vicinity. Adequate compensation would be made to the hospitals supplying the fetuses to cover expenses, including supplies and staff time necessary for maintenance of the fetus prior to the time it was delivered to the embryology clinic.

Two commentators have disagreed over the ethical acceptability of the research in this case. Robert Morison, a physician who was formerly chairman of the Division of Biological Sciences at Cornell University and is presently a visiting professor at Massachusetts Institute of Technology, defends the research:

> The Committee should have no particular ethical difficulty with this proposal. In the first place, it may be viewed simply as an extension to an earlier stage of the work already successfully accomplished on prematurely born infants. There is, of course, one significant difference. In the earlier cases, the parents of the experimental subjects usually hoped for their survival. In the present proposal, the experimental subjects would be fetuses whose prospective parents will have specifically renounced the responsibility of parenthood.
>
> How does this alter the ethical situation? As a first approximation, it would appear to simplify rather than complicate it since the prior decision to allow an abortion would, in almost all instances, have been based on a prior finding that the right to life of the fetus was outweighed by other considerations. Any further threat implied by the proposed experimental procedure would appear to be trivial in comparison.
>
> Those who follow the thinking of the Supreme Court may also point out that, if a nonviable fetus has not yet reached the compelling point for protection against a clear threat to its life, there should be much less hesitation about exposing it to the minor inconvenience of the proposed experimental procedure.
>
> Those who are nevertheless driven to recognize the fetus as a person would ordinarily base the decision to abort on some weighing of the rights of mother and fetus. In such cases, as long as the fetus survives, it would appear to have the status of a minor child. The matter might then be handled by asking the parents' permission for the experimental procedure in the usual way. Alternatively, in order to avoid ambiguities, such cases might simply be omitted from the series. Once these theoretical matters are out of the way, it may be pointed out in supplemental defense of the proposed experiments that they seem to conform with the principles set down in Nuremberg and Helsinki. The probable harm to the fetus is clearly outweighed by the enormous gain to future generations of parents who may have tried repeatedly to bear a living infant, only to have their hopes dashed by spontaneous abortion. It is clearly stipulated that the auspices under which the research is to be carried out are of the first class, and the experimental design leaves nothing to be desired.

A new and serious problem will, of course, arise as the experiments approach success. The proposal recognizes this in providing for the termination of an experiment on any given fetus prior to the period of normal viability. It would clearly be unethical to employ extraordinary means actually to bring into the world of the living an infant whose parents had already rejected it. In other words, as soon as the experiments give promise of imminent success, they should be limited to those spontaneously aborted fetuses that the parents wish to bring to maturity.

Enthusiastic advocates of abortion might oppose the proposed experiment on the grounds that, by pushing back the moment of viability, the development of a successful treatment would progressively shorten the period during which abortions may be regarded as permissible. I find it simply offensive to oppose the experiments on these grounds. Instead, one may be allowed to hope that in countries advanced enough to provide successful treatment for early stages of prematurity the people would be sophisticated enough to have their ordinary abortions before the fourth month.[9]

Sumner B. Twiss, a professor of religion at Brown University, argues on the contrary that the research is unethical on several grounds:

I shall contend that the research proposal *as stated* raises far too many objections to be appraised as morally justifiable. In order to elucidate some of the significant moral issues I will examine three aspects of the research proposal: 1) the background of the research design, 2) the design of the proposed research, and 3) the objectives of the research proposal.

1) Background of the Research Design
According to a growing consensus on canons regulating medical experimentation, it is necessary to engage in what has been called "the animal work" before going on to engage in "the human work." Since the research proposal omits all reference to this stage of research and talks only about developing an artificial placenta by experimenting on human fetuses exclusively, I must assume that it contravenes this rule of medical experimentation, whether by negligence or deliberate intent I do not know.

2) Design of the Proposed Research
The research, as proposed, raises at least three areas of moral concern: the consent of the research subject, the disposal of the fetuses, and the dilemmatic situation produced by successful completion of the research.

(a) Consent: The question of who, if anyone, should consent to the proposed experimentation is difficult to answer. Is it the woman who voluntarily aborts the fetus? Or is it the fetus itself? It should be noted that the proposed medical intervention at least indirectly interferes with the presumed desires and decisions of women to have their fetuses killed. Although the decision to have an abortion may be construed as a disavowal of any responsibility for the fetus after abortion, the practice of abortion seems to presuppose fulfillment of the decision for feticide. Because of the proposed medical interference with this decision, the women's informed consent for the short-term maintenance and experimental use of their fetuses should be obtained. The women may well be construed as experimental research subjects undergoing a medical procedure for the sake of medical research.

However, the issue of consent to medical experimentation does not end here. While informed consent would relieve the researchers from the allegation of illicitly manipulating the desires of unsuspecting and unconsenting human research subjects, obtaining this consent may not release them from the charge of complicity in the women's willingness to be presumptuous with their fetuses. It can be argued that the fetuses are research subjects—not volunteers. To construe the fetuses' informed consent to the proposed research, to consent on their behalf that they be exposed to the risks of experimentation would not be so much absurd as manifestly immoral. Considering the hypothetical case of bringing such a fetus to term *as a person* possibly suffering deleterious consequences of those experimental risks may help to elucidate the point and logic behind my objection here. I contend that by the canons of medical experimentation, the researchers cannot give such proxy consent for the fetuses *as research subjects*. The logic behind this particular objection for denying the legitimacy of proxy consent does not presuppose or imply the position that the fetus is a human person before being brought to term, although it does argue that the fetus should be regarded as a research subject, particularly when the possibility of longer periods of fetal experimentation is taken into account.

(b) Disposing of fetuses: The matter of disposing of the fetuses after short-term maintenance and experimentation raises some difficult issues. On the view that distinctly human life begins at some time before disposal, the research proposal is obviously vulnerable to the charge that it incorporates an inherently immoral practice. Since the fetuses presumably may be obtained up to the 24th week of pregnancy, a two week experiment would permit life maintenance up to as late as 26 weeks, beyond the time abortion is permitted in the country, and very late for denying distinctly human life.

I would like, however, to probe the practice of disposal more subtly, suggesting problems which may arise regardless of whether the fetus is viewed as human life. Disposal is justified by the research proposal on the grounds that experimentation may cause fetal damage so deleterious that in the judgment of the researchers the fetus ought not to be maintained for more than a short period of time, much less be brought to term. Regardless of whether the fetus is human life it is a research subject who did not consent to the possibly damaging experimentation performed upon it. So, by means of the practice of disposal, it may appear that the researchers are trying to rectify one moral wrong by performing another.

(c) Moral Risks with Success: As gradually improving techniques permit fetal growth to later and more mature stages, then the issue of disposal will be met head-on in the form of the following presently unresolved questions: When do fetuses acquire the status of protectable humanity? When they can be brought to term possibly without damage, what will be the grounds for disposal then? Will the original abortive decisions of their biological mothers be invoked to justify disposal, or should the fetuses be viewed as coming under the aegis of "protectable humanity"? If brought to term, will they finally be admitted into the human community or will they still be considered material appropriate for further experimentation? Who will take responsiblity for their personal and social nurture?

Careful consideration of the later phases of the research design raises the broad question of whether the researchers can ever morally get to know how to perfect the artificial placenta. One view argues that unless the possibility of fetal damage caused by the experimental techniques can be definitely excluded, the research, when viewed in its later phases, is immoral. A second view is that the researchers should be expected only to assess whether the risks accruing from the use of the artificial placenta are at an acceptable level, e.g., roughly equivalent to the risks of a natural pregnancy and birth. In the final analysis any decision must consider the objectives, and not only the internal design, of the research proposal. If the goals of the research are thereapeutic, then the second position may seem more plausible. While if the goals are demonstrably non-therapeutic, particularly for the fetuses being experimented upon, then the first position may pose a conclusive objection.

3) Objectives of the Research Proposal

The stated objective of the research proposal is to aid the plight of those women prone to spontaneous abortion. On the fact of it, this counts as a therapeutic objective. Some would maintain that an important line must be drawn between remedial therapy for a medical condition, on the one hand, and "doctoring" or satisfying desires by biomedical technology, on the other. And they would conclude that medical practice and research should be devoted to the former only. Others would consider acute psychological suffering to justify therapy. I think that the present situation is ambiguous enough that the objective of the research proposal may be legitimately construed as therapeutic, and even if this contention is misguided the beneficiaries of the perfected artificial placenta will include the spontaneously aborted fetuses.

Can the researchers morally get to know how to perfect the artificial placenta under the proposed research design? I contend that the experimental design of the research proposal is, on the whole, *not* morally justifiable, despite its praiseworthy therapeutic goals. It does not propose to experiment for therapeutic purposes directly on spontaneously aborted fetuses; rather it proposes to submit other voluntarily aborted fetuses to hazardous procedures not therapeutic for them.

However, I think that research along these lines should be encouraged and could be redesigned so as to avoid many, if not all, of my objections. Here are just a few suggestions: 1) do all the necessary "animal work" first; 2) obtain fetuses only from those women who spontaneously abort them and are willing to consent to "therapeutic experimentation"; 3) develop a discriminate disposal policy based on the welfare of the fetuses being therapeutically experimented upon; 4) hew to all the relevant canons for medical experimentation; etc. With these and similar modifications, I suspect that a good (moral) case could be argued for researching and developing an artificial placenta. It is most unfortunate that the world famous Institute of Embryology was so short-sighted. With careful planning it would have saved itself (and me) a lot of trouble. As things stand now, it may have lost some of its prestige.[10]

69   ARTIFICIAL INSEMINATION FROM A FATHER-IN-LAW

A woman in her early thirties made an appointment relating to the fact that she and her husband were childless. During the meeting, the following story unfolded: The woman's husband was sterile and insisted that they use his father's semen for artificial insemination. The father-in-law had indicated that he would not recognize a child who was artificially produced as his legitimate heir unless the couple agreed to use his semen. While the woman admired her father-in-law and did not object to the procedure since the insemination would be artificial, she had some reservations. Nevertheless, she asked if the adviser could give her a go-ahead and blessing.

The five previous cases raise a number of questions relating to the new biomedical capacities for intervention in the processes of procreation and formation of human life itself. Our understanding of human nature will determine whether such interventions are an appropriate part of the human character, yet that nature is itself part of what is being manipulated.

The first question asks whether these techniques are compatible with the nature of the human character. Debate rages about the ethics of nontherapeutic experimental manipulation of living fetuses following planned abortions. In 1974 a temporary moratorium was declared on any such research while society came to a clearer understanding of its justification and learned to distinguish ethical from unethical manipulations. The same question is raised in the Del Zios' decision to create life in a test tube and in the Schmidts' decision to clone a genetic replication of Johnny. Even traditional artificial insemination can raise this problem.

Research is in part defended because of the aggregate good that can come from the knowledge potentially to be gained. Some would say that experimental manipulation even of human embryos is acceptable provided it serves a worthwhile purpose and the good to be gained outweighs the harm, moral or otherwise. Of course, making such a calculation requires an assessment of both the value of the knowledge, including the purposes to which it might be put, and the risks, especially the moral risks, in manipulating human embryos.

Another approach would be to abandon the balancing of social goods and harms. Some would say that the purposeful manipulation of human sperm and egg or of human genetic material is just not a suitable behavior for fallible human beings. It is playing God. The counterargument might be that humans have the right, even the obligation, to use their intelligence to improve the human condition. The question really boils down to choosing among the four possible definitions of the nature of the human species.

First, the traditional name that humans have given to themselves, *Homo sapiens,* suggests that the human essence is the possession of a capacity to think. The human is a thinking being, a possessor of wisdom. This might imply that it is part of the human character to think out new solutions to human suffering, and that genetic and other prenatal interventions are therefore acceptable. Yet the human is also a fallible creature. Thinking rationally might lead to the conclusion that there are some areas beyond human capability, and that the wise among us should leave them alone. The view of the human as a thinking animal creates other problems. It ignores the social nature of the species. As Aristotle remarked, the human is a political as well as a thinking animal. It also ignores those who are not thinkers or are not wise. The view of the human as a thinking animal raises special difficulties in the area of genetics and prenatal experimenting. If the human is a thinking animal and sperm and egg cells, embryos, and fetuses do not think, are they essentially nonhuman or prehuman? If so, does this justify genetic and prenatal manipulation to suit the tastes of researchers and potential parents? Can the same implication be drawn for infants and the senile?

A second definition of human character views it in terms of *Homo faber,* or man the maker.[11] This is the view that unabashedly affirms technological interventions. According to it, the human character is essentially manipulative, in the neutral sense of the term. Humans at their best use their rational capacities to reorganize their lives and their environment to improve on fate. Robert Sinsheimer, for instance, affirms the increasing capacity to make the world anew.[12] And Joseph Fletcher maintains: "It is of the nature of man that he is not helplessly subject to the blind workings of physical or physiological nature . . . Invincible ignorance and total helplessness are the antithesis of humanness, and to the degree that a man lacks control he is not responsible, and to be irresponsible to be subpersonal."[13] Addressing himself specifically to the possibility of in vitro fertilization, Fletcher argues: "men are character-ized by technique, and for a human being to oppose technology is 'self-hatred.' A 'test-tube baby,' for example, although conceived and ges-tated *ex corpo,* would nonetheless be humanly reproduced and of human value. A baby made artificially by deliberate and careful contrivance would be more *human* than one resulting from sexual roulette—the reproductive mode of the subhuman species."[14]

There are Biblical foundations for the claim that this is a particularly Judeo-Christian understanding of human nature. When humans were created, according to the creation story, they were created in the image of God. They were told to have dominion over the earth and to subdue it. They are co-creator with God of their own environment and destiny. To fail to be responsible for the improvement of the human condition is to fail in one's ultimate responsibility as a human.

A third definition regards the human as *Homo servus* or man the servant. Lynn White argues that the Judeo-Christian view of the human as maker has created problems, one of them being the current ecological crisis, and has thus given rise to this counter-interpretation of the human essence.[15] In theological terms, the human is not a co-creator but a crea-ture created by God for his own purposes. The human is a servant, a custodian, and a caretaker. The Biblical metaphors show the human as the keeper of the talents or the shepherd watching over the flock. Ser-vant, as well as maker, is another dominant image of the Judeo-Christian tradition.

Lewis Mumford challenges the *Homo faber* image in favor of an image of the human in the "minding" role. Leon Kass joins in the criticism by questioning the new techniques for "making" babies:

A new image of human procreation has been conceived, and a "scien-tific" obstetrics will usher it into existence. As one obstetrician put it at a recent conference: "The business of obstetrics is to produce optimum babies." The price to be paid for the optimum baby is the transfer of procreation from the home to the laboratory, and its coincident trans-formation into manufacture. Increasing control over the product is purchased by the increasing depersonalization of the process . . . The complete depersonalization of procreation (possible with the develop-ment of an artificial placenta), and its surrender to the demands of the calculating will, shall be in itself seriously dehumanizing no matter how "optimum" the product.[16]

There is still another image of human nature, which avoids the reduc-tion of the human to a thinking being and at the same time avoids the extremes of making the human either completely master or completely servant. This fourth image is *Homo ludens,* man the player. The term comes from Johan Huizinga, who saw an analogy between the human's role in life and the human's role in playing a game.[17] As player, the human is both the maker and the follower of the rules, simultaneously creator and creature. A similar image is developed by Harvey Cox in *Feast of Fools*.[18] Humans must realize that they are the product of a long biological, social, cultural, and ethical evolution. If they are to remain human, they must play by some rules of social interaction. The world is not theirs to dominate for their own petty satisfactions. Yet they are also responsible agents who, as both social and thinking beings, have the power and the responsibility to change the rules—to change human nature itself. This blending of *Homo sapiens, Homo faber,* and *Homo servus* suggests another basis for debating the social and ethical basis for genetic and other prenatal interventions. The acceptability of such interventions would depend on more specific evaluations of exactly what is proposed.

If the new biomedical procedures in the five cases are found to be ethical, the next question raised is, Where will they lead? It could be that a new embryo itself has no ethical claims or has insufficient claims to make the research unacceptable, but that there is some obligation to anticipate future stages of research and later clinical applications. Cloning a frog may lead to attempts to clone human embryos—strictly for research purposes. At this point there may be no intention of raising the clone to postnatal life. But then the Schmidts' problem may arise, seeming to be an innocent case justifying the first clinical attempt, and this in turn can lead to another apparently innocent attempt. Once the technique is published and generally available, it may be used for less and less innocent purposes, including the mass production of "carbon copies" of individuals with the desired characteristics, such as ideal soldiers, maintenance crews, movie stars, or intellectuals. This is sometimes called the wedge or slippery slope argument. At issue is the extent to which researchers doing basic work on cloning, in vitro fertilization, or genetic engineering, as well as those charged by society with the responsibility of approving or disapproving such research, have an obligation to take into account the reasonably foreseeable uses of their scientific work.

Another question raised by these five cases is whether there is proper consent for the use of human tissues. Purely research manipulations of human tissues in cloning, in vitro fertilization, and genetic engineering necessitate the use of human tissues. As such, free and informed consent of the tissue donors is required. Many women before Mrs. Del Zio were asked to donate human egg cells in order to study the technique of in vitro fertilization, though it was never intended to let the newly created embryos go to term even if such a technique were to become available. Charges have been made that some of these women were falsely led to believe that they themselves would benefit. They might have been given the unrealistic hope that they would be able to have children if they cooperated.

Still another question posed by these five cases is, must there be potential benefit to the embryo, fetus, or infant? Consent, of course, means consent of the tissue donor or, in the case of the clinical application of the techniques presented in the cases, consent of the present or potential parents. The consent, however, of the direct subject of the intervention—the embryo, the fetus, or the infant— is obviously impossible, although consent is normally required for the experimental use of human beings. One solution to the problem is that the embryo or fetus, and more clearly the sperm and egg cells, are not included in the rules about getting consent, because for moral purposes they are not sufficiently like postnatal humans to have any rights about giving consent. That would not seem to be a good argument, however, in the case of a child who might have a defective gene.

Another answer would compare the embryo or fetus to children who are, without their informed consent, made subjects of medical research. Complex debates involve when, if ever, children can be used as experimental subjects without their consent. One critical distinction in the debate is whether the child potentially stands to benefit from the research. If the child is in need of medical treatment that would require testing of a new drug or a new surgical procedure, then for the child's own benefit the procedure is normally found acceptable, although often the parents' consent is required, possibly to assure that the intervention can be plausibly assumed really to benefit the child.

Applied to the five cases, this principle might justify the genetic engineering experiment on the two girls with hyperargininemia. Some who would normally oppose genetic change experiments as going beyond the limits of acceptable human action would make an exception when there is a possibility that the subject will directly benefit, especially, as in this case, where there is virtually no hope without the experiment. [19] In at least three of the other four cases, however, there is no real subject who could benefit. The purpose of the experimental procedure is to attempt to create a new human life. This is the case in the attempt to clone, to create the conception *ex corpo,* or to perform the artificial insemination. The experimentation on the fetus is a bit more complicated. Potentially one could conduct such experiments for the purpose of attempting to save accidentally premature babies. The specific research proposed, however, is to use purposely aborted fetuses. There is no real intention to save any particular life; the object is rather to develop the technique for future life-saving. In fact, the protocol calls for stopping before life can continue outside the womb.

The principle that experimenting without consent is acceptable only when there is a potential benefit for the specific subject would thus rule out all four of these experiments. It also has the paradoxical implication that the fetal research to develop the artificial placenta would be acceptable on purposely aborted babies, but not on spontaneously aborted ones. Yet the purposely aborted ones were chosen in order to avoid the risk of having to continue treatment that might lead to a damaged but viable life in the case of the still desired babies. The decision of the mother to abort must therefore end any right to continued treatment once the fetus is out of the womb, while the mother's desire for the infant precludes the experimental treatment.

The question remains whether a decision can be made to put a human or a future human at risk when there is no potential benefit to that present or future person. Specifically, the problem is whether experimental conceptions can be attempted to benefit the parents while putting the otherwise nonexistent child at risk. One simple answer is no. Another answer is that the benefit to others—the parents, future children, or society in general—can always justify risk to the one who cannot consent, as long as the benefits are great enough. An intermediate position might be that they can be justified only when in general those to be conceived in the future are likely to be better off than they would have been without the research. Thus, if it were known that a future group of children were at risk because a present group of women with a gynecological malformation were likely to continue having children, this might justify an experimental attempt to find a potentially safer method of conception and gestation. Finally, one might want to justify risks to present and future offspring without any specific argument that they or other future children would benefit, and still place limits on the level of risk. For instance, in vitro fertilization risks might be acceptable so long as they do not exceed the level of risk normally undertaken in a "natural" pregnancy.[20] This argument implies that natural risks and experimentally induced risks are interchangeable, that as long as the level of risk is the same, it does not matter whether the risk occurs naturally or is man-made. However, not only the likelihood of the risk alone but also the seriousness of the risk is a relevant factor. Thus, any debate about the risk incidence rate without consideration of the nature of the risk is out of place. The problem is to decide when, if ever, risk can be justified, especially when it is not for the potential benefit of an existing embryo, fetus, or child.

The final question raised by these five cases is, What priority for funds should these techniques get? The in vitro fertilization procedure requires the services of a large team of physicians, nurses, and other professional hospital personnel. So does the artificial placenta research. The clone, which is not yet at the point of human experimentation, would also. At some point the question must be asked how these experiments compare in funding priority with basic health care for embryos, fetuses, and children. The costs in money and medical personnel for one in vitro fertilization, including the diagnostic, surgical, preimplantation, and in utero support, are enough to deliver primary health care to many normal pregnant women and children. Even if the procedures in these five cases were found acceptable in terms of the previous questions raised, they would still have to meet this test. The era of genetic and prenatal experiments is probably just beginning. It is crucial that these questions be faced long before the day when the immediate clinical decisions have to be made.

CHAPTER 9

Transplantation, Hemodialysis, and the Allocation of Scarce Resources

When on December 3, 1967, Louis Washkansky volunteered to subject himself to the scalpel of Christiaan Barnard, he ushered in what might be called the era of transplantation. The first beat of Denise Darvall's heart inside Washkansky's chest was heard around the world. The moral trauma is one from which people are still recovering. The moral impact of that first heart transplant may be in areas far distant from and more significant than the mere replacement of the human pump of life. The most profound writers on the ethics of transplantation have realized that with the heart far more is at stake, symbolically and culturally, than the mere replacement of machinery which circulates the blood. [1] No one, not even the most crusty, lab-oriented physician, can fail to see the moral revolution in tampering with such crucial human organs. The real impact of that first transplant may therefore be to challenge once and for all the notion that medicine is the value-free application of progress in the biological sciences of the human body, and to reveal that all clinical decisions in medicine incorporate value perspectives which are crucial to the decision-making process.

When organs—hearts or kidneys or livers—are transplanted, they are the scarce and invaluable resources that stand between imminent death and a thread of hope for life. The era of transplantation has thus highlighted another critical moral problem in medicine: the allocation of scarce resources when those resources mean life for some who shall receive them and death for others who shall not receive them. Hearts, kidneys, and hemodialysis machines have become the archetype of scarce medical resources in the public policy debates over what constitutes a just distribution of medical resources. It would be wrong, though, to assume that these are the only scarce medical resources. Others are physicians to serve the physicianless ill and health dollars to finance the inevitable national health insurance of the United States, which fall under the general heading of health care delivery.

Obtaining Organs

Many organs for transplantation are obtained from cadavers. Some traditions raise questions about the mutilation of the corpse for transplant purposes, but when a life can be saved by removing a cadaver heart or kidney, most would not object. Aside from the complex question of the definition of death—when it occurs and whether it may morally be hastened—the ethical issues are relatively minor. It is assumed that competent adults can freely consent to donate one of their paired organs, such as a kidney, to relatives whose organs have been destroyed by disease. Occasionally the question arises of the competent adult's right to donate an unpaired organ or both of the paired organs. Such a case arose when a mother who donated one kidney to a son with chronic kidney disease had a second son develop the same disease who also needed a transplant. Normally, however, the ethical questions arise when the competency of the person from whom the organ would be obtained is in question or absent, as with a mental retardate, a child, or a competent adult who is subject to coercion to consent.

70   THE MENTALLY RETARDED KIDNEY DONOR

Marvin MacLeod was 17 years old, but because of Down's syndrome or mongolism, he had the mental capacity of a 3- or 4-year-old. Otherwise he was healthy. His sister Susan, a 30-year-old divorcée, suffered from chronic nephritis and elevated blood pressure. Because of these, she had lost more than 90 percent of her kidney function, and death could occur within the next few months. She had only two means of surviving to her next birthday: hemodialysis or a kidney transplant. The transplant was preferable from her perspective, because with hemodialysis she would be attached to a kidney machine three times a week for six hours at a time.

Susan's medical condition was complex. There was evidence that she also had a condition known as systemic lupus erythematosus (SLE), a disease of the connective tissue, whose symptoms may include fever, weakness, joint pains or arthritis, and lesions of the skin and internal tissues. At present she could not be treated for SLE because of her hypertension. If there were a kidney transplant, however, the drugs used to counteract rejection of the transplanted kidney might also be helpful for SLE. But the presence of SLE would also increase the risk of damage to the new kidney.

Both MacLeod parents were tested and found unsuitable as kidney donors. Susan had four other adult brothers and sisters, the youngest 22 years old. All but one, who was away, were tested as donors and found to be less suitable than Marvin. The risk of rejection of a kidney from one of them within the next three to five years would be between 20 and 30 percent. A similar test of Marvin showed that the risk of rejecting his kidney would be only 4 or 5 percent.

All members of the family agreed that it would be best for Marvin to be the donor. The risk to him was considered minimal; insurance companies do not even increase the ratings of those with only one functioning kidney. The entire procedure was explained to Marvin, and he said he wanted to help his sister. A case was made that it was in Marvin's own interest for Susan to receive the kidney since his parents, now aged 63 and 56, would not be able to care for him indefinitely. Susan could take care of him after their deaths.

With the family and the transplant surgeon all agreed on this course of action, the hospital advised that a declaratory judgment should be obtained from the court authorizing the parents to consent to the kidney donation on Marvin's behalf. The judge determined that no case like this had ever arisen which could serve as a precedent.

71   THE CHILD AS A KIDNEY DONOR

Diane and Dione DeLeon were identical twins born eight years ago. Dione was now suffering from a progressively serious kidney disease, hemolytic uremic syndrome. On December 8, 1971, she began hemodialysis or kidney machine treatments along with other treatments. By February 1, 1972, her kidney was biopsied for a second time because of the onset of a malignant type of blood pressure elevation. The decision was made that the kidneys had to be removed.

Both Dione's parents volunteered to donate kidneys for transplant but were rejected because of a tissue incompatibility. No other related donors were available except Diane who, being an identical twin, would make the ideal donor. There is virtually no risk of failure for transplants from identical twins, but for transplants from an unrelated cadaver source, which is the only other possibility, the rejection risk after three years is estimated to be about 50 percent.

Mr. and Mrs. DeLeon were horrified at the decision they had to make. They agonized with the alternatives in a long counseling session with their minister. He thought that authorizing the transplant between the twin daughters was a morally sound decision. Pressured by knowledge that Dione's condition was deteriorating rapidly, the parents, together with the physicians, decided they should obtain a declaratory judgment from the court to authorize the donation.

The court appointed an independent guardian for Diane who, after spending a great deal of time talking with the child, concluded that she understood to the limits of her age and agreed with what was being asked of her. The guardian consented to the donation. A psychiatrist examined Diane and found that she had a strong identification with her sister and apparently desired to help her without having received undue pressure from the others in the family.

There had been previous cases involving minor identical twin donations, but these involved teenage minors who had a great deal more capacity to understand the procedure. There had also been a case involving a mentally retarded twin donor. He, however, was 28 years old and so utterly dependent on the brother needing the kidney that a strong case was made that he would benefit more by keeping his brother alive than by having the second kidney. In this case while some possible benefit to Diane was recognized, all agreed that it was not a major consideration. The problem facing the judge was whether to permit the parents to approve the transplant, which would be of immense benefit to the recipient, but of some risk and limited benefit to the donor, who was not herself competent to consent.

Kidney donation by a minor or a mentally incompetent raises many of the same issues as does the consent for medical treatment of those who cannot consent or experimentation that does not benefit the subject. These two cases raise several critical issues. First, should it be assumed that the organ donor candidate will not benefit, or can it be argued that the donors might reasonably benefit—Marvin MacLeod because his sister might care for him, and Diane DeLeon because of the psychological risk from damaging the close relation with her twin sister? In another legal case the possible harm to the donor brother was considered the critical factor in justifying the donation. Tommy Strunk, a 28-year-old employee of the Penn State Railroad and a part-time student at the University of Cincinnati, was suffering from a fatal kidney disease. He was being maintained on a kidney machine, but according to the physician's opinion, the treatment could not be continued much longer. Cadaver transplant was considered, but his 27-year-old brother Jerry had a highly compatible tissue match. Both parents and collateral relatives were ruled out as medically unacceptable. Jerry, however, had been committed to the Frankfort State Hospital and School, an institution maintained for the "feebleminded." He had an IQ of approximately thirty-five—the mental age of approximately six years. He could not communicate well with those not well acquainted with him, yet he was the ideal kidney donor.

The Department of Mental Health evaluated the case and made the following report:

Jerry Strunk, a mental defective, has emotions and reactions on a scale comparable to that of a normal person. He identifies with his brother Tom; Tom is his model, his tie with his family. Tom's life is vital to the continuity of Jerry's improvement at Frankfort State Hospital and School. The testimony of the hospital representative reflected the importance to Jerry of his visits with his family and the constant inquiries Jerry made about Tom's coming to see him. Jerry is aware he plays a role in the relief of this tension. We the Department of Mental Health must take all possible steps to prevent the occurrence of any guilt feelings Jerry would have if Tom were to die.

The necessity of Tom's life to Jerry's treatment and eventual rehabilitation is clearer in view of the fact that Tom is his only living sibling and at the death of their parents, now in their fifties, Jerry will have no concerned, intimate communication so necessary to his stability and optimal functioning. [2]

This case represents the extreme of the claim that the donor might benefit from the donation. Questions remain, however. Must there be a benefit to the donor to justify the transplant? Can a legitimate case be made for a donor benefit in the cases of Marvin MacLeod and Diane DeLeon? Would it be more honest to argue for the moral possibility of the donation authorization even without the grounds of donor benefit? If so, should such a decision be made simply by the parents, or should it be reviewed by some other authority, such as a court or a transplant review committee?

A second issue in these cases is the problematic consent of the donors themselves. What should their role be? Is it possible for them to give a meaningful, voluntary, and informed consent in any sense? In contrast with these cases, in the first twin transplant cases involving minors, the minors were teenagers—nineteen in one case and fourteen in two others. Can one rely on their consent for the procedure independent of the benefit to them? If so, what is the difference between their cases and the DeLeons', where the twins were eight years old, or the MacLeods', where the donor was older but mentally incapable of understanding? What should be the response, for instance, if the donor child of five or six says no to the operation even though the parents, psychiatric consultants, social workers, and courts all determine that the donor child does not comprehend his choice and will in the long run seriously regret it?

72   THE ADULT KIDNEY DONOR: CAN SHE CHOOSE FREELY?

Dr. Maxwell Firman was medical director of the Scheller Kidney Center, one of the most distinguished kidney research centers in the country. For some time he had been seeing Audrey Poland, a middle-aged woman, for chronic renal disease. She was almost to the point where some medical action would have to be taken. He had discussed both transplantation and dialysis with her many times. Mrs. Poland, like many patients in kidney failure, strongly preferred a transplant, not wanting to spend the rest of her life attached to a dialysis machine six hours a day, three days a week.

At the most recent visit, Mrs. Poland seemed happy and said that her sister, Ruth Hamill, had volunteered to donate a kidney to her. Dr. Firman explained to her again the importance of tissue typing in a sibling-to-sibling transplant; that is, if the typing is identical, the chance of a successful transplant is about 90 percent, but if the match is less close, the chance of success is less. Poor matches will have no greater chance than with a cadaver graft, or about 50 percent. In that case Dr. Firman would not recommend such a procedure. Mrs. Poland said that she would arrange for her sister to accompany her on her next visit and have the requisite tests performed.

The following day Dr. Firman received a telephone call from the potential donor's husband, who wanted urgently to see him that day. He arranged for an appointment. Mr. Hamill said that he understood that his sister-in-law had spoken to the doctor about Ruth being a kidney donor. Dr. Firman indicated that Mrs. Poland had said Mrs. Hamill was considering such a donation. Mr. Hamill replied that he was glad she had said "considering," because she certainly was nowhere close to making such a decision. Mr. Hamill thought that it would be the completely wrong decision to make. He explained to Dr. Firman the active life that his wife led, with several young children at home to take care of and a deep involvement in other activities, some of which were reaching a professional culmination for her. He described some medical problems that he thought might rule her out as a donor in any case. He vividly contrasted his wife's life style with that of the patient, who was sedentary owing to her chronic disease; and he saw no reason why his sister-in-law would not do well on chronic dialysis. Mr. Hamill said that his wife was deeply disturbed at the prospect of having to confront her sister with a decision not to donate a kidney for her.

Dr. Firman reassured the potential donor's husband that the medical team would do nothing against his wife's wishes in terms of her decision to donate or not to donate, and that if her decision was not to donate, they would make every effort to explain the situation to Mrs. Poland in such a way that it would not jeopardize their relationship.

During the next appointment Dr. Firman had an opportunity to discuss the donation privately with Mrs. Hamill, the potential donor. She expressed great concern about her sister's health and indicated she wanted to do what she could to help. She asked repeatedly about the risks involved in the donation. She seemed tense during the long conversation. She brought up the subject of the suitability of cadaver kidneys for transplant and at one time said, "Would the kidney machine really be that bad for her?'' Later consultation with a psychiatrist indicated that Mrs. Hamill seemed anxious, but there was no evidence of present or past mental disturbance. Still Dr. Firman had real doubts about her willingness to give the kidney freely.

Dr. Firman considered four alternatives when he got back the tissue-typing, which indicated an ideal match: tell Mrs. Hamill of the good match; tell Mrs. Hamill of the good match but express a willingness to suggest to her sister that the match was not acceptable; tell Mrs. Hamill that the tissue match was unacceptable; or tell Mrs. Hamill that the match was good but that he refused to perform the transplant at this time because he was not convinced of her willingness to give the organ freely.

Receiving Organs or Machines

In addition to the dramatic problems of deciding who is acceptable as an organ donor, there are equally serious moral dilemmas faced in receiving organs or dialysis treatment alternatives. One problem faced by the potential recipient is whether he is demanding too much of his fellow human beings—demanding not only the organs of life themselves but the resources—monetary, material, and human—which might otherwise be used for the benefit of other sick and suffering humanity. Even if there are no others competing for the scarce resources consumed, the psychological and moral dilemmas for the potential organ recipient can be excruciating. Key problems are whether an organ can be so much a part of a person as to make its transplant a moral offense, and whether a medical procedure can inflict so much pain and suffering, mental and physical, as to make it morally expendable even though it may well save the patient's life.

73   THE OVARY TRANSPLANT

The patient, Amanda Young, was a 24-year-old Mexican who had been married but childless since the age of 19. Infertility during the five years of marriage was attributed to diseased ovaries. Dr. Raul Hernandez and the reproductive biology team at a major hospital in Mexico City had been studying the problems of infertility for some time. They had experimented with the implantation of ovaries for the purpose of correcting hormonal problems in already pregnant women, and their success in such implants had now led them to consider the actual transplantation of the ovary. This would involve removal of the ovary of a donor, placing it into a recipient, and connecting the circulatory and reproductive vessels in the hope of permitting the woman to have a baby through natural means.

A willing, unrelated donor was obtained for Mrs. Young. The identity of the donor would at no time be revealed to the potential recipient, nor would the identity of the recipient be revealed to the donor. The research team felt that this was necessary because the female contribution to the genetic endowment of the offspring would come from the donor rather than from the woman who was receiving the transplant.

It was recognized that there would be serious psychological risks in such a procedure. Therefore, a team of psychiatric consultants had thoroughly examined both the donor and the recipient, as well as the husband of the recipient. This psychiatric team was given the responsibility of making sure that there would be no significant psychological damage. They were also given the responsibility of convincing the donor that she could have children normally despite the removal of one of her two ovaries.

The recipient, the donor, and the clinical research team had only a short time before the decision must be made.

The case for transplanting lifesaving organs such as the heart, kidneys, and liver is obvious. Even the case for the ovary transplant is clear: a woman strongly desiring a child of her own issue can have that basic wish fulfilled through the marvelous intervention of medical technology. Medical progress, which now permits the replacement of diseased or destroyed body parts, is so much a part of the technological era that it is sacrilege to cast doubt on its desirability. Yet the case for such heroic, humane, and lifesaving intervention also poses problems.

First, in spite of technological man's instinctive homage to the miraculous feat of an ovary or a heart transplant, some may ask whether there are any limits to remaking the human body from spare, or not so spare, parts salvaged from other human bodies. Are some organs or tissues so much a part of the person as a whole that transplanting is somehow a moral assault in and of itself? The question could be posed in the case of the heart transplant. The heart is not simply a pump, a part of the plumbing of the human machine. To claim that the heart is the "seat of the soul" may be without scientific foundation, and to claim that it is the center of the emotions may be poor neurophysiology. Yet the placing of psychological or philosophical significance in certain body functions or organ parts is not refutable by scientific demonstration. The black South Africans who served as the donors of Dr. Christiaan Barnard's hearts or the white middle-class Americans who are horror-stricken at the thought of finding another's heart in their chests may not share the philosophical and psychological biases of *Homo faber,* who sees the transplant of the heart as an elementary task in human plumbing. Cases have been reported where recipient families have asked if the heart of the donor was "saved" or if "Jesus was in his heart." Some questioned putting the "black heart" of Clive Haupt into the "Jewish body" of Philip Blaiberg.[3] At a more profound level the cultural, religious, and philosophical significance of certain organs must be recognized.[4] The fact is that the cultural differences in the significance attached to different organs are radical, and all humans attach special significance to some parts of the body. The transplant of the human brain, even if technically feasible, would probably be repulsive to the most crusty, hard-nosed transplanter.

The same problem—the moral legitimacy of transferring an organ closely identified with the essence of one person to another person—may be raised in the case of the ovary. Not only is the ovary the repository of the sex cells which transmit the genetic endowment of the donor, but it is also responsible for certain hormonal activity which may in a less direct but still significant way be identified with the donor. The first problem, then, with the ovary transplant may be the legitimacy of the organ transfer itself. The attachment of the ovary of one woman to the reproductive system of another is certainly "unnatural." Whether that in itself makes it immoral is arguable.

A second problem raised by the ovary transplant case is more evasive. In discussing this case, some have argued that the woman who would subject herself to the medical risks of such an experimental procedure must have a peculiar psychological commitment to forming children within her own body. Other options are open to her: adoption, childlessness, waiting for possible medical intervention to produce fertility from the damaged ovaries. Unlike the typical woman in her condition, however, Mrs. Young rejects these options.[5] The psychological risks of the transplant are certainly present. New hormonal inputs from the transplanted ovary might add to these risks. Most significant of all may be the psychological impact on the potential future child, who would run both the unusual risk of being monitored as a research specimen and the more traditional risk of having a genetic endowment that did not come solely from his "parents." It has been argued that humans have no moral right to act to inflict potential harm on a "patient" who at the time has nothing to gain because he as yet does not exist.[6]

The problem of the moral obligation to avoid risk to the unconceived future child by experimenting with the means of conception is a serious one. Some would argue that the psychological background of the woman requesting an ovary transplant is not the business of the researchers. Others might claim that the researchers are taking advantage of her unusually intense psychological drive to gain research material. Still others could claim that the physician's only duty is to provide medical help to patients who are in medical need. Evaluation of the motives or psychological make-up of the patient requesting the ovary transplant may not be a legitimate concern of the medical personnel or others concerned with the case, whereas the expenditure of resources—time, talent, and funds—for this purpose may be a question that cannot be avoided.

74   SAYING NO TO HEMODIALYSIS

Karen was a 16-year-old Catholic girl, the second oldest of seven siblings. She was first hospitalized in September 1968, after a three-week course of nephrotic syndrome, or kidney disease. She did not respond to medical treatment. A renal biopsy in April 1969 revealed "chronic, active glomerulonephritis," and by the spring of 1970 a rapid decrease in renal function prompted the decision to plan for dialysis and transplantation. A bilateral nephrectomy, removal of the kidneys, was performed in August 1970, and Karen received a transplant of her father's kidney the following month. The transplant functioned well initially, but several months later proteinuria became increasingly severe, and suddenly in March 1971 the kidney completely ceased to function. Prior to surgery and following the transplant's failure, thrice-weekly hemodialysis was performed. Karen tolerated dialysis poorly, routinely experiencing chills, nausea, vomiting, severe headaches, and weakness.

In April 1970 and prior to transplantation, a child psychiatrist had been asked to evaluate the family. Karen was found to be experiencing a reactive depression, but this response was considered appropriate to her medical condition. The father responded to his daughter's illness by immersing himself in his profession. The mother evidenced suspicion of Karen's medical management. Referral of the mother for psychiatric outpatient treatment was recommended but never accomplished.

The child psychiatrist was again consulted in July 1970. Karen and her parents met regularly with the social worker and the child psychiatrist prior to and after the transplant. The family did well psychologically during the immediate posttransplant period, but as Karen's new kidney failed, she became moderately depressed and the parents became increasingly distraught. Marital difficulties developed because the family could not deal directly with their disappointment at the transplant failure. The marital problems lessened with open discussion of the parents' feelings.

In early April 1971, after it became clear that the kidney would never function, Karen and her parents expressed the wish to stop medical treatment and let "nature take its course." The medical staff was upset and could not agree on the proper course of action. The social worker and psychiatrist attempted to have the girl and her family explore their decision in the hope that with further understanding, they would reject it. Most other staff members conveyed to the family that such wishes were unheard of and unacceptable, and that a decision to stop treatment could never be an alternative. The family decided to continue dialysis, medication, and diet therapy. Karen's renal incapacity returned to its pretransplant levels, and she resumed a life of social isolation, diet restriction, chronic discomfort, and fatigue.

On May 10 Karen was hospitalized following ten days of high fever. Three days later the transplant was removed. Its pathology resembled that of the original kidneys, and the possibility of a similar reaction forming in subsequent transplants was established.

On May 21 the arteriovenous shunt placed in Karen's arm for hemodialysis was found to be infected, and part of the vein wall was excised and the shunt revised. During this phase of the hospitalization, Karen and her parents grudgingly went along with the medical recommendations, but they continued to ponder the possibility of stopping treatment. The child psychiatrist was out of town from the end of April, and the social worker was now counseling Karen as well as her parents. On May 24 the shunt clotted closed. Karen, with her parents' agreement, refused shunt revision and any further dialysis.[7]

Karen's predicament is not designed for the benefit of systematic philosophers of ethics, for her case raises complex issues of death and dying, suicide, refusal of treatment, informed consent, and the locus of decision-making. Three distinctions are critical for understanding the case. First, any competent patient has the right to refuse any medical treatment whatsoever, for any reason no matter how foolish it appears. When cases involve matters of life and death, however, the refusal becomes much more critical.

Second, cases where medical intervention will merely prolong an inevitable dying process must be separated from cases where it will preserve a relatively stable life for an indefinite period, although this distinction is not often made in either law or ethics. Refusing the last surgery for a cancer that has already destroyed half a face is far different from refusing surgery for an appendectomy or refusing a blood transfusion when it will restore normal health. In fact, it can be argued that the refusal of hemodialysis or other truly life-preserving treatments is more a form of suicide rather than is "passive voluntary euthanasia," a term sometimes restricted to those who are inevitably dying from a specific, progressive illness. Yet many ethical traditions insist on the moral significance of the distinction between suicide and the refusal of a treatment that will be lifesaving at the expense of extreme pain and suffering.

Even the tradition of Catholic moral theology appears to treat a refusal of dialysis as a case of rejecting "extraordinary means." The position of Pope Pius XII, which explicitly charges the moral duty "in

case of serious illness to take the necessary treatment for the preservation
of life and health,'' goes on: ''But normally one is held to use only
ordinary means—according to circumstances of persons, places, times,
and culture—that is to say, means that do not involve any grave burden
for oneself or another. A more strict obligation would be too burden-
some for most men and would render the attainment of the higher, more
important good too difficult. Life, health, all temporal activities are in
fact subordinated to spiritual ends. On the other hand, one is not forbidden to take more than the strictly necessary steps to preserve life and
health, as long as he does not fail in some more serious duty.''[8] The
agony of chronic hemodialysis is often given as an example of a treatment that under some circumstances would involve a ''grave burden for
oneself.''

The agony of the hemodialysis treatments should not be under-
emphasized. Several studies have documented the severe mental strain.[9]
F. Patrick McKegney and Paul Lange describe a 40-year-old married
mother of four who began chronic dialysis in April and by May was
expressing the feeling of wanting ''to give up,'' of being ''worthless and
helpless.'' By September there were episodes of dyspnea, agitation, and
screaming, and she was put on tranquilizers. By February admission to
the rehabilitation unit was recommended, but the patient was stating, ''I
want to die; leave me alone; there's no hope.'' Both she and her husband
refused admission for rehabilitation.[10] The suffering is real and excruciating in many such cases. Yet there is also evidence that the mental
suffering may itself be produced by the kidney disease. It is thus possible
that forced treatment might lead to a change of heart on the part of even
an adamant refuser.

A third morally relevant distinction between this case and other
treatment refusals relates to the competency of the patient. The patient
who may die is sometimes incompetent to accept or refuse treatment.
Because of Karen's psychological status and age, her competency to
make the decision for herself is debatable and raises serious questions.
What is the relative significance of her own refusal and the supporting
refusal of her parents? Is it possible that Karen or some other teenager
could be too young to be given the full right to make judgments as an
adult and yet be old enough to contribute and even dominate certain
decisions, especially those that are sufficiently critical that she should be
given the time and counsel to help her understand the alternatives? If so,
how can one determine when the older minor's judgment is adequately
informed and reflective?

Allocating Organs and Machines

The problem of allocating scarce medical resources is first one of determining who the allocators should be. This is the critical issue, for

example, when deciding the composition of a kidney transplant recipient selection committee. The more fundamental question is then what should be decided. Is it "worth it" to spend scarce medical resources so that a woman can have an ovary transplant to bear children within her body? Is it "worth it" to expend the time of medical personnel searching for an adequate dialysis program for a social outcast who in all likelihood has little time to live? How can one square such a decision with the suffering and indifference to mothers with screaming babies in the emergency room of that same hospital? Should the government spend its funds performing exotic procedures on a relatively small number of citizens at great expense even if those procedures will be lifesaving? These are the critical questions of social justice that the techniques of transplantation and hemodialysis finally force upon modern medicine.

75 THE HEMODIALYSIS PATIENT

Oliver Johnson, a 57-year-old black man, was presented to Methodist Hospital intensive care unit in an obtunded state with focal seizures on March 17, 1971. His admission diagnoses were uremia and hypertension. The patient had worked as a steeple jack until 1950, when he was dismissed from his job, and since then he had been unemployed. He was on welfare and was partially supported by his wife.

His significant medical history had begun in 1965 when he entered another hospital for six months with a subarachnoid hemorrhage which was successfully treated with a craniotomy and evacuation of a hematoma over the left temporal lobe. His course of treatment was prolonged by congestive heart failure, urinary retention secondary to bulbourethral strictures, and psoriatic arthritis. In addition, there was a history of alcoholism. After recovering from that admission, he had limited his activities to his apartment. He went out only to a local tavern and only with his wife, who was a nurse in a children's psychiatric ward. Three days prior to the present admission Mr. Johnson became lethargic and anorexic and developed a broad-based gait. He was anuric for twenty-four hours before admission.

On admission, his seizures were initially controlled with diazepam and paraldehyde. A psychiatric consultant noted indications of a severe organic brain syndrome of undetermined duration. The record indicated that Mr. Johnson "couldn't cope." His first course of peritoneal dialysis was begun on March 19 and successfully lowered his blood urea nitrogen and creatinine. His mental status improved dramatically, and he was able to answer simple questions. This dialysis directly into the peritoneal cavity, however, could only be performed for a short period. The patient needed to get into a hemodialysis program.

A urological evaluation was carried out by a resident who was the current Renal Fellow. She found a stricture at the bulbourethral area, but no evidence of prolonged obstructive uropathy showed up on an IVP. His uremia was felt to be either secondary to his hypertension or the result of chronic nephritis.

Following Mr. Johnson's dramatic improvement and completion of his renal status, evaluation efforts were initiated to find a hemodialysis program for the patient. There being no hemodialysis available at the hospital where he had been admitted, an intern inquired about possible admission to the unit of an affiliated hospital. It was discovered that the affiliated hospital accepted hemodialysis patients only if they were candidates for transplantation. There was general agreement that Mr. Johnson was not a candidate. Discussion with the affiliated hospital was terminated. On March 29 the patient and the medical student traveled by ambulance to the clinic of a major teaching hospital in the city, where they were told that only ambulatory patients who could carefully follow instructions were considered for their program. At that time the patient was neither ambulatory nor able to demonstrate motivation for hemodialysis.

During the next three weeks the patient's BUN climbed to 153, his mental status deteriorated, and he became fluid overloaded. The decision was made to return the patient to the intensive care unit. Since the unit had no available bed, the resident decided to move another of her patients out of the unit to make room for Mr. Johnson. Afterward there was substantial debate over whether this had been an appropriate decision. Some, pointing out that the patient had a very short life expectancy in any case, doubted that another patient's care should have been compromised. One person commented that Mr. Johnson was "too much of a boozer" for hemodialysis even if the temporary procedure of peritoneal dialysis was performed. After the patient was transferred, however, a second dialysis was performed. This lowered his BUN to 117, and his mental status improved, though not to the same extent as it had following the first dialysis.

During the next week Mr. Johnson developed congestive heart failure, pulmonary edema, pericarditis, cardiomegaly, and anemia. Peritoneal dialysis was attempted for a third time without success, owing to difficulties in passing the catheter.

The medical student felt that there was still a possibility of finding a suitable hemodialysis program for Mr. Johnson. He realized, though, that it could take hours, even weeks, away from other patients who might benefit from his attention. It would also mean missing out on an important segment in his medical education.

---

1. Should efforts have been made to find hemodialysis for the patient?

2. What is the role of the social characteristics of a patient in determining treatment?
3. What are the criteria for allocation of scarce resources, such as intensive care unit beds or medical personnel? What should be the criteria for entrance into a hemodialysis program? What should be the basis of allocation when a limited number of dialysis machines are available: potential social contribution of the patient, medical need, medical prognosis, or chance?
4. Should the patient have been admitted to the affiliated hospital's dialysis unit? Should he have been admitted to the program of the hospital that accepted only ambulatory patients?
5. Who should make the decision in such cases: the resident, intern, attending physician, medical student, professional committee, or some other agency?

76 THE ARTIFICIAL HEART

On August 21, 1972, the Artificial Heart Assessment Panel held its first meeting at the National Institutes of Health in Bethesda, Maryland. A totally implantable artificial heart (TIAH), the panel learned, is simple in conception: a synthetic pump with a power source designed to be implanted in the human chest to replace an irreparably damaged natural organ. Since 1948 research and development had been underway, and four-chambered pumps with external controls had been implanted in hundreds of animals. In the experiments on calves, supporting pumps had maintained life for periods up to seventeen days. Current technology did not yet permit testing the TIAH in man, but the research was progressing rapidly, and it seemed technically feasible that within perhaps ten years what was once thought to be the seat of the soul and the dwelling place of the emotions would be replaced in a human being by a plastic machine rhythmically pumping the fluid of life.

The TIAH had been developed largely with funding by the United States government. Now a panel had been formed by the government, made up of three physicians, two economists, two lawyers, a sociologist, a priest-ethicist, and a political scientist. The panel's charge was ominous: "detailing the economic, ethical, legal, medical, psychiatric and social implications of clinical application." They were given the task of recommending among other things who should receive the heart as it first becomes available for human testing.

The panel spent months learning the relevant facts. Between 16,000 and 50,000 Americans per year might benefit from a TIAH. This includes a group between the ages of sixty-five and seventy-four that was excluded from earlier estimates of heart transplant recipient candidates because of age. The cost per implantation would be between \$15,000 and \$25,000. Younger recipients might require replacement devices should their first TIAH's wear out. Three power sources are being considered: a biological fuel cell using energy derived from the body, a system using an external electrical source transmitting energy across intact skin, and plutonium-238 which would provide a reliable source of energy for perhaps ten years. Plutonium would be the best source from the standpoint of reliability and the convenience of the patient, but there are disadvantages relating both to cost and to the risk to the patient and those around him created by radioactivity.[11]

One of the tragedies of modern medicine is that physicians now have the capability to save lives and prevent suffering, yet the money, personnel, and will are lacking to apply some of that capability. The costs of life-saving are enormous. The plea that the resources are available if only people were willing to commit them may be true. But to argue that funds should be shifted from highway construction or military budgets to health care, while powerful, may be naive. Even assuming that there were major shifts in priorities, which those committed to health care consider essential, the problems of allocation will still exist. Despite the critical importance of shifting resources from other sectors, the more difficult question in the cases of Mr. Johnson and the Artificial Heart Assessment Panel is how to allocate scarce resources within the health sector.

The costs of the two programs, hemodialysis and artificial heart transplantation, are terribly high, in terms of both money and personnel. Monetary costs are difficult to establish. For hemodialysis it is estimated that about 50,000 people die from kidney failure each year in the United States alone. Of these, between 5000 and 10,000 are suitable for hemodialysis. Kidney transplantation is the only feasible alternative, and it raises its own allocation problems: kidneys are scarce, the procedure is expensive, and in many cases the graft is rejected. To illustrate the potential cost of hemodialysis, one has to make assumptions about the number dialyzed and their potential survival time as well as the cost for the dialysis. Costs vary with the location of the treatment, whether in a hospital, at home, or in a mobile unit. Labor costs may be less at home, but equipment costs are greater there because the unit is normally used for only one patient. A start-up cost of \$20,000 for the first year (it can range from \$10,000 to \$50,000) and a cost of \$5000 for subsequent years would lead to an eventual yearly cost of \$960,000,000 if 8000 patients entered the program each year and the average patient lived twenty years on the treatment. This estimate is consistent with the published estimates of one-half to one-and-a-half billion dollars per year.

This is a great deal of money. The entire American national health budget is only approximately $110 billion per year. Yet the cost is small in comparison with the defense budget, and a valid moral claim can be made for a public duty to save 8000 human beings a year. The question remains as to why the expenditure should be limited to saving American lives, and why it should be limited to lives lost to kidney disease.

The Artificial Heart Assessment Panel's economic problem may be even bigger. Cost estimates range from $15,000 to $25,000 and probably somewhat more for a nuclear-powered heart. It is estimated that there are between 17,000 and 50,000 candidates per year, producing a total cost, conservatively estimated, at between $255,000,000 and $1,250,000,000 per year. This figure would have to be multiplied by the number of hearts needed per person, for it is probable that there will be some mechanical breakdowns. One estimate is that the life span of the heart might be five to ten years. This figure also accounts only for American heart recipient candidates. The same calculations should be made for other potential recipients of the approximately twenty-five different kinds of organs and tissues that have now been used in human transplantation, for hemophiliacs, for cancer patients needing chemo-therapy, and even for psychiatric patients. The total will certainly far exceed the present national health budget even if it is limited to American cases—a limitation hard to justify. In short, even the financial restraints are major. While the answer that the money can be found is no doubt true, it may be unrealistic. Even if the money were found, competition for time, talent, and attention would still force the question of how scarce resources should be allocated.

A number of alternatives for allocating scarce medical resources have been proposed. The debate over the alternatives resembles the classic debate over the meaning of justice. The first alternative, reflected in the present system, relies at least in part on the ability to pay, or to have the right connections. This is probably one of the least defensible means of allocating lifesaving technology.

The second alternative is implied by the physicians in Mr. Johnson's case who argue that he is "too much of a boozer" for hemodialysis. Somehow they think they should take into account the patient's "social worth." The physicians who oppose spending hours and perhaps weeks of their time to find a dialysis program for him also feel that they have a duty to the other patients on their ward. Here, they would argue, is a social outcast, a man who has not worked for twenty years, who con-tributes nothing to society, and who takes away valuable time and bed space from others who would really benefit society.

The dangers of this approach are obvious. Yet if forced to choose between John F. Kennedy and some hypothetical senile alcoholic who happened to need medical attention on that fateful day in Dallas, some would feel compelled to turn their attention to the President. Treating a mother supporting three small children may seem more compelling than caring for another person without dependents. A case can be made that it is dangerous to consider social worth at all in allocating medical care. Patients whose social characteristics resemble those of the medical staff may get a higher priority, which would be hard to explain on the grounds of justice alone. In the long run there may be more justice in ruling out social worth as a criterion altogether, but it would be dangerous to do so if that simply permitted such social judgments to reappear in some other guise. One such guise is the suggestion that Mr. Johnson is not likely to live very long even if he is treated.

A third alternative often proposed is the use of "strictly medical criteria." According to this principle, those who would benefit the most medically are to be selected. This choice leaves open the question of what constitutes a medical benefit. If it is years of added life, then children would get highest priority; the senior citizen would for all practical purposes be barred. If the problem of definition could be resolved, medical benefit might be a plausible criterion for allocating resources. However, it still masks a fundamental value judgment, which reflects a medical orientation. To select on the basis of "strictly medical criteria" is to argue that any amount of "medical benefit," whatever that may be, is preferable to an even larger gain that is not medical. This assumption is questionable.

A fourth alternative for allocating scarce medical resources, which is suggested by those who are frustrated and dissatisfied by the first three, is by lot. Allocation by lot seems wasteful at first, but people often turn to it when there seems to be no other just method of distributing goods.

A fifth alternative is a modification of the principle of allocation by lot. It is the principle of taking turns or standing in line, according to which artificial hearts or kidney machines are distributed on a first-come, first-served basis. This method has the arbitrariness of a lottery, but in medicine it may be particularly unattractive, for if kidney or heart patients have to wait their turn, each will deteriorate while queued up.

Other alternatives are often proposed in more general discussions of justice. In the race to the lifeboat, the standard is "women and children first." If the principle underlying this practice is that the weak and helpless deserve special consideration, then a sound moral claim may be involved, but in a day of consciousness of equal rights for women and for children, such labeling can in itself be dangerous as well as invalid. In some cases a claim of "compensatory justice" may be made. Mr. Johnson could have a claim to special care, for instance, as compensation for the miserable ghetto health care he received through his fifty-five years—care which in all likelihood was responsible for his kidney failure. Finally, some have argued that in certain cases when not all who are in need can benefit, then none should. Edmond Cahn, for instance, claims that in a matter of life and death, as the ship is sinking, so to speak, "If none sacrifice themselves of free will to spare the others—they must all wait and die together."[12] Another conscientious thinker, worried over the allocation of the artificial heart paid for by all through government funds, makes the same argument. No one should receive such hearts until there are enough for all to receive.

These are some of the alternative principles for allocating resources. One way or another, dialysis machines and artificial hearts will be allocated. To ensure that they are distributed wisely, it is essential to understand the moral foundations for such actions.

CHAPTER 10

Psychiatry
and the Control
of Human Behavior

Among the more exotic and provocative issues in medicine is the use of medical skills for the purposeful modification of human behavior. Since the beginning of time, humans have sought the magic potion, the soma of the gods, to give them happiness, or at least to remove their ills. Now that medical science is approaching the skill necessary to control behavior and experience with some degree of specificity, it is not so certain that the ability will prove a panacea.

Many of the social and ethical dilemmas stemming from the ability to control behavior are not unique. For example, consent, or the refusal of consent, for treatment by the psychiatric patient is a perplexing subclass of the general medical consent problem. The question itself falls into two parts: the role of the therapist and the role of the various techniques.

The Role of the Psychotherapist

The role of the psychotherapist in the use of behavior-controlling techniques presents specific ethical problems. Among them is whether the psychotherapist ought to impose a particular set of social values on a client, or whether he ought to offer his psychotherapeutic skills in order to produce the behavioral and psychological effects desired by the patient independent of the therapist's moral evaluation.

77   PSYCHOTHERAPIST AS SERVANT OR TEACHER

The client was a white, 35-year-old advertising executive who had never been married and lived alone in a bachelor apartment in a large Eastern city. He presented the following story to the psychotherapist:

> I am homosexual. I'm lonely. I'm tired of the isolation. I live in continual fear of being discovered. My job would go out the window if they knew. I'm so intimidated that I haven't had a contact in years. Now and then I cruise the bars, but just as I'm about to score, I panic. But it's not just the cops I fear. I regret to say that I don't think much of myself, wanting a guy. Seems to me that anyone with self-control could overcome this perversion. I've been in therapy before, but to no avail—I just couldn't change. But that was 'talk' therapy. I've read how behavior therapists can really get people to change their sexual orientation. I'm willing to try anything, even shock therapy. I think that's what I need, maybe even what I deserve. If you don't help me, I frankly won't know where to turn. I'm estranged from everyone I meet —afraid either that they'll find out or that I'll turn on to them and show myself. It's a living hell.

During the first several interviews the behavior therapist gathered some historical information. The man could not recall ever having been sexually interested in women. His sexual life in early adolescence included masturbation, male fantasies, and looking at suggestive pictures. Social pressures made him date women, but he always maintained a friendly rather than a lover relationship, even though he had numerous chances for intimacy with women. He did not dislike women. Being a sensitive, introspective person, he had read widely in the psychiatric literature and had come to the conclusion that his sexual "perversion" was caused by an arrest in psychosexual development. He attributed the anxieties he had felt throughout college and then increasingly in his advertising work to his mental disorder, which convinced him even more that he was emotionally disturbed and that psychological peace would come only with a change in his sexual preference.

During college, he did have a lover, a young man with whom he roomed during his junior and senior years. He described their relationship as a good one, characterized not only by much orgastic satisfaction but also by an emotional closeness he had heard could be achieved only with a woman, preferably one's wife. The quality of this relationship began to make him believe that maybe loving one's own sex was not sick. Unfortunately for him, his lover during their last year in college became involved with a young woman, whom he eventually married. While it was never said, the client concluded that his lover had somehow straightened himself out, leaving him behind for a normal relationship.

On the job, he play-acted the single "stud," and being personable and good-looking, he had no trouble showing up at social functions with an attractive woman by his side. This deception, however, made him feel even more excluded from the "normal," straight world and contributed mightily to his self-hate.

During the fifth interview, the therapist and client discussed goals. The client expressed a desire to try to change, to become uninterested or less interested in men and to become sexually aroused by women. The therapist, however, made clear that in his opinion and that of most other behavior therapists, homosexuality is a learned behavior, just as heterosexuality is, and that it is not abnormal, sick, or perverted per se.

After the session, the therapist considered two possible alternative strategies on how to proceed. Like the overwhelming majority of behavior therapists, the therapist could adopt the hetero-strategy and agree to work toward the client's goals; that is, to accept that the client truly wanted to change. A therapeutic regimen could be proposed consisting of three parts: "playboy therapy" or graded masturbation exercises at home, enabling the client to ejaculate while looking at photos of attractive women; instructions on heterosocial and heterosexual techniques, to fill the gaps caused by the client's lack of experience with women; and covert sensitization, an aversive conditioning procedure whereby the client imagines homosexual situations while at the same time being induced to feelings of nausea and disgust.

Or, like a small minority of behavior therapists, the therapist could adopt a homo-strategy and question the client's apparent desire to change. Such an approach rests on certain assumptions: sexual preferences probably cannot be eliminated; the client can be better helped by reducing his feelings of self-disgust and social anxiety; any program of aversion therapy is problematic, both because experimental evidence is lacking to warrant its use with humans and because the imposition of negative consequences following homosexual thoughts and feelings would only add to the client's self-hate and reinforce his belief that homosexuality is perverted, regardless of the therapist's stated liberal attitudes about unconventional sexual patterns; there are growing social support systems, like the gay liberation groups, which can provide the needed reference groups for the client; and any sexual relations between consenting adults are acceptable provided they do not generate self-hate or other psychological or physical injury.

The therapist was at first inclined to follow the hetero-strategy, the more usual course for behavior therapy. He felt uneasy, however, so he first debated in his mind the arguments against the homo-strategy. First, homosexual behavior is against the law. He would therefore be encouraging illegal behavior and the client might lose his job. This risk, however, is problematic. Therapists, at any rate, already counsel illegal activities, such as oral-genital contact. After all, all therapy is political. The problem was whether the client would be best served by saving his job while maintaining his misery.

The second problem in connection with the homo-strategy is that the client had asked for change, not adjustment, in the matter of his homosexuality. There is no evidence, however, even in the behavior therapy literature, that enduring the elimination of homosexual feelings is possible, so that to offer such a promise is itself ethically questionable. Moreover, the therapist, himself a straight male, was likely to convey to the client the greater desirability of wanting to change in the direction of heterosexuality and hence to make the client reluctant to admit his wish for the acceptance of his homosexuality, if such a wish were present. Failing to change, the client might blame himself even more and lose more ground than if no therapy had been attempted at all.

The third problem of the homo-strategy is that it puts the therapist in the position of teaching a new set of values rather than simply serving the client's expressed wishes. The therapist had always thought of himself as one who contracted with his clients to produce behavior changes according to their own desires. Yet if a therapist believes a client is really doing nothing wrong and is simply suffering because of social prejudices, and if the therapist further believes that he has the skill to relieve that suffering by getting the client to accept the behavior he has been socialized into believing is wrong, the therapist must have an obligation to influence his client to consider the new alternative.[1]

This case presents in an unusual form the dilemma of the health professional who, on the one hand, wants to exclude his own personal values from his therapeutic relationships with his clients and, on the other, feels obliged to get his client to consider new alternatives—including new value alternatives—which might lead in the long run to the greater happiness or adjustment of the client. Often the moral response to homosexuality is revulsion. Had the behavioral therapist been completely convinced that it is the proper response, he probably would have had no conflict when requested by the client to use behavior modification techniques to change his behavior to that of a heterosexual. In mentally reviewing the problems with the homo-strategy, however, the therapist does not express serious moral objections to homosexuality per se. In fact, he seems to believe that the behavior itself is acceptable. He goes on, however, to raise different problems. Homosexuality is illegal, it is not what the client is seeking, and to offer it as an alternative thrusts the therapist into the role of teacher of values. While the therapist seems to accept a value system that includes the homosexual alternative, he is seriously disturbed with the use of the therapist role to teach a new value system.

One level of debate would challenge the apparent acceptance of homosexuality on the part of the therapist. The dilemmas raised about the role of the therapist, however, are even more interesting. In order to clarify those dilemmas, it is helpful to bracket the question of homosexuality per se and to focus on the therapist's problems, assuming his own evaluation of homosexuality. All three objections he raises to the homo-strategy center on one basic issue: the relation between the therapist's value commitment to producing a satisfactory adjustment on the part of the client and the values of others who may not share that basic commitment.

The therapist's first problem is the conflict between client adjustment and the laws of the state. Apparently the state finds homosexuality so objectionable that it has made the behavior illegal. The therapist recognizes that "all therapy is political," that is, all therapy is based on a social and value framework, and that therapists sometimes counsel illegal acts when they believe these will serve the client's psychological adjustment. The question is whether the counseling of civil disobedience is called for in this case. The response seems to be that client adjustment would justify overriding the moral obligation to conform to a law established by due process.

The second conflict focuses more directly on the client. He asks for change, not adjustment. The therapist's reply is once again rooted in the principle of adjustment. The change strategy will not work, because there is no evidence that aversion therapy can really produce lasting elimination of homosexual feelings, because the therapist himself is heterosexual and therefore cannot adequately convey the acceptability of the homosexual alternative, and because failure will lead to even greater self-blame. Therefore, in adjustment terms, the heterosexual modification program is self-defeating.

But the problem posed is that the client wants change, not adjustment. To respond with the argument that change is not acceptable because it will not produce adjustment is fallacious. One cannot argue against the change course and for the adjustment course by claiming that the adjustment course will produce better adjustment.

The third conflict is a moral conflict within the therapist himself. He raises the question of whether he is a value-free servant of his client, bringing to the client potent techniques for behavioral change according to the expressed instructions of the client, or whether his real task is to pose to the client new alternatives, new interpretations, which will resolve his problem in a new and more effective manner. The therapist once again seems to opt for what he thinks will benefit the client. In the long run the client will be psychologically more satisfied and possibly even physically better off if he learns to accept a new set of values which see homosexuality as an acceptable life style. This is the classical principle of the ethics of the medical profession—doing what one thinks will benefit the patient—even if the principle is in this case expressed in a very different behavior outcome, which might have been abhorrent to the Hippocratic physician, and even if it is not now a physician but a behavioral therapist who is leaning toward the principle of doing what he thinks will be beneficial rather than what the client has expressly requested.

With all three problems, the therapist seems to be wrestling in his own mind between two views of the client-therapist relationship. One view emphasizes the importance of contractual obligations: both the citizen's social contract with the state to obey its laws, even if they are not completely acceptable, and the personal contract with the client to fulfill his expressed needs. The other view emphasizes client adjustment, even at the expense of violating laws and refusing to accept the values and beliefs of the client.

78   THE PSYCHIATRIST'S ROLE IN WAR

The following report appeared in an Air Force *Newsletter* about the psychiatric treatment of an Air Force sergeant while on duty in Vietnam in 1966:

> Fear of Flying: A 26-year-old SSgt AC 47 gunner with 7 months active duty in RVN, presented with frank admission of fear of flying. He had flown over 100 missions, and loss of several crews who were well known to the patient precipitated his visit. He stated he would give up flight pay, promotion, medals, etc., just to stop flying. Psychiatric consultation to USAF Hospital, Cam Ranh Bay, resulted in 36 days hospitalization with use of psychotherapy and tranquilizers. Diagnosis was Gross Stress Reaction, manifest by anxiety, tenseness, a fear of death expressed in the form of rationalizations, and inability to function. His problem was "worked through" and insight to his problem was gained to the extent that he was returned to full flying duty in less than 6 weeks. This is a fine tribute to the psychiatrists at Cam Ranh Bay. (633 Combat Spt Gp Dispensary, Pleiku AB)[2]

This news story raises difficult issues about the role of the psychotherapist. Three commentators have focused on different dimensions of the case. Robert G. Newman, a physician with a master's degree in public health and a consultant on drug abuse, makes clear that there are dangers in labeling behavior that is socially unacceptable according to particular standards as a medical or psychiatric problem:

> This case illustrates the inherent dangers of psychiatrists' equating deviance with psychopathology and proceeding unquestioningly from

the premise that "curing" such deviance is a universally valid goal. In fact, the clinicians in this instance display precisely the type of symptomatology they ostensibly seek to treat: an inability to recognize and respond appropriately to reality, sublimation, and escapism.

1. The reality which confronted the patient in this case made "fear of flying" a reasonable, appropriate, and psychologically healthy response. The corollary is also true: the use of psychiatric intervention in overcoming the fear elicited by such a situation leads to a condition which might best be termed iatrogenic psychosis.

2. Instead of recognizing the extraordinary dangers which the patient somehow managed to survive during seven months of combat, and accepting his right to refuse to participate further, the Cam Ranh Bay psychiatrists determined that the cause and the cure of the "problem" lay in the head of their patient.

3. In "blaming the victim," the medical officers avoided the conflict which would have been created had they refused to accept the patient as a psychiatric referral.

In retrospect, this case history generally elicits incredulity and laughter. The great threat to civil liberties is easily overlooked. The awesome power vested in psychiatrists, despite recent court challenges, is frightening. It is virtually impossible to refute a psychiatric diagnosis, and the harder one tries, the more the attempt is viewed as additional confirmation of the severity of the "mental illness." Involuntary "treatment" can follow, in which case the individual must either adopt conformity or suffer the consequences. One can only speculate on the consequences for the unfortunate sergeant had he not been able to "work through" what was termed *his* problem and conquer his fears.

It must be conceded that the article does not unequivocally indicate whether the sergeant was referred to the psychiatrists voluntarily or not. It would certainly appear, however, that he presented his superiors with a statement of fact, with a rational decision that the enormous risks inherent in continued air combat outweighed the material benefits of increased pay, the added privileges of higher rank, or the pride which might be derived from commendations. What appears to be inappropriate under these circumstances might indeed have been laudatory if he had expressed a wish to continue flying instead of announcing a decision to stop.

An analogous area in which the conflict between practitioner and patient is most prevalent today is the field of drug abuse. Drug users are increasingly being forced into treatment programs under the threat of prosecution, and as a condition for release from prison after sentencing. This approach, which has been heralded as a humane alternative to applying criminal sanctions for the violation of laws, is in fact a perversion of the physician-patient relationship. As with the Air Force sergeant, the illness and the criteria for successful treatment are determined unilaterally by the psychiatrist, frequently in direct opposition to the expressed views of the patients. Addict-clients are considered to be successfully rehabilitated when they accept whatever grim reality others have determined to be their lot, just as the sergeant was hailed as a therapeutic triumph when, after being subjected to "psychotherapy and tranquilizers," he resumed as gunner in an AC-47.

When the patient does not have the unequivocal option to refuse treatment, one must proceed from the assumption that voluntarism is lacking. Under these circumstances the concept of success and failure loses all meaning. Whether the "problem" is fear of flying, drug abuse, homosexuality, masturbation, or any other behavior, it must be left to the individual to decide if it is acceptable or not, and whether change is a desired goal. The attitudes of the psychiatrist regarding the behavior, and the value which the psychiatrist may personally place on modifying that behavior, are irrelevant. The circuitous logic evidenced in this case history, which cites as proof of success the fact that the patient ultimately came to share the psychiatrists' views, must be rejected. Nor does the self-righteous assertion that the psychiatrists' motivation is benevolent mitigate the invidiousness of involuntary treatment. As Thomas Szasz has pointed out in *Law, Liberty and Psychiatry:* "Treating patients against their wishes, even though the treatment may be medically correct, should be considered an offense punishable by law . . . Let us not forget that every form of social oppression has, at some time during its history, been justified on the ground of helpfulness toward the oppressed."[3]

The second commentator is E. Tristram Engelhardt, a physician and philosopher who teaches at the Institute for Medical Humanities, University of Texas, who apparently agrees that serious problems are created by the use of the disease label, but separates this problem from the more general problem of using medical skills for the service of debatable political goals:

In reading this case, one might be tempted to consider it simply an example of the misuse of medicine in the service of a political goal. That would be an oversimplification because the individuals concerned, the psychiatrists, the persons who asked for their consultation, and in the end perhaps the patient, probably saw themselves as acting in accord with reality. The case illustrates the role that value judgments play in the concept of disease. The judgment that someone has a disease presupposes, among other things, (1) that the person afflicted is the subject of phenomena that are abnormal and (2) that those phenomena are explainable in terms of the laws of pathophysiology and psychology. That is, the statement that some condition is a pathological state presupposes more than a mere description. The condition must be held in some sense to be a state of suffering and to be abnormal, where "abnormal" means other than "usual." Even if most persons had some cardiovascular disease at age seventy, one could still term the condition a disease condition. It would be "abnormal'' where ''normal'' expresses an ideal of function. Thus one will term diabetes, menopause, alcoholism, etc., diseases depending on what one judges proper to the human condition. Similarly, one will term angina a disease state because it is a painful and incapacitating condition, while one will not term teething a disease, because the latter is held to be a normal and proper state of pain, since it is closely bound to achieving a normal human goal—having teeth. Similarly, polydactylism and vitiligo will be held to be deformities or diseases on the basis of a judgment about what human form should be like. In contrast, an intelligent or very beautiful person will be held to be above normal, because of a set of human judgments about what humans should be. Finally, as Talcott Parsons has indicated, calling people sick assigns to them a social role which excuses them from blame for their condition. One may blame a cigarette smoker for becoming ill with brochogenic carcinoma of the lung, but not for being ill. Consider in this regard the disease of alcoholism or drug addiction; consider as well the history of diseases which we now in retrospect can see to have reflected particular cultural judgments: the disease of masturbation and draepetomania (the pre-Civil War disease of slaves running away).

In ''Fear of Flying,'' the flier was appreciated as being ill in that he was in distress (that is, suffering—afraid that he would be shot down in combat) and was unable to function normally. Normal function was here defined as the ability to engage in combat. Moreover, the failure to function was held to be caused rather than to be a chosen pattern of conduct. To consider a state of affairs a disease is to hold that it is caused by pathological processes, not freely willed action. Diagnosing the flier as ill with a ''Gross Stress Reaction'' thus authorized (1) the use of medicine to restore health and the ability to function normally, and (2) excused the individual from responsibility for not having functioned.

One should notice that once one chooses to consider the condition a disease condition, the description of the ''facts'' of the matter changes. The facts become embedded in a theory which then infects them with a special valence. The individual who is the focus of concern becomes a ''patient,'' his judgments concerning the risks associated with flying become ''rationalizations,'' his refusal to fly becomes an ''inability to function.'' It is not clear from the material available whether the individuals seeking treatment for the gunner actually thought he was ill, or whether someone used the disease model in order to avoid court-martial for the flyer. In either event, this case illustrates the social role of ''disease'' concepts and the ways in which they presuppose value judgments about norms for humans and the human condition. This is inescapable. The best we can do is to amend those concepts of disease which conflict with our more general human values concerning freedom and individual responsibility.

One should recognize this case as a flamboyant example of the generally value-laden character of talk about disease and health. It is not as if one could simply isolate those diseases which are objectively disease categories and those that are not. Rather, some disease concepts fail (and should fail) because they conflict with general human values.[4]

The political uses of psychiatry hinted at in Engelhardt's comments force consideration of the role of the psychotherapist in another way. If the physician—and psychiatrists are a special group of physicians—has an obligation to benefit the patient and exclude from consideration broader social and political concerns, the employment of a psychiatrist by the military or any other governmental agency may seriously compromise that obligation. Can a psychotherapist justifiably combine service to the patient with service to the state? Perry London, a psychotherapist and professor of psychology and psychiatry at the University of Southern California, thinks that in principle one can:

As the *Newsletter* says, success in returning the gunner back to duty is a fine tribute, indeed, to psychiatrists' efficiency as technicians. The question is: does it also testify to their deficiency as moralists? Proper morality, in some views, would have made them work against the official position of the government and the military in the Vietnam war; and holders of such views are outraged that physicians would sell their services in such an unjust cause. Since we lost the war only recently, and therefore still blanch doubly at having fought it altogether, it is easy to be seduced into moralistic "right-think." Losing a war is forgivable, and time dulls the bitterness of unjust victories; in those cases the moral imperatives are not so clear and obvious. Israeli doctors who returned gunners to their tanks and planes in 1973 or their counterparts in the Mexican-American War in 1845 are not subjected to the same scrupulosity. And perhaps a century from now, Wehrmacht doctors will be seen as no more evil than they must have felt in 1941. Even the Nuremberg trials may seem, like Magna Carta, a celebration of the victors' power. Might may not *make* right, but it certainly influences comment on it.

Outrage at the Air Force doctors reflects what I call the "new conventional morality." The old conventional morality said, simplistically, that a soldier's duty was to uniform, mission, or country via chain of authorized command; the new morality implies that soldier-doctors should themselves define where their duty truly lies. "Right-think" adherents assume the psychiatrists would have decided to subvert the government by preventing the gunner's recovery, or by treating him and at the same time trying to persuade him to alter his public position from one which would produce an "unfitness" or "disability" discharge (with full veteran's benefits) to one which would subject him to general court-martial (with full prison sentence). If the psychiatrists were themselves to define their moral duty, and then do exactly what they did because they supported the Vietnam war, the new morality would be hoisted on its own petard. But moral outrage may blind us to this fact, as it blinds us to the fact that there are people who actually believe in Nazism, racism, and paganism as moral imperatives. So much for logic. Even more to the point is the psychologic fact that psychiatrists, like most of us, are not much cut out for the practical heroics of subversion or rebellion, or even for pondering too much about them. To argue that most people can, or should, be routine arbiters of their own morality, I believe, slaps harshly in the face of reality.

Individual morality is built on the bedrock of social norms, and is sustained by reinforcements in social custom. It perishes slowly but surely when social norms change and the rewards and penalties of erstwhile good and bad behavior are changed to meet new rules. Most Nazis, I fancy abhorred cruelty to dumb animals (not the same as Jews); most Arab terrorists love their children (not my children); most air force gunners don't like to kill people (and still less to get killed). Most psychiatrists try to do the jobs expected of them—on the couches of Fifth Avenue, in the Cuckoo's Nest, and at Cam Ranh Bay. Some people in all these groups change their minds and try to leave the field, generally quietly, keeping a low profile to ward off retaliation; but sometimes noisily, almost begging for martyrdom. Yet most of humankind, most of the time, are too busy trying to manage the routines of daily living to spend much energy on moral calculations. Most morals get borrowed from the neighbors, the organization, or the big shots of our other-directed society. Just as politics is the exercise of leadership, and most of us are rather passive followers, morality is the exercise of normative behavior, and most of us are rather passive actors in the creation of our norms. The Children of Israel liked Egypt and did not mind slavery in principle; it was the beatings, the strawless bricks, and the baby snatchers that did them in. So it is with most of us, most of the time.

I do not mean to argue that people should never be held individually accountable for their acts, or that the Vietnam war was a just one. I do mean to say that a decent society makes the individual the last arbiter of morality, not the first one. In 1966 (when the *Newsletter* was published), I thought, like many others, that we were on the right side of the Vietnam war. By 1969, like many others, I had changed my mind. In 1975, it is unseemly, if not immoral, to retrospectively condemn the doctors of last decade's war for doing what then looked like their duty in a cause which they probably supported. Physicians are no more ignorant, or ill-intentioned, or immoral, than the rest of us. The case is a study in tragedy, not morality.[5]

Behavior Control Techniques

The techniques available for the control of human behavior raise social and ethical questions beyond the more general ones of the role of the therapist and the extent to which he ought to incorporate his values in the therapeutic relationship. All of the basic themes of medical ethics—

patient benefit, social benefit, justice in distributing health resources, confidentiality, truth-telling, and consent—arise in the context of psychotherapy and behavior control. Some behavior control techniques, however, raise special problems or raise them in special ways. Whenever an individual is a candidate for psychotherapy or other behavioral change interventions, it is an open question whether he has the capacity to consent to or choose for himself the mode of therapy he prefers. The consenting organ itself, the brain, is the locus where there may be pathology. Moreover, the very value system upon which choice might be based is often the target for change. To try to resolve the medical conflict by appealing to the value framework of the patient will not solve the problem unless there is a preliminary determination that the patient's own values will be the basis for intervention.

The several behavior modification techniques available at present are psychosurgery, psychotherapy, and chemotherapy. Or a case could be interpreted as falling completely outside any medical model and more in some other context, such as criminal deviancy to be treated by traditional penal methods. The first problem is to choose among these possible intervention strategies.

79 PSYCHOSURGERY OR PSYCHOTHERAPY FOR THE VIOLENT ALCOHOLIC

A man in his late thirties, who had been convicted of a series of petty offenses, all of them alcohol-related, was found standing over the dead body of a friend, holding a bloody hammer. He was charged with murder. Conviction would have been difficult because of his chronic alcoholism and the fact that the only evidence available outside of circumstantial evidence was that of his wife, which was inadmissible in court. He was sent for a diagnostic evaluation to Ettinger Institute, the state facility for the criminally insane. On their recommendation he was declared a defective delinquent, and given an indeterminate sentence to be served at Ettinger.

He had been there for nine years undergoing their standard treatment program, primarily group and individual psychotherapy at weekly intervals. According to the staff, he showed no change over the nine years, and the parole board had denied his standard yearly applications for parole. The therapeutic staff was somewhat discouraged by the lack of progress. However, their attitude was that they should never stop trying and that they should be willing to keep him there indefinitely, even for the rest of his life, continuing to send him to weekly psychotherapeutic treatments in the hope that there would be some kind of change. They were convinced that his alcohol-related violence would show itself again on the outside if he ever had the opportunity to drink. They were also convinced that their responsibility to the patient and to society was to keep him in the institution.

One psychiatrist, after seeing the man in a group therapy session, concluded that there was organic damage, probably from the alcohol, although she could not convince the other staff members that a complete workup by a neurologist would be fruitful. A senior psychologist suggested that one possible alternative to indefinite incarceration with little hope of improvement would be a psychosurgical procedure, whereby the man could continue to drink without going into violent rages. The other staff members wanted nothing to do with the suggestion, insisting that psychosurgery had never been done and would never be done at Ettinger.

Another staff member proposed the use of disulfiram as a way of freeing the man from prison. Disulfiram interferes with alcohol metabolism so that individuals on the drug who ingest alcohol experience a transient illness, including nausea, vomiting, rapid heartbeat, and occasionally unconsciousness, which is followed by drowsiness, sleep, and complete recovery. According to other staff persons, however, the man had refused any kind of disulfiram therapy because he liked to drink and did not want to be put in the position of never being able to take a drink without becoming ill.

At one point in the staff conversation a young, politically active social worker shocked the group by arguing that he was not so sure the man was sick at all: "We've got an alcoholic on our hands, and we should face up to it. I don't know any evidence that this fellow couldn't control his drinking if he wanted to. The more we tell him he is sick and can't control himself, the more he is going to believe it. There is something inhumane about the way we look on all our so-called patients as if they were children who can't control their own behavior. We should take care of the physical damage from all his drinking the best we can and send him back to Harrison (the state penitentiary) to serve his time. At least that way he won't be strangled by this indeterminate sentence."

There were now advocates for psychosurgery, drug therapy, and imprisonment, but most of the staff were still convinced that some form of psychotherapy was the answer. Even among that group, however, there was disagreement. One faction supported continuing the group therapy sessions, even though they had not been very effective. Another faction advocated behavior modification through classical conditioning techniques, including the establishment of a "token economy" at the institution. According to such a plan, rewards for appropriate behavior would be given in the form of tokens, which could be used to buy snacks, cigarettes, and privileges. Still another faction, led by the analytically trained member of the staff, fought for more individual therapy. The staff was left puzzled, not only by this dispute among the types of psychotherapies but also by the conflict between psychotherapy and the other approaches proposed.

———————

1. How significant a factor is the success of the different treatments? What other factors are important?
2. The argument for psychosurgery seems to grow out of the possibility of organic brain damage. Is organic pathology important in deciding for brain surgery, and if so, why?
3. The treatments proposed differ in the ease with which they can be reversed. Psychosurgery, for instance, is thought to be irreversible, while disulfiram effects can be easily reversed by stopping the drug. What are the other differences in reversibility? Is reversibility an asset or detriment in the treatment for a condition of this kind?
4. The proposed actions differ in the extent to which they presuppose the capacity for free choice on the part of the patient-inmate. What is the significance of this presupposition?
5. Should the same treatment options, including psychosurgery, be available for alcoholics who have not committed violent crimes but are simply dissatisfied with their persistent uncontrollable drinking?

This case of a violent alcoholic highlights the conceptual and moral issues in the choice among treatment modalities for someone who may have mental or neurological damage. Psychosurgery is one option being considered. More and more cases are being proposed for psycho- or neurosurgery. Whereas decades ago prefrontal lobotomy was a crude procedure proposed for remedying patients with sweeping and crude diagnoses, today interventions in the human brain are being proposed for much more specific conditions. The surgery proposed usually has a clearly defined objective and a precise target.

The debate over the morality of the treatment, however, is passionate. Some see psychosurgery as a benevolent surgical tool offering the relief to physical or mental agony that has been sought by mankind for millenia.[6] Others see it as nothing more than the old lobotomy in a new and more sophisticated form. Peter Breggin has attacked psychosurgery as "a uniformly dangerous operation—exactly what one would expect from mutilating normal brain tissue." Breggin is particularly concerned about the blunting of personality; for him, this concern extends even to surgical procedures for the relief of intractable pain:

> While accepting these scientific, ethical and political objections to psychosurgery in general, some well-meaning physicians and laymen still see a use for psychosurgery in the relief of intractable pain and anxiety in terminal illness. But the use of psychosurgery for this purpose borders on euthanasia—a partial destruction of the responsive

"self" or "identity" of the living human being—and therefore suffers from all the dangers inherent in euthanasia. But still more important, to allow its use for this one purpose opens up experimentation on thousands of dying patients and further promotes its future use for other more dangerous purposes.[7]

80   AIN'T NOBODY GONNA CUT ON MY HEAD

A 56-year-old farmer, Wilber Williams, accompanied by his wife, Nellie, consulted the Neurology Service of the Veterans Hospital because of a memory difficulty. For two years the patient had experienced increasing trouble with the technical aspects of his work. More recently he had been talking about his brother George as if he were alive although he had died two years earlier. He identified his own age as 48 and the year as "1960 . . .er, no, 1970." Examination revealed that the patient walked with a wide-based gait, a standard sign of brain pathology, and had a decreased cerebral function but was otherwise normal. The patient had no difficulty with simple coin problems and could repeat six digits.

Pleading pressing business, the patient declined hospitalization to determine the cause of his decreasing cerebral function. His wife tried to persuade him to enter the hospital, but when the physician suggested that she might assume guardianship of her husband through court action, she declined.

Six months later the patient's condition had worsened. Through the urging of the county agent the patient had leased most of his farmland to his neighbors and now did no work. His gait had became so wide-based that acquaintances mistakenly thought him inebriated. He urinated in his pants about once a week but seemed not to care. He sat watching television all day but paid no attention to the program content.

A medical examination showed an apparently alert man without speech difficulty but with considerable mental deterioration. This time the patient gave his age as 38, the year as 1949, the president as Eisenhower, and the location as a drugstore in his home town. He failed to recognize the name Lyndon Johnson, but upon hearing the name John F. Kennedy, he spontaneously volunteered knowledge of his assassination. The patient could not subtract 20 cents from a dollar but could name the number of nickels in a quarter. He could recite the months of the year and could, upon request from his wife, give fairly long quotations from the Bible.

The resident and the attending physician urged hospitalization. They told the patient that they would evaluate him for treatable causes of mental deterioration and memory deficit. In view of his wide-based gait and urinary incontinence in association with dementia, it was likely he had occult hydrocephalus. It was explained to the couple that this disorder causes decreased mental abilities by interference with the absorption of cerebrospinal fluid. The mental deterioration in such patients is partially reversible, as in his case at the present time, or completely reversible, as in his case six months ago when first seen. The treatment is to place a plastic tube through the skull to drain the cerebrospinal fluid from the brain to the vascular system, which was explained to the patient with diagrams. The patient immediately rejected the surgery, summarizing his thoughts with these words: "Ain't nobody gonna cut on my head."

The patient's wife again attempted to persuade the patient to accept hospitalization and, if tests confirmed the clinical impression, surgery. The attending physician argued to the wife that the patient did not have the mental competence to decide his own fate and that the wife should become the patient's legal guardian through court action and force his hospitalization. The wife politely but vigorously rejected this course of action, pointing out that in her family the husband made all important decisions.

The resident and the attending physician differed in opinions at this point. The resident thought the patient should be followed in the outpatient clinic until he perhaps changed his mind. The resident pointed out that though the patient had decreased mental abilities, he still retained enough intelligence to decide his own fate. The attending physician wished for court action to make the patient the ward of one of his relatives or, if necessary, the temporary ward of the hospital, and to force hospitalization and therapy.

This case emphasizes the dilemma of getting consent for surgical intervention when the consenting organ itself is apparently diseased. It also reveals that psychiatric and ethical dilemmas can arise even in a situation normally thought of as neurological rather than psychiatric. Two commentators have addressed the case. James Gustafson, a professor of theological ethics at the University of Chicago, defends court intervention to force the surgery against the instructions of the patient and his wife:

> The principal substantive moral issue in this case is the status of the right of the patient to determine his own bodily destiny. He refuses to consent to a procedure which is likely to relieve his disability, though apparently he understands in lay terms what is involved in the surgery. At his level of competence he is "informed," but he refuses to give "consent."
>
> The principle of informed consent is based upon one moral assumption and upon one philosophical judgment. The moral assumption is that individuals have a right to refuse treatment even when in the judg-

ment of others that treatment is in the patient's own best interests. A person has a right to determine his or her own destiny. The ground of this assumption is historically located in the libertarian tradition of Western culture; it stems from the same tradition that values civil liberties, that believes that the state exists properly only on the basis of the consent of the governed, and so forth. The philosophical justification for the individual's right to self-determination has been made in various ways: the right is "natural"; capacity for self-determination is what makes humans distinctive as a species and from this is derived both its value and the right; individual rights are conferred by God; excessive incursion on self-determination leads to repression and in turn to social unrest, and for this reason the right is to be protected.

The serious philosophical judgment on which the principle of informed consent is based is that persons actually have a capacity to determine their own destinies. Every case of this sort opens the historic debate about "free will" if the case is carried beyond the immediate clinical circumstances.

This case can be analyzed on the basis of two questions which follow from the two previous paragraphs. 1) Are there *moral* grounds for exerting persuasive, or legal and coercive, measures to override this man's presumed right of self-determination? Do his obligations to his family and to the community (or, to make the point in a weaker way, do the interests of his family and the community) provide a sufficient basis for intervention without his consent? How one would answer this question would depend upon the status of the right of self-determination in relation to the claims of communities (his family, the neighbors, etc.) to limit and even override that right. 2) Are this man's capacities to judge rationally and to act in accordance with a rational judgment impaired by his illness to the extent that he cannot properly exercise his moral right to self-determination? Is he, to use the common term, really "competent?" Does his impairment provide "excusing conditions" so that just as he is not held accountable for his wide gait, so he is not accountable for his rejection of the proposed therapy? Given the assumption of "free will" in the consent procedure, can his will be judged to be "less free" than is necessary and sufficient to make a sound judgment? The attending physician could justify his "wish" for court action on the basis of either or both of the matters raised by these questions.

In this case I would argue in favor of the attending physician's "wish." My principal argument would be on the basis of the patient's limited capacities to exercise his right of self-determination. Note that an empirical judgment about those limits is involved. A hypothesis (and that is all it is) would be required to support the argument, namely, if this man's capacities were not so impaired he would consent to the surgery. Procedurally, I would support the steps taken in the report of the case; that is, first seeking voluntary consent of the patient, then of his family, and only as a last resort seeking a court order. I am prepared also, however, to argue that this man has obligations to his family and to the community that he ought to take into account in making his own judgment. His failure to consent is, it appears, costly to others; others are dependent upon him and thus also have a claim on him to consent to a procedure that would permit him to fulfill his duties to them. Procedurally, if such a line of argument failed to persuade him, and then his family, there would be a moral justification for court action. At the base of my conviction here is a significant qualification of the individual libertarian tradition in the direction of a more "social" view of persons and of duties and obligations of persons to other individuals and to communities.[8]

The second commentator, Francis C. Pizzulli, a lawyer, defends the more libertarian position, favoring the right of the patient and his wife to refuse the surgery and emphasizing the long-term consequences of the court intervention:

At first blush, the attending physician presents a fairly convincing case for initiating state intrusion into the patient's brain. As the title of the case implies, the proffered therapy is fairly characterized as "brain surgery" and thus avoids categorization as "psychosurgery," replete with its politically value-laden premise of experimental treatment for the purpose of controlling socially deviant behavior. If, indeed, the preliminary diagnosis of occult hydrocephalus is sound, the operation would be tailored to rectify an accepted organic brain pathology. Though this entails the concomitant effect of controlling aberrant behavior (e.g., urinary maintenance and dementia), the presence of excess cerebrospinal fluid calls into play a well-defined medical/disease model which makes less persuasive the need to inquire into the motives of the physician as a check against the potential transmogrification of psychiatrists into thought-controllers.

If one were to accept the physician's evaluation of the mental incompetency of the patient, coerced institutionalization and treatment could be defended on a number of grounds. The procedure is relatively non-intrusive; to wit, it is a safe, non-experimental operation which involves no destruction of brain tissue and is intended to control behavior that ranks rather low on the continuum of volitional and autonomous functions. Not only is this intrusion minimal, but an array of humanitarian and utilitarian impulses militate for intervention. Does not the state have a moral obligation to the patient's former self to restore it? Or an obligation to construct a new self for the person, at which point he would be released to exercise his autonomy to its fullest potential? And would not this restoration to optimal functionality redound to the benefit of his family and community?

Even if we were to assume the patient's competency, the cost of overriding his competent judgment would be measured in terms of a single interference with personal autonomy at a particular time, presumably to be outweighed by the personal and social interest in a long-term increase in autonomy achieved by effective treatment.

Is there a decisive rebuttal to the physician's benevolent despotism? From a traditional legal perspective the case for involuntary commitment (i.e., enforced hospitalization) in this instance is rather weak. There is no mention of anti-social activities by the patient, which would warrant a finding of "dangerousness to others." To say that occasional urinary incontinence and mindless fixation upon the boob tube—behavioral traits found in many "normal" persons—constitute dangerousness to oneself reflects a most extreme paternalistic bias.

Even if the criteria for involuntary commitment are met, the case against intervention by no means fails. We cannot conclude that because an individual may no longer be competent to care for himself generally (e.g., due to memory deterioration), he is thereby incompetent to pass informed judgment upon such an intrusion as the proposed organic therapy. The notion of limited competency, besides having legal recognition, is rooted in the empirical observation that certain mental illnesses do not completely obliterate a person's ability to make decisions. While the patient may no longer recall dates and ages, it is hard to envision how memory deficit can totally discredit the capacity to understand the consequences of an operation, and to immediately summarize the resident's explanation and conclude with a refusal, as the patient has done. Even if we were to adopt the simplistic view that there is no competency where the refusal only occurred because of the mental deterioration, there is no evidence to indicate that the patient is other than strongly individualistic, and would not have decided likewise prior to the onset of deterioration. Moreover, the competent spouse's concurrence in his decision might be construed as evidence of agreement with his life-long views on brain surgery.

To respond to the invocation of a classic Benthamite calculus that would override limited, albeit informed, judgment to refuse therapy, we might profitably view the case from a rule-utilitarian perspective. While it may be true in this particular case that only a minimally intrusive operation is needed to arrest mental deterioration and partially restore memory function, we should ask what the consequences would be of a practice of substituting the state's judgment for individual informed consent in order to achieve the incremental gain in utility involved in curing those who suffer from marginal mental impairment. Is it too far-fetched to conclude that the result would be a society in which democratic values of personal autonomy, freedom, and privacy would be subjugated to the ideal of state control over various kinds of behavior?

There is one final barrier to coerced surgery, assuming for the sake of argument that there are grounds for civil commitment and that the patient does not have the limited competency to give informed refusal to treatment. Shall the next-of-kin be designated as the proxy, with the power to give or withhold consent? To argue in the negative, because it is suspected the spouse will only rubberstamp the incompetent's decision, conflicts with the legal presumption of identity of interests among kin. Likewise, to propose a third-party guardian who will rubberstamp the physician's decision, on the ground that it will enhance the well-being of the patient and his family, arrogates to the physician the right to define that well-being, instead of allowing it to be defined within the privacy of the family.

In sum, only a highly paternalistic society could tolerate the intrusions upon autonomy and privacy that would flow from a practice of coercion in cases such as that at hand.[9]

81   AMPHETAMINES AND THE PHYSICIAN'S RIGHT TO PRESCRIBE

John Ludlow, a 28-year-old physician, was employed in the student health service of a large state university. In the course of his work, he often saw students who requested pills for a variety of psychosomatic disorders related to anxiety or stress, such as insomnia, nervousness, and headaches, but he refused to prescribe dangerous psychoactive drugs with the potential for abuse because of his generally conservative attitude toward medication.

On one occasion, however, a friend of his, a graduate student in psychology, requested a prescription for a small number of amphetamine pills to use on the infrequent occasions when it was necessary for him to stay up late studying and he was unable to keep awake. The friend put a lot of pressure on Dr. Ludlow and reassured him that he neither used nor abused drugs and would use the amphetamine only if "absolutely necessary."

Dr. Ludlow looked up amphetamine in a standard reference text for drugs and learned that there were only three FDA-approved indications for the use of amphetamines in routine office practice: relief of narcolepsy, a condition in which the patient has uncontrollable spells of falling asleep; control of hyperkinetic behavior in children with "minimal brain dysfunction"; and weight reduction, a condition in the process of being withdrawn by the FDA.

Dr. Ludlow wrote out a prescription:

dextroamphetamine sulfate 5 mg. #6
sig.: 1/2 tab p.o. q 6 hours as needed

The state triplicate narcotics prescription blank required that he also list the pathological condition for which the controlled drug was being prescribed.

82   PRESCRIBING FOR THE AGGRESSIVE CHILD

Elvin Bradley was a 10-year-old who had recently entered the fourth grade at Benjamin Franklin School. He had been in a special education program since second grade, when he began to be inattentive, hyperactive, and aggressive in class and was found to be seven months behind in his reading level. For the last two years he had the same teacher, trained in special education, and was assigned in a small class where he received a lot of individual attention, which seemed to help his behavior problems somewhat, though not entirely. This September he was given a new teacher, who was older and not as patient with Elvin as his former teacher had been, and the class size was increased because of overcrowding and insufficient funds in the school system. His behavioral problems—hyperactivity, short attention span, and aggression—had gotten somewhat more serious.

Melvin Green, Elvin's teacher, called in his parents and, after discussing his hyperactive behavior, suggested that they take Elvin to his pediatrician to "see about getting some pills prescribed to calm him down." The teacher explained that Elvin behaved like many children who are found by their doctors to be "suffering from minimal brain damage" and that when these children are treated with amphetamines, they calm down and are able to pay better attention, become less disruptive, do better in class, and behave better at home.

Mrs. Bradley brought Elvin to the pediatric neurology clinic at Mount Zion Hospital and Medical Center, where he had been followed for four years for his hyperkinetic behavior. He had always been a very active child, who was easily frustrated and difficult to manage at home. After a thorough neurological evaluation at the age of six had revealed no abnormalities, the parents had been counseled to be especially patient and understanding with Elvin in order to give him the attention he needed. For the past several years he had continued to be hyperactive but did well at home and in school with only occasional relapses into aggressive behavior.

Mrs. Bradley now brought Elvin back to the doctor, concerned that her son did have something wrong with his brain and wanting to know if he should in fact take the pills his teacher had suggested. She explained to the doctor: "Elvin's teacher said that often the doctor can't tell by tests whether or not a person has minimal brain damage, but that if he improves when he takes the pills, that means he has it. He says there are over 200,000 children taking these pills for hyperactivity and that they really help and have no side effects. If that's all true I guess we should start Elvin on those pills."

———————

A more traditional and widespread way than psychosurgery to change human behavior is through drugs. While the use of drugs, at least through orthodox medical channels, is debated with much less passion than is psychosurgery, the proliferation of psychopharmacological agents in the 1960s and the expansion of their use for the amelioration of relatively mild psychoneurotic complaints had dramatized the ethical and social ramifications of their use. Diazepam, the antianxiety agent, is currently the largest selling drug in the United States. The other so-called minor or mild tranquilizers, such as chlordiazepoxide and meprobamate, the antidepressants, and the central nervous system stimulants are all major drug categories. Their use depends on a particular view of the world, a particular value system, or a particular attitude about the use of chemical agents to modify human behavior and experience.

Although these two cases are quite different, they pose a similar set of questions about the social and ethical foundations of drug use to modify behavior and experience in situations where controversy rages over the correct model for interpretation of the intervention. The first question that must be addressed to any problematic medical intervention is whether it will work, or better, how sure one must be that it will work. In the case of amphetamine use as a stimulant to increase productivity, as requested by the graduate student, the evidence of its effectiveness is clear. The main doubt is whether the side effects—the risk of nervousness and inability to concentrate that are sometimes reported with central nervous system stimulants—might interfere with the graduate student's work. In the case of the child with reported hyperactivity, the evidence also seems to be accumulating, although the mechanisms of action are not clear.[10] There are consistent reports of the paradoxical calming effect of stimulants like the amphetamines, possibly by increasing the arousal level of the central nervous system.[11] There is also clear evidence, however, that the effects of stimulant drugs vary from child to child, and some reports question the effectiveness of the drug in hyperkinesis.[12] Side effects are also reported, the most common of which are inability to sleep and loss of appetite.

The question of whether the drug will produce the desired effect is particularly critical in the case of the hyperactive child who cannot knowledgeably consent to the drug use. It leads to the second question raised by the cases: is informed consent necessary and is it sufficient? The graduate student would seem to have both the right and the responsibility to know the effects of any drug he is taking. If the university physician decides to write the prescription for him, he at least has a corollary obligation to make sure the student knows the effects of the drug.

Consent for the hyperactive child is more problematic. Most would hold that the parents must consent to any medical treatment for their child, especially one as controversial as the use of stimulant drugs for hyperkinesis. Consent, however, is a strange term for what the parents give. Unless the child is thought to be the property of the parents, consent might not be the parents' to give. Some have begun using the term "proxy consent" for such ambiguous situations. Here the presumption is that the guardian will act in the interests of the one who cannot himself give the consent. Doubts have arisen whether parental permission or refusal must be taken as definitive. There are cases in which parents have been found to be so unreasonable in refusing a medical treatment for their child that the courts have ordered the treatment, using the guise of taking temporary custody on the grounds of parental negligence.[13] These arguments presume that in most cases consent is a necessary condition for the use of behavior-modifying drugs, although it is clear that, especially in the case of parents, the consent itself raises serious problems. The exceptional case might be one where it is necessary to authorize treatment for children over the parents' expressed objection. The question is whether the use of behavior-modifying drugs could ever be authorized in this way.

Another question is whether consent or parental permission is always a sufficient condition for authorizing drug use, which directly forces the issue of the substantive legitimacy of drug use. In the case of the graduate student desiring amphetamines for a so-called nonapproved use, the doubts are particularly acute. Can two freely consenting adults acting in private agree to use a drug for a purpose that they take to be justified on balance after considering all of the risks and the benefits? If they can, why should the physician be involved in the decision at all? Assuming that the law required clear labeling of all the risks of amphetamine and permitted sale only to adults capable of reading the label, would this be a sufficient control on drug use among adults, or may society decide that some drug usages are so inconsistent with its mores that they can be forbidden? This question is particularly critical in the case of a proxy consent. The child cannot make an informed judgment. The question is whether society, acting through its agents, can at least forbid parental discretion for some kinds of drug use.

A fourth question is raised by these two cases. Both make use of drugs for social-behavioral purposes rather than for the more traditional medical purposes in the narrower sense. Is behavioral change, especially without direct evidence of an underlying physiological pathology, a legitimate use of chemicals, and if so, should those trained with medical skills be the gatekeepers? Why should the physician be the one who can consider prescribing the amphetamine for the purpose of increasing the graduate student's work capacity or for the purpose of changing the child's behavior? One response would be that drugs, as well as medical interventions in general, should be reserved for clear-cut medical problems. Another view, however, is that even for clear-cut medical problems people intervene when and only when behavioral or experiential change is desired. Thus there is no reason not to make use of such tools for behavioral purposes even when there is no evidence of physiological pathology.

No memory.

83 BEHAVIOR MODIFICATION
IN A LIFE-AND-DEATH SITUATION

In June of 1966, American psychiatrist Dr. Lloyd Cotter, an unpaid participant in an AMA-sponsored program to aid the medically-neglected South Vietnamese civilians, arrived at the Bien Hoa Mental Hospital to join the three Vietnamese psychiatrists working there. It was located on physically beautiful grounds, but the patients' conditions within the wards varied from good to deplorable. No treatment program other than custodial care existed for more than three-quarters of the 2000 patients.

More disturbing, about one patient per day was dying—six times the usual mortality rate owing to inflation and the inability of the hospital director to convince the South Vietnamese government of the importance of increasing the hospital's food money. The patients were aware that the poor quality of the food was killing them and were asking that something be done. When all other attempts to better the food situation came to naught, the psychiatrists decided that the only recourse was to have the patients grow food on the hospital grounds. That this activity would probably benefit the patients insofar as their mental illness was concerned was considered a secondary benefit.

Asking the patients to work to better the food situation produced only a few volunteers no matter what reasonable rewards were promised. It became apparent that a massive behavior modification approach was required. Difficult decisions were then made concerning the techniques to be used which would not have been made if physician inactivity relative to the high mortality rate had not been considered an immoral alternative. An aversion to the idea of depriving malnourished people of their food, even for a short period of time, resulted instead in the initial decision to use electroconvulsive treatment or ECT as a negative reinforcer for work. Generally, behavior modifiers prefer to use only positive reinforcers. When negative reinforcers are used, the least aversive which will produce the desired results is, of course, preferable. On the other hand, starting with an ineffective reinforcement and gradually increasing its intensity may foster adaptation on the part of the patients and thus the ineffectiveness of other reinforcers which if used initially would have achieved desired results. The quick elimination of the unnecessarily high death rate was the goal which strengthened the resolve to choose effective reinforcers immediately.

The 120 nonvolunteering patients on the first ward were told: "People who are too sick to work need treatment. It is not painful and is nothing to be afraid of. When you get well enough to work, let us know." ECT was continued on a three-times-a-week schedule. Gradually there began to be evident improvement in the behavior of the patients, the appearance of the ward, and the number of patients volunteering for work.

However, for many, the option of terminating shock treatment did not prove to constitute a sufficient incentive for them to begin work. For these patients, with some trepidation and reluctance, a second proposal was set forth: "Look. We doctors, nurses, and technicians have to work for our food, clothes, rent, money, etc. Why should you have it any better? Your muscles are just as good as ours. After this, if you don't work, you don't eat. Who is ready to start work immediately rather than miss any meals?" About twelve patients made this choice; the others received nothing to eat. During the next three days, with no food for the non-workers, all the remaining patients volunteered for work. A sigh of relief was breathed that none had held out to the point of starvation or death.

Thus, all the hospital patients who were not physically ill were motivated to assume the work role and were paid one piastre for each day's work. They were in a routine roughly approximating their functioning outside of the hospital. Functioning as normal is usually of great assistance in the development or return of the patient's feelings and thoughts to a more healthy state. The patients in the field working to alleviate the food shortage displayed good spirits and made comments which indicated that they were more satisfied with themselves in their more productive and useful role and grateful for having been pushed into it.

Long-term patients who had failed to respond to other treatment modalities were included in a program which could be expected to result in better adjustment and probably in more rapid recovery for a satisfying percentage of such patients. More important, since most crops grow rapidly in the tropics, the food problem was soon resolved and the death rate returned to the normal rate of about one death per week.

In his conclusion Dr. Cotter shares his conviction that those mental hospitals which feed, clothe, and shelter schizophrenics without effectively demanding anything from them in the way of productivity are perpetuating rather than treating the schizophrenic illness with its sick needs for withdrawal, regression, and dependency. If faced with the same situation again, he would certainly not waste time with the only partially effective ECT. He states, "If the less effective, but more usually relied on reinforcements of productive behavior do not work, then a more effective reinforcement, such as food for hungry patients, will produce the desired results . . . [their use] should not be neglected due to misguided ideas of what constitutes kindness."[14]

----

1. Was the behavior modification effort successful? What factors must be taken into consideration to judge a program successful?
2. How important is success in evaluating the ethical implications of a behavior modification program? Is it possible to be successful and yet

wrong, in the moral sense, or is a program that produces the most good on balance necessarily right?

3. What were the other options available in this case and how do they compare?

4. Should psychiatric treatment choices which do not involve patient consent be excluded despite the fact that patient deaths or chronic illness may result from no treatment or failure of other treatments? Is the violation of a mentally ill person's civil rights ever justified? Should not mental patients be allowed to die with their rights intact if that is their apparent choice?

5. Should mentally ill patients ever be denied regular scheduling of that most basic necessity, food? Can the end justify the means? Did it in this case?

6. If an increased mortality rate had not been a factor in this case, would the techniques used have been justified?

CHAPTER 11

Experimentation
on Human Beings

Some of the most dramatic and complex problems in medical ethics arise in the context of experimenting on human subjects. In one sense medicine has always experimented. From the time of the shaman, medical practitioners have at times tried something out on a patient when his disease has appeared unusual or resistant to the currently accepted treatment. Classical medical systems, including the Hippocratic, developed new treatments, and in some cases these were even organized in a rudimentally rational fashion. The concept of a "medical experiment," however, is a uniquely modern phenomenon. If the term refers to a procedure systematically designed and controlled for the purposes of gaining information instead of or in addition to curing a particular patient, the practice did not arise until the modern period. By tradition, Harvey, who in 1628 published his research on circulation, is given the title of father of systematic medical research. In fact, the clearly differentiated concept of the medical experiment did not emerge until the nineteenth century. There is no specific mention of the ethical obligations of the researcher in the Hippocratic oath, the oath of Maimonides, or other classical codes prior to the nineteenth century.

As long as the notion of medical manipulation of the patient-subject primarily for the purpose of gaining knowledge had not emerged, the Hippocratic ethic could still apply. According to the oath, the physician's moral obligation is to do what he thinks will benefit the patient according to his "ability and judgment." Strict adherence to the oath flatly prohibits nontherapeutic research and even procedures during therapy primarily for the purposes of research, such as taking an extra milliliter of blood for an experimental assay.

Consent of the subject for experimenting has recently become the central focus of debate. The issues, however, are much more complex, and they shade into questions not limited to the experimental context. These include: the relationship of therapeutic to nontherapeutic procedures, the relation of subject risk to societal benefit, the degree of organization that qualifies a procedure as an experiment, the duty to continue a successful experimental procedure, the right of a patient to be an experimental subject, the problem of privacy, the researcher's responsibility for harmful consequences, and the publication of unethical research.

Justifying the Decision

Several factors are involved in justifying a decision to experiment on humans. One is the possible benefit to the patient. Another relates to the adequacy of the consent of the subject. Still another concerns the limits, if any, on the risks a competent adult should be allowed to take, whether for therapeutic or nontherapeutic reasons. And finally it must be determined what rights the patient has to demand experimentation for his own sake.

84 PSYCHOSURGERY FOR A SEXUAL PSYCHOPATH

This case came to this Court originally on a complaint for a Writ of Habeas Corpus brought by Plaintiff Kaimowitz on behalf of John Doe and the Medical Committee for Human Rights, alleging that John Doe was being illegally detained in the Lafayette Clinic for the purpose of experimental psychosurgery.

John Doe had been committed by the Kalamazoo County Circuit Court on January 11, 1955, to the Ionia State Hospital as a Criminal Sexual Psychopath, without a trial of criminal charges, under the terms of the then existing Criminal Sexual Psychopathic law. He had been charged with the murder and subsequent rape of a student nurse at the Kalamazoo State Hospital while he was confined there as a mental patient.

In 1972, Drs. Ernst Rodin and Jacques Gottlieb of the Lafayette Clinic, a facility of the Michigan Department of Mental Health, had filed a proposal "For the Study of Treatment of Uncontrollable Aggression."

This was funded by the Legislature of the State of Michigan for the fiscal year of 1972. After more than 17 years at the Ionia State Hospital, John Doe was transferred to the Lafayette Clinic in November of

1972 as a suitable research subject for the Clinic's study of uncontrollable aggression.

Under the terms of the study, 24 criminal sexual psychopaths in the State's mental health system were to be subjects of experiment. The experiment was to compare the effects of surgery on the amygdaloid portion of the limbic system of the brain with the effect of the drug cryproterone acetate on the male hormone flow. The comparison was intended to show which, if either, could be used in controlling aggression of males in an institutional setting, and to afford lasting permanant relief from such aggression to the patient.

Substantial difficulties were encountered in locating a suitable patient population for the surgical procedures and a matched controlled group for the treatment by the anti-androgen drug. As a matter of fact, it was concluded that John Doe was the only known appropriate candidate available within the state mental health system for the surgical experiment.

John Doe signed an "informed consent" form to become an experimental subject prior to his transfer from the Ionia State Hospital. He had obtained signatures from his parents giving consent for the experimental and innovative surgical procedures to be performed on his brain, and two separate three-man review committees were established by Dr. Rodin to review the scientific worthiness of the study and the validity of the consent obtained from Doe.

The Scientific Review Committee, headed by Dr. Elliot Luby, approved of the procedure, and the Human Rights Review Committee, consisting of Ralph Slovenko, a Professor of Law and Psychiatry at Wayne State University, Monsignor Clifford Sawher, and Frank Moran, a Certified Public Accountant, gave their approval to the procedure.

Even though no experimental subjects were found to be available in the state mental health system other than John Doe, Dr. Rodin prepared to proceed with the experiment on Doe, and depth electrodes were to be inserted into his brain on or about January 15, 1973.

Early in January, 1973, Plaintiff Kaimowitz became aware of the work being contemplated on John Doe and made his concern known to the Detroit Free Press. Considerable newspaper publicity ensued and this action was filed shortly thereafter.

With the rush of publicity on the filing of the original suit, funds for the research project were stopped by Dr. Gordon Yudashkin, Director of the Department of Mental Health, and the investigators, Drs. Gottlieb and Rodin, dropped their plans to pursue the research set out in the proposal. They reaffirm at trial, however, their belief in the scientific, medical and ethical soundness of the proposal.

Upon the request of counsel, a Three-Judge Court was empanelled, Judges John D. O'Hair and George E. Bowles joining Judge Horace W. Gilmore. Dean Francis A. Allen and Prof. Robert A. Burt of the University of Michigan Law School were appointed as counsel for John Doe.

Approximately the same time Amicus Curiae, the American Ortho-psychiatric Society, sought to enter the case with the right to offer testimony. This was granted by the Court.

Three ultimate issues were framed for consideration by the Court. The first related to the constitutionality of the detention of Doe. The second is after failure of established therapies, may an adult or a legally appointed guardian, if the adult is involuntarily detained at a facility within the jurisdiction of the State Department of Mental Health, give legally adequate consent to an innovative or experimental surgical procedure on the brain, if there is demonstrable physical abnormality of the brain, and the procedure is designed to ameliorate behavior, which is either personally tormenting to the patient or so profoundly disruptive that the patient cannot safely live or live with others?

Finally the court addressed the question "If the answer to the above is yes, then is it legal in this State to undertake an innovative or experimental surgical procedure on the brain of an adult who is involuntarily detained at a facility within the jurisdiction of the State Department of Mental Health, if there is demonstrable physical abnormality of the brain and the procedure is designed to ameliorate behavior which is either personally tormenting to the patient or so profoundly disruptive that the patient cannot safely live or live with others?"

After a long hearing on the issues of the case the court ruled that informed consent cannot be given by an involuntarily detained mental patient for experimental psychosurgery and that although guardian or parental consent may be legally adequate when arising out of traditional circumstances, it is legally ineffective in the psychosurgery situation. The court held that the guardian or parent cannot do that which the patient, absent a guardian, would be legally unable to do.

The "informed consent" form signed by John Doe and submitted to the court read as follows:

Since conventional treatment efforts over a period of several years have not enabled me to control my outbursts of rage and anti-social behavior, I submit an application to be a subject in a research project which may offer me a form of effective therapy. This therapy is based upon the idea that episodes of anti-social rage and sexuality might be triggered by a disturbance in certain portions of my brain. I understand that in order to be certain that a significant brain disturbance exists, which might relate to my anti-social behavior, an initial operation will have to be performed. This procedure consists of placing fine wires into my brain, which will record the electrical activity from those structures which play a part in anger and sexuality. These electrical waves can be studied to determine the presence of an abnormality.

In addition electrical stimulation with weak currents passed through these wires will be done in order to find out if one or several points in the brain can trigger my episodes of violence or unlawful sexuality. In other words this stimulation may cause me to want to commit an aggressive or sexual act, but every effort will be made to have a sufficient number of people present to control me. If the brain disturbance is limited to a small area, I understand that the investigators will destroy this part of my brain with an electrical current. If the abnormality comes from a larger part of my brain, I agree that it should be surgically removed, if the doctors determine that it can be done so, without risk of side effects. Should the electrical activity from the parts of my brain into which the wires have been placed reveal that there is no significant abnormality, the wires will simply be withdrawn.

I realize that any operation on the brain carries a number of risks which may be slight, but could be potentially serious. These risks include infection, bleeding, temporary or permanent weakness or paralysis of one or more of my legs or arms, difficulties with speech and thinking, as well as the ability to feel, touch, pain and temperature. Under extraordinary circumstances, it is also possible that I might not survive the operation.

Fully aware of the risks detailed in the paragraphs above, I authorize the physicians of Lafayette Clinic and Providence Hospital to perform the procedures as outlined above.

	/s/
Date	Signature
	/s/
Witness	Signature of responsible relative [1]

The striking thing about the proposed psychosurgery experiment is that, in spite of the fact that it is one of the most dramatic interventions in man's biology and has potentially horrendous consequences, it probably passes the ethical test of the Hippocratic oath. According to the ability and judgment of the researcher-physician, the experiment is evidently judged beneficial to the patient-subject. Granted that the researcher has other purposes in mind, including the gathering of knowledge about the treatment of uncontrollable aggression, it seems plausible for him, or at least for some researcher somewhere in the world, to conclude that in his judgment in the procedure on balance can be conducted because of the potential benefit to the patient, given the alternatives open to that patient.

There is clearly something wrong with a moral requirement based solely on the researcher's personal judgment about what will benefit the patient rather than on what will "really" benefit him, as some modern codes of ethics for medical professionals have recognized. The general codes of medical ethics, as well as the more significant codes on experimentation, reveal the great confusion surrounding the conflict between patient risk and possible societal benefit (see Appendices). The International Code of Medical Ethics, for instance, requires: "Under no circumstance is a doctor permitted to do anything that would weaken the physical or mental resistance of a human being except from strictly therapeutic or prophylactic indications imposed in the interest of his patient." Such a requirement, if applied to John Doe, candidate for psychosurgery, would eliminate justifying the procedure simply because the researcher thinks it will benefit him, but it still requires that the subject benefit. It also raises the question of who will decide whether he will indeed benefit.

Some, however, remain uncomfortable with the requirement that every medical procedure be justified by its potential benefit to the patient. The World Medical Association itself, which authored the International Code of Medical Ethics in 1949, began to have second thoughts. By 1954 their "Principles for Those in Research and Experimentation," refering to experimentation on both sick and healthy subjects, emphasized that healthy subjects should be "fully informed." By 1964 in the Declaration of Helsinki, the World Medical Association felt it necessary to make a positive case for the necessity of research, including that which does not benefit the subject directly: "It is essential that the results of laboratory experiments be applied to human beings to further scientific knowledge and to help suffering humanity." The recommendations include a set of guidelines for "non-therapeutic clinical research." The patient-benefiting principle, at least in some cases, has fallen to claims of more societal needs and interests.

85   CAN OVERWHELMING RISKS BE JUSTIFIED?

In December 1964, 155 subjects were tested and interviewed to determine if they would be suitable candidates for an experiment on the individual's personality. The subjects were recruited from an advertisement for experimental subjects to be paid at a rate of $2 per hour. Of the 155, 12 percent knew a considerable amount about LSD, 15 percent had never heard of it, and the remainder had only casual knowledge. Fourteen percent were enthusiastic about participating in the experiment, while 23 percent expressed concern over the safety of LSD. The rest were simply curious and "had no expectations of lasting effects, either beneficial or detrimental."

Of the 155 subjects, 34 were disqualified because of a previous experience with LSD or peyote, a history of psychosis in the immediate family, or a doubtful interview or psychological profile. Another 24 withdrew for other reasons, such as school or job load. In addition, 25 withdrew because of concern over the dangers of LSD.

Before receiving the test drug, each subject was given a battery of tests, including tests of anxiety, attitudes and values, aesthetic sensitivity and creativity, and projective tests. He was also given the Minnesota Multiphasic Inventory for psychological screening and the Myers-Briggs Type Indicator and Aas' Hypnotic Susceptibility tests for matching experimental and control subjects. He received a one-hour interview with a clinical psychologist in which he was told he might or might not receive LSD. The psychologist "attempted to establish rapport with the subject, allay anxiety, assure him that he would be well cared for, and that no surprises, tests, or other demands would be introduced during the drug session . . . Questions pertaining to safety of LSD were answered, but no mention was made of possible personality or other changes resulting from the experience." The experiments were double-blind; that is, neither researcher nor subject knew whether an active drug was being given until the drug symptoms were sufficient to identify the drug. The subjects were divided into three groups, to be given either 200 ug. LSD, 20 mg. amphetamine (5 mg. immediate and 15 mg. sustained release), or 25 ug. LSD per subject in three separate day-long sessions during the first eight months of 1965. The last two groups, though expected to produce some effects, were considered control groups for the purpose of the study.

The drugs were administered to all the subjects at 8 AM in a room specially designed to enhance the drug experience. A psychologist in the background did not initiate interaction unless the subjects appeared to require support. At 5 PM a graduate student took the subjects to dinner and then to their homes. Arrangements were made for the subjects to be in the company of a friend during the evening. They were given a sedative to take if needed on retiring.

In the 200 ug. LSD group, six subjects withdrew after the first session. Three of these probably would have continued had they not been influenced to withdraw by wives or friends. The other three suffered frightening anxiety reactions. A seventh subject was terminated by the researcher after a "prolonged unrealistic reaction with some grandiose paranoid tendencies which slowly subsided." All subjects were given a follow-up testing two weeks and six months after their last drug session.[2]

In this case, in contrast to the psychosurgery case, no plausible argument can be made that it is conducted for the benefit of the subjects. There seem to be serious problems about the nature of the consent. A substantial majority of the subjects, at least those in the original subject pool, had no more than casual knowledge of LSD and "had no expectations of lasting effects, either beneficial or detrimental." No information was given to the subjects about the possible long-range personality changes.

Suppose, however, that the researchers had decided to inform the subjects specifically of those risks. There are still two problems. First, the knowledge would seriously jeopardize the results of the experiment itself. Such information might change results as fragile as psychological profiles. This possibility suggests that the class of experiments that would be destroyed if risks or purposes were disclosed either must be banned entirely or must be conducted with something less than full consent.

Even if there were full disclosure and some way were found to disclose without destroying the experiment, a fundamental question remains. Can society permit subjects knowingly and voluntarily to accept serious experimental risks merely because for some reason, whether selfish, humanitarian, medical, or financial, the subject and the researcher are both willing to proceed? Should an unlimited right to experimental medicine be granted to fully competent and mutually consenting adults for nontherapeutic purposes?

In the case of the LSD experiment, the calculation of risk involves a choice of life styles. If the subjects were indeed informed of the risks, it would seem that societal disapproval should not, in itself, be enough to forbid the experiment. One function of a review committee, besides monitoring research and assuring adequate consent, must be to decide when the potential consequences of the experiment are so harmful in proportion to the risks that the experiment must be banned even in the face of a consenting researcher and subject.

86   EXPERIMENTING OR JUST FOOLING AROUND

George Martin, a second-year medical student working in the clinical chemistry lab in the summer, was running the glucose machine when he noticed that the lab had received from the clinic five samples of amniotic fluid, the fluid surrounding a fetus, for glucose tolerance tests. He knew from his summer's experience that they usually received about one a week from the clinic.

He mentioned the extra tests of amniotic fluid to his supervisor, who seemed upset and said she would speak to the clinic about it. The next week when the student was back in the lab, he noticed that this time they had received no amniotic fluids from the clinic, which he remarked to his supervisor. She told him that someone had again sent five amniotic fluid samples that morning from the clinic and the clinic director had told him to stop. A physician in the clinic had simply had an idea about the relation of the glucose tolerance to some aspect of fetal health and thought he would try out his idea on a small scale before designing a formal experiment on the idea.

----

1. When does an experiment become an experiment? If the physician had simply asked about and recorded some special aspect of the women's

diet solely for the purpose of trying out an idea of his, would that procedure have been more acceptable?

2. Who is the subject of the experiment? The consensus of medical opinion at the time these fluid samples were taken was that there is probably a small but nevertheless real risk to the fetus in each removal of amniotic fluid. If the fetus is put at risk for purposes unrelated to its own medical benefit, does this constitute unacceptable experimenting on the fetus? If so, since a fetus can never consent to experimentation, does this mean that all procedures not potentially beneficial are banned for all those who cannot consent?

3. What is the role of the medical student, nurse, lab technician, and others in subordinate positions when they discover medical procedures raising ethical questions?

This case raises the problem of risks to nonconsenting subjects, including possibly nonconsenting unborn children. It also raises the question of recognizing a medical experiment when it occurs. Because of such cases, a distinction has been drawn between experiments that are potentially beneficial for the subject and those that are not. The first instinct is to require rigorous control for experiments that have no potential for benefiting the subject. This is probably a much overemphasized and even misleading distinction, however. It is clear that a patient must consent for medical treatment whether or not it is experimental. Older codes of experimentation propose the alternative of "benefit or consent." The British Medical Association in 1963 approved a code on experimentation which specifies: "No new technique or investigation shall be undertaken on a patient unless it is strictly necessary for the treatment of the patient, or, alternatively, that following a full explanation the doctor has obtained the patient's free and valid consent to his actions, preferably in writing." The Public Health Council of the Netherlands adopted a similar position, as did the authors of the 1955 version of the "Ethical and Religious Directives for Catholic Hospitals." The 1971 revision of the "Directives" modified the benefit or consent formulation, saying simply that experimentation on patients without consent is morally objectionable. In fact, a case can be made that those who can potentially benefit from a medical treatment are in the greatest jeopardy in the experiment situation. They are in a weakened condition and are also in need of continued services from medical personnel. If such is the case, the hospital patient who is a candidate for research unrelated to the disease for which he is hospitalized is in the worst possible position. A ban on all nonbeneficial research on hospitalized patients has been seriously proposed by some concerned about protecting those patients.

87 BENEFITING MENTALLY RETARDED CHILDREN BY GIVING THEM HEPATITIS

Willowbrook State Hospital is an institution for the care of the mentally retarded in Staten Island, New York. In 1972 there were 5200 residents, 3800 severely retarded, with IQ's of less than 20. In 1954 Dr. Saul Krugman was appointed as a consultant in pediatrics and in infectious diseases. When he began work, he discovered that such diseases were very prevalent at Willowbrook, including hepatitis, measles, shigellosis, parasitic infections, and respiratory infections. Dr. Krugman and his colleagues began a number of studies of those diseases, including research on measles vaccine and hepatitis.

In 1956 Dr. Krugman, together with Drs. Joan Giles and Jack Hammond, began studies on hepatitis. Four times a year from then until 1970 they admitted approximately 12-15 children into their research unit, for a total of 700-800 children out of the 10,000 admissions to the hospital. The researchers injected infected serum to produce hepatitis in the patient-subjects in their research unit. The objective was to gain a better understanding of the disease and possibly to develop methods of immunizing against hepatitis. The research was approved by the Armed Forces Epidemiological Board, one of the funders of the research, the executive faculty and the Committee on Human Experimentation of New York University, where Dr. Krugman held a faculty position, and the New York State Department of Mental Hygiene.

The researchers defended their decision to expose the children to strains of hepatitis virus on the following grounds:

(1) they were bound to be exposed to the same strains under the natural conditions existing in the institution; (2) they would be admitted to a special, well-equipped, and well-staffed unit where they would be isolated from exposure to other infectious diseases which were prevalent in the institution—namely, shigellosis, parasitic infections, and respiratory infections—thus, their exposure in the hepatitis unit would be associated with less risk than the type of institutional exposure where multiple infections could occur; (3) they were likely to have a sub-clinical infection followed by immunity to the particular hepatitis virus; and (4) only children with parents who gave their informed consent would be included.[3]

---

1. Was the experiment designed to protect the mentally retarded at Willowbrook? Was the best medical care of the time, such as gamma globulin injections, given to the children on the research ward? Were all the exposed children really going to get hepatitis?
2. Why was the United States Army one of the funders, and what kind of review did they provide? Were the reviews by the army, the university with whom the researchers were affiliated, and the state Department of Mental Hygiene adequate, or is a more rigorous review necessary in cases where research involves institutionalized patients who by the very nature of their condition cannot give informed and voluntary consent?

3. Were some parents coerced into the experiment by offering their children a place in the research ward when no places were open in the general facilities? Was the parental consent for such a study adequate in the first place? Were there other possible subjects, such as adults about to receive blood transfusions, who could have given valid consent to be subjects of the research?

All things considered, there is the possibility that the patients in a research project such as this, who are undergoing controlled exposure to hepatitis but are receiving high-quality general health care, might be better off than their peers in the general institutional wards. Independent of problems of consent and research alternatives, there is a remaining question. Is it ethically acceptable to justify an experiment on the grounds that the subject will benefit from the research, when he will benefit from it only because of the social condition in which he finds himself? In this case it is clear that if the residents at Willowbrook received optimum health care and lived in minimally sanitary conditions, the argument that the subjects in the research unit would on balance be better off by receiving the intentional exposure to hepatitis would collapse.

Upon reflection, most subjects would appear to volunteer for experiments because their social condition has created a situation where, on balance, they are better off in the experiment than fending for themselves. Prisoners with no outside means of earning money volunteer for risky drug testings. Clinic patients volunteer when they fear, rightly or wrongly, that they have no other means of getting needed medical care. Except in cases where the experiment provides real hope for treating a medical condition that cannot be remedied by a change in the social condition of the patient, as with subjects for trying new cancer treatments, "volunteers" are always recruited because of the social alternatives open to them.

What are the ethical options? The Hippocratic ethic of being concerned only about benefiting the patient may justify ignoring the sociopolitical conditions of the hospital that make hepatitis rampant in the first place. To rechannel attention from the subjects in the research ward to the primary health needs of those in the general wards would improve the health of the group in toto, but perhaps not so much that those who are research ward residents would be any better off than they would be if the research continued. Does that justify and in fact generate a moral obligation to continue the research rather than shifting attention to the more general hospital conditions? This might be the implication of a duty to do only what will benefit one's patients. The individualism of the Hippocratic ethic could conceivably justify a duty to ignore the broader social conditions.

If, however, broader social conditions are indeed relevant to the debate about the justification of the experiment, what options remain open? At one extreme one could argue that the moral duty of any researcher encountering a group of subjects who will volunteer only because of their social condition is to improve that condition rather than take advantage of it. Certainly the ordinary random individual in society does not have a strict moral duty to alleviate every case of suffering in the world, but this is a special relationship. Researchers, presumably physicians trained with the skills needed for care, have a specific institutional affiliation with the group of patients needing medical care. One might argue from a morally rigorous position that there is always a duty to alleviate social conditions producing suffering when one has the skill and is directly involved in a relationship with those suffering. This view is "rigorous" in that it has a utopian quality. Everyone would certainly be better off if all in such positions throughout the world indeed fulfilled their obligation, but in a less than utopian world there will always be those in need for whom research on, say, hepatitis immunization might, once developed, relieve much suffering. A rigorous moral position might lead to the conclusion that it is impossible ever to develop drugs to treat a socially caused disease, just as research on a "clean" nuclear bomb might be considered inherently unacceptable.

At the other extreme is the argument that one can trade off a medical service to the general group in need of medical help for the privilege of experimenting. In a prison, for instance, a physician might trade the offer of twenty hours of work in the prison infirmary for the right to test a drug on a group of the prisoners. This proposal has a crassness, however, suggesting that the individual may be sacrificed for the good of the group. The end results might benefit the whole group, but the benefit to the subject certainly cannot justify the experimental risk. When patients, such as mentally retarded children, cannot consent, it seems hard to defend the trade-off.

What then is the solution? Is there an intermediate position, such as research designed to benefit the subjects vis-à-vis their other alternatives combined with a commitment to alleviate the underlying conditions of the group from which the subjects were drawn? The conflict is a fundamental one between an ethic that compromises with the evil of the world and an ethic that refuses to condone an intentional evil even if that evil may on balance prevent more harm in the real world.

88 THE DUTY TO EXPERIMENT

The patient, Martha Ambrose, was a 47-year-old who had entered the gynecological clinic three years before her current admission with a mass in the lower right quadrant. In surgery the medical team had cleaned out as much of the tumor as could be seen. A year before this admission Mrs. Ambrose had had a second operation also for the carcinoma. Since then she had been treated with radiation and chemotherapy.

At the time of the second operation the patient had signed herself out of the hospital after a heated dispute with the attending physician. She in fact had a long and unpleasant relationship with the hospital. She was first seen by the gynecological service at age 17 for treatment of gonorrhea. She had an arrest record for prostitution, petty shoplifting, and bizarre public behavior including assault. She had been seen in the psychiatric clinic on a number of occasions for the aggressive street behavior. She had an IQ of 85-90, and there was the unconfirmed possibility of organic brain damage. She had had two brief marriages and was currently unemployed.

The present hospitalization began four months previously with severe pain in the pelvic area. There were now secondary metastases to the lungs and possibly to the central nervous system. She was being maintained on meperidine to relieve the pain. Her condition changed from day to day. There were periods in which she was semicomatose intermixed with periods of hyperactivity, anxiety, and hostility in which she demanded treatment. The surgeon was considering a radical, experimental surgical procedure which had a minute chance of giving survival for a year or possibly even longer. Without the surgery the woman was given at most a few weeks to survive.

The medical team was divided on the proper course. The surgeon wanted to try the surgery but admitted that he might better spend his time with other patients in the overcrowded ward. The physicians who would be responsible for her care after the surgery were reluctant to invest the time and resources in what was admittedly a long-shot procedure. The patient was heard shouting, "I demand that you operate on my cancer."

There is one more dimension to the ethics of justifying the decision to undertake an experimental procedure. Possibly in the case of mentally retarded children at risk for hepatitis, but more probably in the case of the sexual psychopath tormented with the fear of uncontrollable rage, some patients may want to claim a right to receive an experimental treatment. It is normally assumed that no physician is obligated to take on a patient without his consent. Certainly the notion of a physician being required to perform a particular medical treatment when he does not approve of that treatment seems abhorrent. Yet health care is also beginning to be seen as a right. In Wyatt v. Stickney the courts recognized that the confined mentally ill have a fundamental right to needed health care. Further, the patient has a right to control over decisions, including medical decisions, that affect his own body. To complicate the matter, while a physician is not normally obligated to accept a patient without his consent, it seems both reasonable and legally required that a physician cannot abandon a patient under his care without making suitable arrangements for the patient and giving proper notice to the patient.

What does all of this mean for a patient who is demanding an experimental procedure from a physician who is unwilling to render it? One major body of medical ethical opinion holds that neither the patient nor the physician is required to use "extraordinary" medical treatments. Whatever the definition of extraordinary, it would appear that experimental, radical surgery with only minute hope of limited success would qualify. If, however, the patient is not obligated to undergo the experimental surgery, does she have a right to? When the ethical tradition states that neither patient nor physician is obligated to participate in extraordinary treatment, does this include those cases where the patient is pleading for the treatment and the physician is reluctant?

In cases such as the woman demanding an operation for her cancer, there is certainly a right, in principle, for the physician to perform the surgery, if he is willing. Or fulfilling her right may take a careful referral of the patient to another physician willing to perform the surgery or even case-by-case adjudication in the courts to determine if the treatment desired by the patient must be given and, if so, by whom. In some classes of patients, however, there is danger of removing any semblance of a right to consent to experimental treatment. This may be the implication, for instance, of the court decision in the case of the sexual psychopath who at first consented to the experimental psychosurgery. If the courts, the law, the medical profession, or some practitioners within that profession declare that, in principle, no incarcerated, mentally ill, or minor person can consent or have proxy consent for certain classes of experimental treatment, are they depriving patients in those classes of the right to participate in potentially therapeutic experiments to the same degree as competent adult patients? An experiment may be justifiable in a specific case because the patient insists he wants it, even if the procedure cannot be more generally accepted for the general class of patients.

The Research Process

The ethical issues that arise before the experiment can begin—such as consenting to overwhelming risk, justifying patient risk by countervailing social benefits, benefiting patients because of their miserable social condition, and agreeing to a patient's choice of an "extraordinary" procedure—may all seem to differ from the ethical issues that arise in the conduct of the experiment or after the experiment is concluded. In the end, however, the distinction may prove artificial. It may well be that some experiments cannot be justified in their inception simply because there is no conceivable way for the researcher to deal with the envisioned moral implications at some point in the research process. For instance, in the case of protecting the privacy of subjects when gathering potentially incriminating information, even if the criteria of consent and acceptable benefit-harm ratio are met, a research project may be morally unacceptable if there is no conceivable manner of protecting the confidentiality of the data.

Another question which arises during the course of some experiments but which should be considered ahead of time involves the ethical obligations that are generated should the experiment prove successful. In many cases the object is to produce a short-term cure. The results are either successful and the patient is cured, or unsuccessful and the patient dies. In other cases, however, the object is to develop a long-term treatment which the researchers can anticipate will be both scarce and expensive. The question is whether the researchers have a duty to continue a successful experimental treatment.

Conversely, ethical obligations may be incurred by the researchers when an unsuccessful experiment produces unexpected harm. A moral dilemma is involved when unethical research produces needed findings.

89 PRIVACY AND EXPERIMENTATION

The emergency room of State Hospital was the city's primary referral institution for medical emergencies. Of the scores of crises dealt with on a typical day, several were psychiatric episodes. The city police, as well as friends and relatives acting in a private capacity, often brought in bizarrely behaving individuals for emergency attention prior to more permanent disposition in the psychiatric ward of the hospital, in private hospitals, or, for police cases, in the city penal system. The emergency room was staffed by State Medical School, which had authority over medical affairs at the hospital. In addition to the regular nursing and physician personnel on duty in the emergency room, available for consultation were a psychiatric nurse, a resident, an intern, and usually two medical students, one third-year, the other fourth-year. A staff attending psychiatrist was on call.

A person brought to the hospital in acute crisis was normally seen first by the nursing staff and then by the available psychiatric resident or intern. Medical students generally handled a part of the intake interview, but occasionally, when the emergency room was particularly crowded, they had to do the entire workup.

Dr. James Warton, chief of the psychiatric service, and Dr. Emily Branton, a senior staff psychiatrist, were concerned that such inexperienced staff were often handling patients in extremely serious condition.

They recognized the importance of the experience for the young physicians and medical students, and were convinced that they usually handled their cases competently, but doubt remained. The two psychiatrists also recognized that, given the present funding problems, the alternatives were very limited. They decided to undertake a research project to evaluate the quality of interaction in these initial intake interviews. The most effective way to conduct the research, they reasoned, would be to videotape the interviews and evaluate them systematically. Under study would be three groups of medical personnel and two groups of patients. The residents, who had from two to five years of hospital experience, would be included in one group, the interns, who were one to two years out of medical school, would be in the second group, and the medical students would be in group three. The patients were initially divided into two broad groups: those in acute reactions to psychoactive drugs, and all others. This selection was made because the researchers believed that the personnel were probably more adequate in the former group. Later, if it seemed worthwhile, the patient groups would be broken down further on the basis of more specific diagnoses.

In order to get the most realistic assessment of the medical personnel and patients, the two psychiatrists decided that they would have to tape the interviews without the consent of patients or professionals. This was arranged for by placing a videotape camera and microphone in the radiator grate. Drs. Warton and Branton were disturbed about the resulting invasion of privacy. They first considered asking for permission, but concluded that it would invalidate the results. They were driven on to conduct the experiment by their fear that some patients were getting less than optimum care. They were convinced that only with hard evidence of such inadequacy, evidence that might come from the proposed study, could they persuade the state Department of Health of their desperate need for additional staff. Furthermore, the tapes would be monitored personally by one of the two researchers, who could then intervene, as soon as was possible without revealing their project, so as to counteract any errors made by the young personnel. By this procedure they felt that patient care would possibly be better than at present.

---

1. To what risks, if any, are the subjects of the experiment exposed?
2. Are the risks justified by the potential benefits to the subjects?
3. Are they justified by the potential benefits to others, such as future patients in the emergency room and in other emergency rooms similarly staffed?
4. Who are the subjects in the experiment?
5. Is the invasion of privacy that concerned the researchers better thought of as a "risk" or as an ethical concern independent of risk?
6. What steps should the researchers consider if they want to assure

themselves that others will not have access to the tapes and the data taken from the tapes?

7. The situation is one where police are at times linked to the cases and where some patients, those who are in acute psychotic reaction to psychoactive drugs, have probably engaged in illegal behavior. Are the risks and the invasions of privacy more serious in these cases? If so, what can be done with the research design and the storage of data to protect against unintended consequences?

8. If researchers acquire by whatever means evidence that patients have engaged in illegal behavior, what is their obligation to the patient and to society? What reasons, if any, would justify using information gathered for research purposes to facilitate law enforcement, protection of the interests of third parties, or other goals?

90   THE DUTY TO CONTINUE EXPERIMENTING

In the late 1940s medical researchers were discovering the pharmacology of the cortisone compounds and testing their use in a number of conditions, including rheumatoid arthritis. A 41-year-old had been suffering some symptoms of rheumatoid arthritis and rheumatoid spondylitis since 1936. Both conditions were chronic after 1944. He was admitted to the hospital on September 5, 1948. At the time many peripheral joints were swollen and tender. There was a flattening of the lumbar region, an abnormal curvature, and marked limitation of motion of the spine. His right knee was flexed ten degrees, and movement of the left arm was limited. Other treatments had been ineffective.

After being withdrawn from aspirin, the patient was given 100 mg. of cortisone for seventy-five days, which caused marked improvement in his condition. Within two days he had lost much of his stiffness. He was able to walk and climb stairs. By November 16, swelling and pain at rest had disappeared from all his joints with the exception of the right knee.

Without the knowledge of the patient or the clinical researchers, cholesterol was given for seventeen days from December 19 to January 4 to see if the absence of cortisone could be detected. Stiffness returned. On January 5, cortisone was resumed again without the knowledge of the patient or clinical researchers. Within thirty-six hours the response to the cortisone was noted. The patient was continued on cortisone or cortisone acetate from January 5 until May 25. During the course of the treatment minimal side effects were noted, including mild transient dizziness, increased energy and restlessness, some difficulty focusing his eyes when reading, which was corrected by glasses, and possibly a more rapid growth of hair. The researchers noted on a follow-up examination after the end of the experiment: "In June, about two weeks after the patient's dismissal, the condition of right knee flared up moderately; other joints were unchanged. Then arthritic activity increased slightly. Moderate exhaustion occurred for three or four weeks. Late in August (three months without cortisone) he visited the clinic. He thought that he had lost 15 to 20 percent of his maximal improvement. The right knee was moderately swollen and slightly tender."[4]

This case is from a previous generation of medical experimentation and must be evaluated in that context. The purpose of presenting it is not to debate what the researchers did or should have done for the patients who were apparently benefiting from cortisone treatments. Rather, the question is what moral obligation contemporary researchers have to the patient when they undertake research that will, if successful, provide a treatment for chronic conditions. Remarkably little attention is given to this dimension of experimentation ethics involving the duty to continue treatment. No mention is made, for instance, in the current guidelines of the Department of Health, Education, and Welfare or in any of the public and professional codes on experimentation.

Does there exist a duty to the patient to continue a treatment once it appears to be successful? If stopping the treatment would lead to death, as in the development of insulin, is there an obligation to continue the experiment as therapy? If the researchers do not have a special obligation to treat the patient before the experiment begins, do they acquire such a duty by way of temporarily saving the subject's life or relieving his suffering? Does any such duty continue when the product becomes available on the market, as insulin did quite rapidly after the initial clinical trials? How is the responsibility divided for any continuation of therapy? Is the funding agency, the clinical researcher, the researcher's institution, or the individual subject responsible for continuing costs?

91 THE RESPONSIBILITY FOR HARMFUL CONSEQUENCES

Compound HR-7724 had just received approval from the Food and Drug Administration for investigational use in human beings. Both the research and the marketing divisions of Houston Pharmaceuticals were excited. They sensed that they were on the verge of a treatment for atherosclerosis which would be both a money-maker to them and a help to mankind in fighting the leading chronic killer of adults in the world.

Compound HR-7724 had gone through thorough animal tests: two years in rats, two six-month trials in two species of dogs, including beagles, at two dosage levels selected for the production of toxic effects, and one year in monkeys. In the group of fifty rats, one registered a weight loss in the final two months and one died of undetermined causes. One of the control group of rats also died. In the dogs and monkeys no toxicity could be demonstrated even at dosage levels ten times the effective dosage calculated on a per kilogram basis. The first phase of the trials in human beings had been completed on healthy patients at the State Prison with no observed toxicity.

Dr. Nathan Barnes was a leading internist in Houston. He contracted with Houston Pharmaceuticals to conduct the second phase of clinical trials in human beings. Phase two trials are the first tests in patients who might themselves potentially benefit from the drug being tested. The trials would be conducted at the research ward at Jerome Hospital. It had been built by Houston Pharmaceuticals and was the site of many of their early stage clinical trials. Dr. Barnes had tested HR-7724 in four previous subjects. All had been patients of his suffering from advanced coronary artery disease. All were given meticulous details of the risks envisioned: minimal risk of build-up of precursors of cholesterol with little known effect, minor hair and skin changes, and possibly nausea. The patients were also informed that an earlier compound designed for similar purposes (MER/29) had produced cataracts, but the mode of action of HR-7724 was substantially different. No cataracts or other effects on the eye were found in any animal species and none were anticipated in humans. The subjects signed a detailed consent form after being given a chance to ask additional questions.

In the fifth patient, symptoms began to appear approximately two weeks after initiation of the drug trial. First there was a loss of appetite, nausea, and some vomiting. Jaundice developed rapidly, together with upper abdominal pain and tenderness. A diagnosis of acute toxic hepatitis led to an immediate suspension of the trial. After a week of intensive treatment in the research unit, the patient was transferred to Community Hospital where his general practitioner had privileges, and where the costs of his care would be covered by his own group medical insurance policy.

---

1. This case raises another aspect of continuing responsibility, namely, responsibility for unanticipated harm in an experiment. Who should bear the responsibility for the care of the patient-subject: the medical insurance, the research doctor, the local physician, or the drug company?
2. If it can be shown that the drug is the cause of the liver damage, does that shift the locus of responsibility?
3. If the subject is a paid subject for a phase one trial, that is, a normal subject for the purpose of testing toxicity, does this shift the locus of responsibility?

4. What if the subject for the phase one clinical trial is a nonpaid volunteer?

5. Current HEW regulations require that for HEW-funded research "the agreement, written or oral, entered into by the subject, should include no exculpatory language through which the subject is made to waive, or appear to waive, any of his legal rights, or to release the institution or its agents from liability for negligence." Should this requirement be extended to research conducted under auspices other than HEW-funded research?

6. Should the ban on a waiver of liability be limited to cases of negligence, or should it apply to all damage resulting from the experiment whether negligent or not?

7. Should there be a positive requirement to tell the patient who will be responsible for damage done rather than simply a ban on the waiver of liability?

92   PUBLISHING UNETHICAL RESEARCH

Dr. Jefferson Oxford, senior editor of the distinguished medical journal *Biomedical and Pharmacological Research,* had just received a manuscript for review and possible publication in his journal. The research involved giving the drug Chloridomide to four hundred pregnant women scheduled for abortion at a major medical center. Chloridomide, an anti-anxiety agent distantly related to thalidomide, was being developed by Webster Pharmaceuticals and had recently been approved for use in psychiatric practice for all but pregnant women. Following the thalidomide scare, Webster and the Food and Drug Administration had been particularly cautious in permitting the use of such drugs for pregnant women.

Drs. Frank Hyman, Joseph Polk, and Lois Victor, the three senior attending physicians in the obstetrics service of the hospital where the study had been done, were concerned about the use of the drug in pregnant women. They had obtained a supply of Chloridomide from Webster and let it be known in the community that the obstetrics clinic would perform pregnancy tests on women seven days after a missed period and would perform abortions on those who requested it if the woman was found to be pregnant. This permitted them to administer the drug to four hundred women coming to their service for abortion during the years 1971-1973. The scientific paper under consideration reported that three of the abortuses of the women given the drug had gross anatomical defects similar to the thalidomide babies. The report included the fact that in order to avoid any possible psychogenic effect on the pregnancies, the women were told simply that they were being given vitamins to prepare them for the abortions. In fact, the Chloridomide was placed in a capsule that did contain vitamins as well. The "vitamins" were begun immediately, so that if there was an effect on the fetus, it would be likely to be seen. The women were told that hospital scheduling problems required a delay of approximately five weeks before the abortion could be performed and that in the meantime they should take their "vitamins" daily.

Dr. Oxford knew that effective August 8, 1975, about a month before the journal received the manuscript, such research would have been prohibited by HEW guidelines. Those guidelines specify:

(a) No pregnant woman may be involved as a subject in an activity covered by this subpart unless: (1) The purpose of the activity is to meet the health needs of the mother and the fetus will be placed at risk only to the minimal extent necessary to meet such needs, or (2) the risk to the fetus is minimal.

(b) An activity permitted under paragraph (a) of this section may be conducted only if the mother and father are legally competent and have given their informed consent after having been fully informed regarding possible impact on the fetus, except that the father's informed consent need not be secured if: (1) The purpose of the activity is to meet the health needs of the mother; (2) his identity or whereabouts cannot reasonably be ascertained; (3) he is not reasonably available; or (4) the pregnancy resulted from rape.

Dr. Oxford contacted Dr. Hyman by telephone to raise what he thought were serious ethical problems in the research. Dr. Hyman responded that the research was done during 1971-1973, before the guidelines were in effect. Moreover, the research was not conducted with a grant from HEW but with funds of the drug company and the Department of Obstetrics, so that even if the guidelines had been in effect, they would not have applied to this research.

Dr. Oxford replied that he was arguing not that the research was illegal but rather that it was unethical to entice these women into the clinic for the pregnancy test, give them the experimental drug under false pretenses, and delay their abortions for research purposes. Dr. Hyman countered that the research was ethical because the Chloridomide might have been therapeutic for the women, combating the anxiety of the unwanted pregnancy and the abortion. In any case there was no risk to the fetuses, according to Dr. Hyman, because they were to be aborted anyway. Even if every fetus had gross physical malformations, it would mean nothing to an abortus. Finally, Dr. Hyman argued that it would have been unethical to inform the women, thereby increasing their anxiety and possibly their guilt feelings for having taken the experimental drug. Not only might it have destroyed the validity of the experiment, because of the experimental artifact of the anxiety caused by fear of the drug, but more important, according to Dr. Hyman, it would have been cruel needlessly to expose these women to the added trauma when they were already undergoing a great burden. The physician's duty is to benefit the patient, not to create needless anxiety.

Dr. Oxford was not convinced. He conceded that there was ambiguity in the HEW guidelines. They did not make clear whether a fetus scheduled for an abortion could justifiably be considered at minimal risk when exposed to a drug that would be a high risk for a baby going to term simply because the fetus would in all likelihood never reach postnatal life. More significantly, he was convinced that women have a right to consent to such experimental manipulations or at least a right to consent to the delay in the abortion.

Dr. Oxford was also convinced, however, that the findings were important. If he were to refuse to publish the paper on ethical grounds, women taking the drug and unexpectedly becoming pregnant could bear more thalidomide-like babies. Furthermore, if he refused to publish the paper, some other journal probably would.

There are at least three options that Dr. Oxford ought to consider. The traditional view of editors of scientific journals is that their journals were created to disseminate scientific findings. They should not get involved in making ethical or other value judgments about the work of their contributors. This value-free approach to scientific publishing has encountered serious problems, however. Even the defenders of value-free science, such as Max Weber, recognize that for certain steps in the process of scientific investigation value inputs are necessary.[5] One of these is the selection of "valuable" subjects to investigate and report. One of the crucial functions of an editor is to select from among the scientifically accurate studies submitted those that are most important or most valued for purposes of publication. The selection criteria depend not only on the validity of the conclusions but also on the worthiness of the subject. Values necessarily play a role in making those decisions. The remaining question is whether an ethical evaluation of the data-gathering process should be considered or whether the choice should rest entirely on other ethical and value considerations.

A second option for Dr. Oxford to consider is the refusal of the manuscript on ethical grounds if he decides that the research is unethical. This judgment recognizes the moral and logical impossibility of excluding value considerations. It is a judgment reached by Dr. Franz J. Ingelfinger, editor of *The New England Journal of Medicine,* who takes the position that "reports of investigations performed unethically are not accepted for publication."[6] The decision not to publish can be defended on the grounds that one should not participate in an unethical act, even indirectly and even if that act produces good results. If subjects are treated as means to an end without their consent, then the research is unethical even if good results follow. Another defense rests on a judgment about the long-term consequences of the practice of refusing to publish such research. It is conceded that useful information will be lost by refusing to publish, but if researchers are dissuaded from conducting unethical research in the future because they know that their research publications will be refused, then the policy of refusal might produce more good consequences than bad.

There are objections to this second position as well, however. For one, it is likely that Dr. Hyman and his colleagues will find another journal to publish their study. If the refusing journal were as prestigious as *The New England Journal of Medicine,* the researchers might suffer from having to publish in a lesser journal, but they would still get most of the benefits of publication. Furthermore, no one would know of the ethical stand taken by Dr. Oxford. The policy of refusing to publish work considered unethical also requires dependence on the editor's personal ethical judgment or that of his editorial board. Some research considered unethical by the reasonable person might not be rejected on ethical grounds by particular editors no matter how high their moral standards. If a work is published in a journal with a policy such as Dr. Ingelfinger's, however, it implies that a positive ethical judgment has been made. In that case presumably the broader public would eventually be able to enter into the ethical evaluation. If the reverse happened, however, if the editor judged unacceptable a piece of research acceptable to the broader community, the research would be lost and not available to public scrutiny unless published elsewhere.

These problems have led to a third option. Robert J. Levine, editor of the journal *Clinical Research* and a professor of medicine at Yale University, has advocated the policy that "Manuscripts describing research conducted unethically but which satisfy the usual scientific criteria for acceptability should be published along with editorials on which the ethical deficiencies are exposed and criticized."[7] Such a plan raises the ethics of the research to a level of public debate. It makes the useful data available, but in a context where the publisher makes clear his ethical reservations. It has also been proposed that the author be given space to reply to the editorial criticism.

This plan still leaves difficult questions unanswered. Does publication imply that the editor is furthering unethical actions? Does it sacrifice or enhance the deterrent effect of the no publication policy? Do editors, especially those who are members of a professional group such as physicians, have an additional ethical responsibility beyond deciding whether to publish or whether to editorialize? Most professional groups impose a duty on their members to report evidence of unethical conduct to an appropriate professional board for review. A confidence that members of the profession will fulfill this responsibility is the only justification for the public's reliance on professional modes of discipline. Especially in the case of the editor who refuses to publish, it can be argued that he is suppressing the unethical conduct of a colleague when he has a duty to expose it. The same duty to initiate professional disciplinary action might well rest on an editor who takes the stance that his journal is a value-free vehicle for scientific communication, or even on the editor who editorially exposes his ethical reservations about a piece published in his journal. The only alternative would seem to be a special exemption from the general duty to initiate disciplinary proceedings for any member of the profession who is filling the role of editor. The basis for such an exemption has never been articulated.

CHAPTER 12

Consent and the Right To Refuse Treatment

Consent is becoming one of the major issues in the ethics of experimentation on human subjects. Traditionally there has been a radical separation between the principle of consent for experimentation and consent for nonexperimental therapeutic medical treatment. The notion of consent is relatively new in human history. Traditional medical ethical principles required that the physician do what he thought would benefit the patient. Not only was it not until the modern period that the notion of rational and systematic experimenting in medicine for the purpose of gaining knowledge emerged as a dominant principle to separate the medical experiment from medical treatment, but the modern period has produced the emphasis on individual freedom and self-determination which is at the root of the principle of consent. The Lockean principles of individualism and autonomy which form the basis of Anglo-American political philosophy also lie behind the emergence of the principle of reasonably informed consent.

Percival wrote a code of ethics for the Manchester Infirmary which, when published in 1803, was to become the foundation of professional medical ethics for the English-speaking world. In it he recognizes that when ordinary modes of medical practice do not help in a particular situation, it is essential that ''new remedies and new methods of chirurgical treatment should be devised.'' He warns that the physician undertakes such innovation at his own peril and even that no such trials should be instituted without a previous consultation with other physicians and surgeons, but there is nary a word about consulting the patient.[1] American court cases of the late nineteenth century follow the same principle. As late as 1895 a judge could argue: "When a particular mode of treatment is upheld by a consensus of opinion among the members of the profession, it should be followed by the ordinary practitioner; and, if a physician sees fit to experiment with some other mode, he should do so at his peril. In other words, he must be able, in the case of deleterious results, to satisfy the jury that he had reason for the faith that was in him, and justify his experiment by some reasonable theory."[2]

There is not any reference to patient consent even for experimental procedures. By 1914 Judge Benjamin Cardozo was applying the principle of individual self-determination to medicine, arguing that "every human being of adult years and sound mind has a right to determine what shall be done with his own body; and a surgeon who performs an operation without his patient's consent commits an assault, for which he is liable in damages."[3] Not until the 1960s, however, did the radical implications of the principle of patient consent really begin to be recognized, both for experimentation and for the more normal therapeutic patient contact.

The problems of consent for both medical experimentation and nonexperimental medical treatment can involve either normal adults or subjects who cannot give free and informed consent either because they are unable to comprehend the implications of the experiment or because they are in a position, such as a prison or mental institution, where free choice is problematic. No consent, of course, can ever be completely free or totally informed. To attack the notion of "fully informed" consent is to attack a straw man. The real question is when consent is "reasonably free and informed," that is, sufficiently voluntary and knowledgeable that the reasonable person would judge it adequate. In acutal cases these judgments can be infinitely complex.

Consenting to Experiments

Of all the cases involving consent, that of the healthy, mentally competent adult volunteering for a medical experiment is probably the simplest. The issue of whether the subject is sufficiently informed and sufficiently free to consent, however, is still sometimes difficult to resolve. It is important to realize that consent can be either voluntary and not informed, or vice versa.

93 HOW INFORMED IS INFORMED CONSENT?

Walter Halushka was a summer school student at the University of Saskatchewan in 1961. Applying for a job at the student employment office, he was told that no jobs were available but that he could be paid $50 by

serving as a subject in an experiment at the University Hospital. Drs.
G. M. Wyant and J. E. Merriman were conducting tests of an experimental general anesthetic, Fluoromar, to measure heart and circulatory
response. It had not previously been used or tested by these researchers in
any way.

On August 22, 1961, Mr. Halushka went to the anesthesia department
at the University Hospital. He was told that the experiment involved
making an incision in his left arm and inserting a catheter or tube into his
vein. It would take about two hours. He was given the following consent
form:

Consent for Tests on Volunteers

I, Walter Halushka, age 21 of 236 3rd Street, Saskatoon hereby state
that I have volunteered for tests upon my person for the purpose of
study of

[Blank filled in] Heart & Blood Circulation Response under General
Anesthesia

The tests to be undertaken in connection with this study have been
explained to me and I understand fully what is proposed to be done. I
agree of my own free will to submit to these tests, and in consideration
of the remuneration hereafter set forth, I do release the chief investigators,

[Blank filled in] Drs. G. M. Wyant and J. E. Merriman,

their associates, technicians, and each thereof, other personnel involved in these studies, the University Hospital Board, and the University of Saskatchewan from all responsibility and claims whatsoever,
for any untoward effects or accidents due to or arising out of said
tests, either directly or indirectly.
Witness my hand and seal.
[Signed] Walter Halushka
[Signed] Iris Zaechtowski (Witness)
Date: Aug. 22/61

According to the court record, Mr. Halushka was told that the test was
"perfectly safe" and that it "had been conducted many times before."
He asked the researchers what was meant by "accident" in the consent
form and was told that it meant things like falling downstairs at home
after the test.

During the test, which was performed the next day, a catheter was inserted in the vein and pushed toward the heart. As it approached the
heart, Mr. Halushka felt some discomfort. The anesthetic was administered and the catheter tip was advanced through the chambers of the
heart and out into the pulmonary artery. After about fifty minutes there

were changes in cardiac rhythm, suggesting to the researchers that the anesthesia level was too deep. Five minutes later the subject underwent complete cardiac arrest. The heart was resuscitated by manual massage. An incision was made from the breastbone to the line of the armpit and two ribs were pulled apart. A vasopressor was administered to stimulate heart heat, as well as urea, a drug used to combat swelling of the brain. After one minute and thirty seconds the subject's heart began to function again. Mr. Halushka remained unconscious for four days. He was discharged ten days later, after having been given $50 by the researchers.

Mr. Halushka claimed that afterward he felt a considerable amount of pain in the chest area and that a portion of his left arm was numb for approximately six weeks. The next fall at school he became very tired every day and had to rest for about three hours before doing his homework. He failed six or seven subjects that year and did not try to continue his university education.

Mr. Halushka brought suit against the university, claiming a lack of informed consent. Testimony at the trial established that the use of any anesthetic agent involves "a certain amount of risk." Cardiac arrest can result in temporary or permanent brain cell damage sometimes leading to death. A consultant could find no abnormality at the time of the trial, some four years later, but stated that he knew of no equipment which could unequivocally determine whether there had been minor brain damage. While the consultant gave the opinion that the insertion of a catheter into the heart is not a dangerous procedure, other competent experts at the time claimed that the risk of catheterization of the right side of the heart is about one death per thousand cases.[4]

This case is a landmark in understanding the meaning of informed consent. It is clear that Mr. Halushka signed a piece of paper called a "Consent for Tests on Volunteers" but also that the information transmitted about the risks of the test was not adequate to call the consent reasonably well informed. The question growing out of the case is just what information the subject would have needed to make his consent reasonably informed. The Department of Health, Education, and Welfare used this particular case as the basis for its formulation of guidelines for consent:

> Informed consent is the agreement obtained from a subject, or from his authorized representative, to the subject's participation in an activity.
>   The basic elements of informed consent are:
>   1. A fair explanation of the procedures to be followed, including an identification of those which are experimental;
>   2. A description of the attendant discomforts and risks;
>   3. A description of the benefits to be expected;

4. A disclosure of appropriate alternative procedures that would be advantageous for the subject;

5. An offer to answer any inquiries concerning the procedures;

6. An instruction that the subject is free to withdraw his consent and to discontinue participation in the project or activity at any time.

In addition, the agreement, written or oral, entered into by the subject should include no exculpatory language through which the subject is made to waive, or appear to waive, any of his legal rights, or to release the institution or its agents from liability for negligence.[5]

There is little in this list with which to quibble. The more difficult question is whether these requirements are all that is needed to make a consent reasonably informed. Those who are insisting on the most rigorous standards for informed consent demand that additional information be transmitted to the subject before the consent can be called informed. The Nuremberg Code requires that the purpose of the experiment be explained. In the test of Fluoromar this might not have created a serious problem, although if Mr. Halushka had been told that the purpose was to test a general anesthetic for the first time, it might have given him pause. In other experiments, especially psychiatric, psychological, and social ones, the entire experiment might be destroyed if the purpose is revealed.

The Nuremberg Code calls for the disclosure not only of discomforts and risks but also of "inconveniences" reasonably to be expected. While inconveniences might be thought of as a risk, many researchers would not include them.

The consent form signed by Mr. Halushka contains language by which he appears to waive any claims against the researchers, their agents, or the university. Such waivers do not always stand up in court, but often subjects may not realize the fact. The HEW guidelines ban exculpatory language by which the subject is made to appear to release the institution "from liability for negligence." There is still the problem of liability for damage done during an experiment where the researchers are not negligent. Suppose that the researchers inform the subject that there was one chance in a thousand of permanent heart damage which would require continual medical attention. Who should be liable for the costs? Some have suggested that an institution be banned from asking for a waiver of any liability whether from negligence or not. Others have proposed that the requirement be put more positively. In order for consent to be informed, the subject should be told who will be responsible if something goes wrong. If the institution and the researchers are not willing to be responsible for damages, then the subject must be told. This is not now required in the HEW guidelines. For research not conducted with HEW funding none of the guidelines apply, even the banning of a liability waiver.

Other possible requirements include the name of the chairman of the human experimentation committee or someone to whom the subject can turn if he has questions. If the experiment is one in which the subject might benefit medically, he might have to be told explicitly whether there is a placebo in the research design, whether he will be able to continue getting the medication if the research is designed to test a drug for possible chronic use, and whether he has the right to obtain the best available treatment from the institution if he chooses not to participate in the experiment.

94   NONBENEFICIAL RESEARCH ON THE CHILD

The Protection of Human Subjects Committee of a major teaching hospital had just been submitted a research protocol for a prospective study of ten infants at high risk of allergic diseases. A paired group of ten infants not at high risk would be followed as controls during the same period. The committee had a flat policy, with respect to those who cannot give informed consent, of never permitting research that was not potentially beneficial to the subjects themselves if the research could be done on consenting adult subjects. The committee had another policy for experiments on those who cannot consent of considering each case individually, both when the research might possibly be more beneficial to the subjects than to the normal population, and when the subject was no more likely to benefit than the normal population and the risk to the subject was viewed as minimal.

According to the proposal, a pediatrician specializing in allergic diseases planned a five-year study on the development of allergy, especially asthma. Allergy tends to occur in families: if both parents have allergic symptoms, there is a 75 percent chance of allergy in the children; if one parent is allergic, a 50 percent chance of allergy in the children; and only 30 percent if allergic patients have no family history of allergy. Consequently, the investigator proposed to study children at high risk from families in which both parents and a sibling had allergy, along with a control group of children from families with no history of allergy.

Asthma and other allergies are widespread in the American population, which includes seven million chronic asthma sufferers and another seven million with a history of asthma that could recur at any time. Asthma is the leading chronic disease in children, accounting for 25 percent of school absences annually. An additional seventeen million Americans suffer from other allergic diseases of sufficient severity to cause them to seek professional care; thirty million more treat themselves with over-the-counter antihistamine medicines for minor allergic symptoms. The study sought to advance the scientific understanding of allergic diseases by focusing on the early developmental stages and possible isolation of environmental events that tend to turn on the allergic sensitization mechanism.

Ten families in the high-risk group and another ten controls would be selected in the first year of the study. It was hoped that four or five families would remain throughout the entire five-year period. Substitute families would be sought for those that dropped out. Procedures on the infant and child subjects would consist of: blood samples, 10-15 ml. each, drawn quarterly during the first two years of life and twice annually in succeeding years; and evaluation of allergic status by metabolic and skin tests and by inhalation of a substance known to provoke asthmatic attacks twice each year during the first two years of life and annually thereafter. Additional evaluations would be performed if appropriate.

The proposed procedures involved certain risks. Venipuncture carried the remote possibility of infection and the more immediate danger of hematoma or a swelling caused by the accumulation of blood at the puncture site. The intradermal injection of 1 ug. acetylcholine for sweat tests could also cause an infection or hematoma, as could the epinephrine tolerance test. Airway resistance tests using a mask and body box could cause crying, leading to a rise in blood pressure with the possible bursting of a blood vessel, or cold air inhalation, leading to a reflex bronchospasm.

The allergic families would be chosen mainly from among those who had been referred to the principal investigator for help in managing allergic problems in the siblings. The control families would be selected from scientific personnel, that is, mostly or entirely from members of the university's faculty and staff. The primary physician of the selected families would not be a member of the investigating team. Each procedure was assigned a reimbursement figure arrived at by estimating transportation and baby-sitter costs and inconvenience to the family routine. The reimbursement schedule could amount to up to $300 per family per year, but in practice would probably amount to $50 a year or less.

The procedures and their attendant risks were set out in a written consent form to be signed by the parents. The investigators proposed to interview both parents, together if possible, during pregnancy. During the interview the project would be explained in detail and the goals clearly stated. The primary goal of the study was a possible benefit to society. The possible personal benefit to the individual infant or child would be presented as clearly secondary. The principal investigator would also seek an interview with the potential subject's primary physician to explain the study and enlist his or her cooperation as an independent medical advisor to the family regarding its participation in the study.

The proposed study touches the heart of the question of the use of child subjects in medical experimentation. The infants and children are put at risk in order to gather data which it is hoped will be useful to a reasonably large segment of the American population—victims of allergic diseases—for whom this and other studies may provide more effective therapy. The infant subjects will be studied before they are known to have or not to have allergic disease. And they obviously cannot personally consent to their participation in the study. In addition, the question of unfair inducement is raised regarding the consent of the parents.

Two schools of thought exist on the question of research on children and others who cannot consent, such as prisoners or the mentally ill, when the research is no more likely to benefit the subjects than the normal population. The Protection of Human Subjects Committee, by deciding to examine this proposal including research on a control group of infants who are not at abnormal risk for allergy, has implicitly taken the position that at least in some cases such experimenting is acceptable.

A radically different position is implied in the Nuremberg Code. Though it does not refer to children explicitly, it charges that "the person involved should have legal capacity to give consent." Although there is a generally held belief that research on children which will be of no direct benefit to them is forbidden by English common law, William Curran and Henry Beecher argue that English law actually reveals no authoritative support for such a flat conclusion. They do, however, recognize that the British Medical Research Council has published a statement opposing all such research, and they quote Sir Harvey Druitt, who advised the council in formulating its position. Druitt's interpretation is: "a parent's right to assault his child is in law strictly limited. No doubt the parent has the right to consent to a doctor carrying out upon his child medical procedures which are thought to be for the child's benefit. But I am confident that the parent has no legal authority to consent to medical procedures being carried out on his child for the advancement of scientific knowledge or for the benefit of humanity, if those procedures 'are of no particular benefit to' the child and 'may carry some risk of harm.' "[6]

American interpretations have not usually been so restrictive. The American Medical Association's Ethical Guidelines for Clinical Investigation, adopted in 1966, permit "nontherapeutic" investigations on minors or mentally incompetent persons only if "The nature of the investigation is such that mentally competent adults would not be suitable subjects," and "Consent, in writing, is given by a legally authorized representative of the subject under circumstances in which an informed and prudent adult would reasonably be expected to volunteer himself or his child as a subject."

Of course, the AMA is a private professional organization and its views do not have the weight of law. Its position raises certain problems. Certainly it should not be sufficient for a parent to be willing to volunteer himself for an experiment in order to justify volunteering his child. Adults may altruistically take risks for the benefit of mankind and be praised for it, but that cannot justify imposing a similar risk on their children.

The only official American public policy on consent for children is contained in the HEW regulations on the protection of human subjects. These guidelines are binding on all research funded by HEW and apply on a voluntary basis to all research conducted at some 750 institutions receiving HEW funds. They require that the "informed consent of subjects will be obtained by methods that are adequate and appropriate," but define informed consent as "the agreement obtained from a subject, or from his authorized representative, to the subjects' participation in an activity." Thus it can be a representative and not the subject himself who is informed and consenting. The guidelines spell out the requirements when the subject himself cannot consent: "When the subject group will include individuals who are not legally or physically capable of giving informed consent, because of age, mental incapacity, or inability to communicate, the review committee should consider the validity of consent by next of kin, legal guardians, or by other qualified third parties representative of the subjects' interests. In such instances, careful consideration should be given by the committee not only to whether these third parties can be presumed to have the necessary depth of interest and concern with the subjects' rights and welfare, but also to whether these third parties will be legally authorized to expose the subjects to the risks involved."[7]

On November 16, 1973, the report of a special study group dealing with the problems of protection of children, prisoners, and the institutionalized mentally infirm was published.[8] Currently their findings are under consideration as official regulations at HEW. The study concludes, "When research might expose a subject to risk without defined therapeutic benefit or other positive effect on that subject's well-being, parental or guardian consent appears to be insufficient." The study proposes the formation of several "Ethical Review Boards" to provide rigorous review of "specific proposals or classes of proposals" submitted to HEW by sponsoring agencies. The board would be required to review all proposals involving children except those where it is determined the children are not at risk. In addition, a local "protection committee" would have to determine whether it is justifiable to conduct a particular investigation on children. Thus for research involving children and others who cannot themselves consent, even when that research will not benefit them directly some research could be approved. This is departure from the traditional medical commitment of working to benefit the patient and not society in general.

---

1. Are the control group infants "at risk"? Is it possible to do an experiment where there is no risk and therefore to exempt the protocol from consent guidelines?
2. Since control group families will be selected from scientific personnel, who can be expected to be unusually sympathetic to medical research, are infants in those families subjected to additional risks?
3. Would the experiment be more or less acceptable if parents were not paid at all?
4. If some potentially valuable experiments can be done only when normal infants or children are involved, are there other methods of recruiting subjects? What about selecting on the basis of fitness, by random choice or lot, or by parent plus public guardian?
5. For research on older children, should they be required to consent as well? How old should a child be before his consent is added to that of his guardian? How old should he be before his consent replaces that of his guardian?

95 CONSENT THAT DESTROYS THE EXPERIMENT

Drs. William Harter, Sidney Weinberg, and Cynthia Martin were staff psychiatrists at State Hospital, a major state-supported mental hospital. Dr. Harter was the chief of staff, and Dr. Martin held a staff position at County Hospital, thirty miles away. They had been engaged in a number of medical experiments testing psychoactive drugs, especially some new antipsychotic agents chemically related to chlorpromazine. These experiments had been done routinely with placebo or sugar pill control groups, so that some of the patients received active drugs while others received the placebo.

The researchers supported requirements to obtain informed consent for the experimental drugs and were quite willing to go into reasonable detail in explaining potential risks to both patients and their guardians. Although these measures were inconvenient, the researchers were committed to the ethical importance of consent.

One risk concerned them, however, which they could not adequately explain to their patients. Some patients would definitely be getting a completely ineffective medication, the placebo, and would thus run a particularly high risk of deterioration of their condition during the time they were not medicated. Some patients, the researchers reasoned, might plausibly decide to exclude themselves from the study, thus continuing to receive the regularly used medications. The subjects were all to be selected from the group for whom the regular medication was not completely satisfactory, but they still received some benefit from those drugs. Only those patients would be selected whose condition was reasonably, but not perfectly, stabilized on existing medication.

Dr. Weinberg took the view that the researchers could simply explain to all the patients, as well as to the psychiatrists directly responsible for the units from which the patients came, that some would be receiving placebos. Dr. Martin objected, claiming this might distort the data with many patients, for those in the experimental as well as the control groups, suspecting they were receiving the placebo, would tend to report inaccurately their perceptions.

Dr. Harter became fascinated with this problem, recognizing that it had broad implications for informing all subjects who might receive placebos in place of active medication. He proposed that they do a study on the effect of informing patients that they might receive a placebo in place of an active experimental compound. He, together with Drs. Weinberg and Martin, suggested adding this research question to an experiment they were developing. They proposed to have two control groups. One group, selected from State Hospital patients, would be told explicitly that they had one chance in four of receiving a placebo which would not be effective for their condition. The subjects were to be told that the researchers could not explain whether they would get the sugar pill or the active drug because that was the only way the researchers could tell if the drug being tested really had a positive effect.

The experiment would be repeated at County Hospital with a similar group of patients. In this setting neither the subjects nor the physicians directly responsible for patient care would be told of the presence of the placebo group. Dr. Harter would arrange the administration of the drug and the placebo so that he would be personally on the floor of the hospital to monitor the patients and could break the code if necessary to provide treatment for patients receiving the placebo.

All the researchers recognized that the subjects in the second group would not be fully informed. They would, however, be told that there was some chance the "new drug" might not be effective in their case, which the researchers concluded was a fair statement of the overall risk. According to the HEW guidelines for experimentation, the purpose of the experiment must be disclosed for consent to be informed. The researchers told the subjects that the purpose was to test new drugs for the treatment of their mental condition. What they did not reveal, because they could not do so without destroying the experiment, was that one of the purposes was to measure the effect of telling a group of patients that they were at risk for receiving a placebo. They defended this omission on the ground that learning whether disclosure of the presence of the placebo made any significant difference in the experiment was crucial for deciding all future drug experiment consents. In the long run, they argued, all researchers would be able to get more fully and fairly informed consent if the subjects could be told of the placebo. Without the deception in this one experiment, researchers would probably continue to offer less information than they should for consent to be reasonably informed.

There was no way of telling the one group of patients what the real risks and purposes were without destroying the experiment.

_____

While voluntary and informed consent is normally considered to be a requirement of research involving human subjects, the research in this instance could in all likelihood not be done validly if all patients were informed of the nature of the experiment. The researchers feel for the same reason that the patients' own psychiatrists at the hospital should not be informed. They might have argued that this would possibly jeopardize the therapeutic relationship arousing suspicion on the part of the therapists, or that the psychiatrists' fears of the placebo could be transferred to the patients. There are a number of experiments and therapeutic procedures where disclosure of the relevant facts about the experiment, especially its purpose could clearly destroy its validity. Screening urine of outpatients in a mental health center would provide useful information, but it would destroy the usefulness of the procedure to get consent.

The problem is even more acute in sociopsychological experiments. The experiments of Solomon Asch demonstrated the effect of group pressure on perception. In one such experiment the task was to match the length of a given line with one of three unequal lines. The task was easily done in a control group situation. In the experimental situation, however, the subject responded after another group who had been instructed beforehand to give the wrong answer on certain trials. The experiment showed that the naive subject was greatly influenced by the incorrect responses of his peers.[9] These experiments, and others like them designed to study authoritarianism, have the potential of being socially useful. They are certainly of scientific interest. Yet to inform the patient of the nature of the experiment would clearly destroy it.

Several solutions have been proposed to this dilemma. First, the experiment can be designed in such a way as to eliminate some of the problems. If a single blood or urine test is to be made, for instance, it might be possible to use specimens collected for normal therapeutic purposes, obtaining subject consent after the sample is collected but before the test is made. Of course, if the study involves behavior such as covert drug use, consent refusals might bias the data. In pain or perception studies involving placebos, although the subject clearly cannot be told that he is receiving a placebo, it might be acceptable to inform him that there is a placebo in the research design and that he has a chance of receiving it. In such cases it might also be necessary to inform him whether he will later have the opportunity to receive the active medication should it prove effective.

Some have proposed that consent can be waived in cases where there is virtually no risk to the subject and consent would spoil the experiment. Risks, however, are difficult to estimate. In the study of placebos, for instance, the physical risk to the subjects is probably negligible. But there may be an impact on the relationship between patients and therapists at the hospital after the study is published. Or in a study of covert drug use there might be an impact on the subjects themselves if the fact is published that a certain percentage of the patients at an identifiable hospital covertly use drugs. Or the experimenter's records might be subpoenaed. Even in states which have confidentiality laws protecting the medical records that a physician obtains from his patients, it is not at all clear that research records are part of such a patient-physician relationship.

A more fundamental problem is whether the absence of risk justifies waiving consent. If the consent requirement has as its purpose the protection of individual self-determination rather than simply the protection from undesired risks, then the absence of risk should not be a sufficient argument for waiving consent. One compromise is available in cases where it is impossible to get consent without spoiling the experiment and the experiment is thought to be important. The implied consent of the real subjects may reasonably be assumed if, and only if, there is good evidence that a reasonable person would consent if he had been adequately informed. A mock subject group can therefore be selected from the same population, using the same criteria as are to be used in the experiment. Without performing the experiment, the experimenters can explain the nature and purpose of the experiment to the mock subjects, including any possible risks and benefits, following the standard criteria for adequate information for consent. Then the mock subjects can be asked if they would consent to the experiment, in this case the urine screening. If virtually all, say 95 percent, decide that they would, it can be assumed that another group selected from the same population would also consent. This limited use of implied consent would still have to be followed with careful debriefing.

Consent for Nonexperimental Therapy

The principles of informed and voluntary consent apply to nonexperimental medical diagnosis and treatment as well as to experimental procedures. Their application, however, is more ambiguous. Only since the 1950s has the profession begun to grapple with the radical implications of the requirement of patient consent. Beginning in 1969, the conflict was made explicit between two potentially conflicting standards for the amount of information which must be revealed to a patient before that patient is adequately informed to consent. According to one standard, called the standard of the profession, the physician should be morally and legally required to disclose only such information about the diagnostic, therapeutic, or preventative procedures as is normally disclosed by other physicians in the community. According to the other standard, called the reasonable person criterion, he should disclose whatever information the reasonable person would want to know.

96   THE PRACTICE-OF-THE-PROFESSION
OR REASONABLE PERSON STANDARD

In 1961 Bernard Berkey fell down an embankment and injured his neck, for which he was treated by Dr. Frank M. Anderson. In February 1962 Mr. Berkey injured his neck again while reaching into the back seat of his car. Dr. Anderson conducted a neurological examination, discovered nothing wrong, but concluded that Mr. Berkey should have a myelogram to examine the spinal cord. According to Mr. Berkey, he asked Dr. Anderson if the myelogram was like the electromyograms he had been having to measure the activity of his muscles. Dr. Anderson replied that the procedure was exploratory and nothing to worry about, that the most uncomfortable thing about it was that he would be harnessed down on a cold table and tilted about. He would feel nothing because Dr. Anderson would order a pain-killing injection for him. Mr. Berkey claimed that he had no other knowledge of what was involved in a myelogram. He also said that the nature of the myelogram was not explained to him by Dr. Rickenberg, the physician at the hospital who actually performed the procedure. Dr. Anderson never contended that he had described a myelogram to Mr. Berkey beyond indicating that it was a further procedure in the diagnosis of his case.

Dr. Rickenberg had performed hundreds, perhaps thousands, of myelograms over a twenty-year period. During this procedure the patient is placed prone on a fluoroscopic table and harnessed so that he does not move when it is tilted. A 20-gauge, 3-1/2-inch spinal needle is inserted into the lumbar area of the spine. The position of the needle can be located at any time by the use of a fluoroscope. After the needle is introduced into the subarachnoid space, 8-10 cc's of spinal fluid are removed and sent to the laboratory for analysis. An opaque substance is then introduced through the needle. Because it is heavier than the spinal fluid, tilting the table makes it flow back and forth in the spine while X-rays are taken.

Mr. Berkey claimed that during the procedure he had felt "a couple of mild sticks I didn't mind at all" and then suddenly a terrific thrust as if someone were jamming an ice pick into his lower spine, that he never felt anything so excruciating before, and that a terribly sharp pain shot over his side and left leg. He was told to rest for twenty-four hours after the myelogram. At the end of that period when he attempted to arise, he found that he had what he called a "rubber leg." When he put weight on it, it buckled. Dr. Anderson examined him some three weeks later and

304 Special Problem Areas

found symptoms not previously observed, consisting of diminished sensation in the front of the left leg below the knee and a weakness in the left foot, sometimes referred to as "foot drop."

In August Mr. Berkey was examined by a Dr. Faeth, who found an irritation or compression of one of the nerve trunks arising from the lower end of the spine, which in his opinion was probably caused by a herniated disk. Dr. Anderson admitted the possibility that a herniated disk could be caused while performing a myelogram but only under special conditions, such as repeated injury with a large bore needle. Dr. Rickenberg claimed that he had never heard of foot drop resulting from a myelogram.

Mr. Berkey brought suit against the physicians, claiming in addition to the charge that the myelogram was performed negligently that it was performed without his informed consent. Dr. Anderson claimed that other physicians in the community would not have explained the remote risk of serious spinal injury. He appealed to an earlier court case on informed consent where a physician was found not to be in error in refusing to give certain information. The question in that case was whether, before giving a patient an injection of penicillin, the physician was required to advise him that in rare instances anaphylactic shock may occur and result in death, when there was no evidence that the standard of practice in the community required a doctor to do so. Mr. Berkey argued, however, that the physician's duty to disclose is not governed by the standard practice of the physicians' community, but by what the reasonable person would want to know about the procedure, even if the risk is extremely small. The issue is what criteria to use to determine whether information should be given to the patient, especially in cases where the risk is rare and might unnecessarily disturb the patient.[10]

This case, which was debated in the courts in 1969, was the forerunner of cases in many jurisdictions, all of which force the issue of what standard to use in determining which information should be given the patient for his consent to be adequately informed.[11] There are, in fact, not two but three standards to which appeals have been made to answer the question. The first is rooted squarely in the principle of benefiting the patient. While the notion of consent for experimental procedures began to emerge in the first half of the twentieth century as a requirement independent of patient benefit, it was commonly assumed for nonexperimental diagnosis, treatment, or preventive procedures that the patient offered his consent for whatever procedures the physician thought were in the patient's interest when he first agreed to enter into a patient-physician relationship. The physician might explain matters to the patient as he went along in the course of treatment, but this could be justified by the patient's probable benefit from knowing something of his condition. The decisive factor, as in the Hippocratic oath, is whether or not the physician thought the information would benefit the patient.

It was not until 1960 in the legal case of *Natanson* v. *Kline* that the notion of an independent requirement for informed consent really began to be recognized. The case deals with the problem that to explain every risk of a procedure, no matter how remote, might alarm the patient who is already upset, resulting in a refusal to undergo the procedure even if the risk is only minimal. This case set the trend for the sixties and is generally thought to establish the principle that the physician should disclose what the "reasonable medical practitioner would make under similar circumstances." The court opinion shares with the earlier ethical tradition a conviction that, "How the physician may best discharge his obligation to the patient in this difficult situation involves primarily a question of medical judgment."[12]

In the Berkey case, Dr. Anderson makes a similar argument. He concedes that he did not disclose the minimal risk of a serious spinal injury, but he claims without evidence to the contrary what is undoubtedly true, that other practitioners in the community would not have mentioned the minute risk. Mr. Berkey appears willing to grant that other practitioners in the community would not mention it, but still maintains that he and other reasonable people might well want to know the rare, but serious, risk involved. The neck injury was apparently not causing great problems, and Mr. Berkey might well have foregone the myelogram had he been aware of the risk. The question is whether it is possible that the reasonable person might want to know something about a medical procedure even if there is a consensus among the practitioners in the community that they would not want to know it or that revealing it might do more harm than good. The court in *Berkey* v. *Anderson* evidently thought it was, for they conclude: "We cannot agree that the matter of informed consent must be determined on the basis of medical testimony any more than that expert testimony of the standard practice is determinative in any other case involving a fiduciary relationship. We agree with appellant that a physician's duty to disclose is not governed by the standard practice of the physician's community, but is a duty imposed by law which governs his conduct in the same manner as others in a similar fiduciary relationship."

In fact, this opinion may not really be different from the 1960 *Natanson* v. *Kline* case, as is often assumed, for the judge in that case remarks: "So long as the disclosure is sufficient to assure an informed consent, the physician's choice of plausible courses should not be called into question if it appears, all circumstances considered, that the physician was motivated only by the patient's best therapeutic interests and he proceeded as competent medical men would have done in a similar situation." It appears even here that informed consent is required independent of the standard practice of the community.

97   CONSENT THAT PRODUCES A HEADACHE

Joyce Roberts, a 48-year-old, was admitted to Woman's Hospital for evaluation of postmenopausal vaginal bleeding and was noted during her physical examination to have an elevated blood pressure. She had never before been told of having high blood pressure. The medical student who performed the admission evaluation decided to dilate Mrs. Roberts' pupils with phenylephrine drops, a safe and routine procedure, in order to examine her retinas for the changes of long-standing hypertension. After ascertaining that she had no history of glaucoma, the only contra-indication to the procedure, he instilled several drops in each eye. He warned her that her normal vision would not return for four to six hours. He also asked her to notify him if she developed a headache, a possible sign of an incipient attack of glaucoma precipitated by the eye drops. This rare complication, when it occurs, generally occurs within minutes of the instillation of the medicine and is promptly reversible with an antagonistic drug.

Six hours later she called the medical student to complain of the persistence of blurry vision and was reassured that it would go away by morning. During ward rounds the next morning she still complained of blurry vision and now also a headache, blaming it on "that medicine." A physical examination by the resident, confirmed by the attending physician, revealed the absence of any signs of glaucoma. They were convinced that the symptoms could not be related to the medicine which the student had given her.

Outside the patient's room the problem was discussed on rounds, and the resident advised the medical student not to warn patients of "all the possible side effects" because the power of suggestion can cause side effects when otherwise they would not occur. The attending physician disagreed. He said that medicolegal precedents have forced the doctor to warn of every possible side effect in order to protect himself, and that if a few patients experience imagined side effects as a result of suggestion, "that is just too bad," but unavoidable. "Patients and their lawyers have created this problem, not the doctors."

To reveal extremely rare risks of diagnostic procedures can produce disturbances for a patient, as suggested by this case. It shows that informed consent for medical treatment is a problem not only for major, complex medical and surgical procedures but for the most routine procedures as well.

98 CONSENT FOR ROUTINE LABORATORY TESTS

Pauline Jaffe had moved to Chicago earlier in the year to become a graduate student at the university, studying anthropology. She thought that she needed a complete physical examination, for it had been over six years since her last one. She discussed it with a neighbor, who referred her to Dr. Mary Vaccaro, a general practitioner whom the neighbor had seen on a number of occasions. Ms. Jaffe called for an appointment and was told that the cost for the physical examination would be $100. She was quite satisfied with the exam, after which Dr. Vaccaro told her she was perfectly healthy except that she should lose ten pounds. She paid Dr. Vaccaro's receptionist by check as she left.

She was surprised when three weeks later two bills came from Diagnostic Labs, Inc., one for $15 labeled "profile number one" and another for $6 labeled "cervical cytology." She assumed that the bills were connected with her visit to Dr. Vaccaro but was troubled because she had not been told that any special laboratory work would be done or that she would be billed separately. Dr. Vaccaro had taken 10 cc's of blood and a pap smear during the exam, telling Ms. Jaffe that they were for "routine tests." Ms. Jaffe called the physician after receiving the bills for an explanation of the additional charge, but also wanting to know what tests had been done and why she had not been informed of the results. Further, she had not authorized the performing of the analyses outside the doctor's office. Dr. Vaccaro explained to her that sending out lab specimens was routine, that the information was kept confidential, that separate billing was required by law, and that there was no reason anyone would want the information anyway.

Ms. Jaffe at this point became more and more distressed. She knew that the right of the patient-consumer to select her own medical providers is considered sacred by the American Medical Association and is a fundamental principle of American business. She also recalled that a student friend of hers worked in some medical lab on a part-time basis, though she was not really worried about disclosure of the data. She wondered why the patient's right to consent to medical treatment would not apply to the choice of lab tests and the lab to perform the tests. While she recognized that she did not have much of a basis to make such a choice, she felt that she should, in principle, be the one to authorize the procedures. The extra $21 medical bill bothered her, but the main worry was that a diagnostic procedure had been done without her consent by a group of people she did not even know.

Ms. Jaffe called the lab and asked for copies of the finding, claiming that if she was paying the bill, she was at least entitled to the results. She was told that the lab could give the results only to the physician who had asked that the tests be done. The regulation, the company explained, was for the patient's own protection. There might be something in the data that might upset the patient. The doctor should be the one to decide whether the patient should be told. Ms. Jaffe was confused. She knew that in theory she should consent for medical treatment or diagnosis, yet she could not recall ever hearing of anyone giving consent for lab tests.

Another problem is to establish the reasonable limits of consent. It is clearly a careless error of omission when Dr. Vaccaro's receptionist says the cost of the physical examination will be $100 without including information on the cost of the lab tests. However, the question is whether the patient's role includes consent to simple, routine medical procedures such as lab tests, or whether a blanket, implied consent for the physician to do whatever she thinks reasonable and within the scope of normal, routine procedure can be assumed. Certainly Dr. Vaccaro must be shocked that the question of consent is raised at all. She could well point out that blood tests and cervical cytology are radically different from open heart surgery for which a patient might now be expected to consent. In the case of open heart surgery the risks are great. The patient might prefer to take his chances without the operation once the risks and alternatives are explained. In the case of blood tests, however, the issues seem trivial. There appears to be no significant risk to the patient. The physician can hardly stop to explain and obtain consent for every move that is made in a routine physical examination.

The problem may be a disagreement between Ms. Jaffe and Dr. Vaccaro on the purpose of consent in the first place. If, as traditionally held in medicine, the physician's duty is to benefit the patient and there is virtually no risk involved in the lab tests, then the grounds for obtaining the consent are problematic. Ms. Jaffe, in the remotest of circumstances, could possibly have a friend who may see her medical data, but realistically, even if that happens she does not really care. As a graduate student, Ms. Jaffe might prefer to forgo the extra expense. Every medical decision involves an economic calculation which can only be figured on the terms of the one paying the bill. But it seems reasonable to assume that if she is willing to pay the $100 for the exam, she would be willing to pay the extra for the admittedly significant part of the exam. She might have been comparing the price quoted by Dr. Vaccaro with another physician who charges $110 for an exam including the lab tests, but it is granted that the patient should be told the full costs. In fact, if patient benefit is the basis of the judgment, a good case might be made against consent for the lab tests. The time involved would increase the cost of the exam or be at the expense of some other procedures. The patient might benefit by making the judgment about open heart surgery, but probably would not benefit greatly from the time spent explaining the diagnostic procedures.

On the contrary, Ms. Jaffe may feel that the purpose of the consent is to permit her to exercise some self-determination over her own medical care. She may feel it is irrelevant whether she would benefit in any direct way from being asked to approve the lab tests and the laboratory. She may see it as part of her right to determine her own medical treatment with the advice of the medical professional. If this is the case, the grounds for consent are very different. It may still be that some things are so trivial that the costs, in time and energy, to get an adequately informed consent for the routine medical procedure outweigh the requirement of self-determination, but the basis is nonetheless different. If this is her position, it explains why she is disturbed when the laboratory refuses to give her the results, insisting that they have to go to the physician—for the protection of the patient. The ethical conflicts of truth-telling and the obligation to disclose information are closely related to problems of justifying obtaining consent or waiving that requirement.

Consent by Psychiatric Patients

Consent and refusal of consent become even more complicated in the situation where the patient may not be capable of comprehending the information necessary to give an adequately informed consent or where there are serious constraints on his freedom to choose, as with prisoners or military personnel. At issue is the ability of the patient to understand the information necessary to give adequate consent.

99 CANCELING CONSENT FOR ELECTROSHOCK TREATMENT

Mary Malone, a quarrelsome and despondent matron in her mid-fifties, was the chief clinical problem on the ward. She had admitted herself to the psychiatric ward of the private hospital in the depths of despair. Her husband had died four months ago after a prolonged and agonizing series of operations for cancer. She had refused an invitation to live with her son, saying she believed that "my daughter-in-law doesn't want to have anything to do with me."

The diagnosis was acute, severe depression. Electroshock therapy was agreed upon by the two psychiatrists and the neurologist who examined her. She was given a careful explanation of the treatment and told that a series of shocks would be necessary. They would be very unpleasant, of which she was aware, but she agreed to the treatment. She said, "I really don't care what happens to me anymore." She readily signed the permission for the series.

On the morning of the first treatment she was given amobarbital for sedation. At the instant of the shock she experienced a convulsion similar to a grand mal epileptic seizure. Two days later she was scheduled for a second treatment. That morning she was very anxious. She broke her fast, begging some food from another patient. The treatment had to be postponed until the next morning.

On that morning she made her stand. In a fit of anxious rage she screamed that she would have no further electroshock treatment. "That machine was torture," she yelled. "I won't let you touch me again." She leaped for the door, but it was locked. She turned to flee from the staff who had gathered around her. The psychiatrist tried to explain to her that the treatments would make her well again, and that even though they were unpleasant right now, they would be best for her in the long run. Every means of persuasion was used, but she was adamant.

In the staff meeting the arguments for continuing the therapy were heated: "Now that she has started the treatments, it would be a disaster to stop." "She really isn't enough in control of her faculties to refuse the treatment." "Certainly we cannot just release her." "I'm not givng her a choice at this point." "It is clear what is best for her even if she is too sick to understand." "We have a signed consent for the treatment." These arguments prevailed. Screaming and yelling, Mrs. Malone was dragged to the electroshock room by the nurses and attendants under the direction of the psychiatrist who was giving the treatment.

100 THE RIGHT TO REFUSE PSYCHOACTIVE DRUGS

Robert Watson, a black 22-year-old, had been studying to become a computer operator but dropped out of school and spent his time locked in his room or taking long walks through the city. About midnight on July 8, two policemen saw him walking down a street near his home swinging a large stick. The police later reported that they stopped him to ask what he was doing and that he gave them inconsistent answers and cursed at them. When they asked for the stick, he first clutched it to him and then started swinging it wildly. The officers further reported that he struck one of the officers with the stick, knocked the other down, and ran from them. They cornered him as he was entering the apartment building where he lived, shot him once in the shoulder and once in the thigh, and charged him with menacing, disorderly conduct, resisting arrest, and assault.

Mr. Watson told his court-appointed attorney a rambling version of the events. He denied hitting the officers and felt the charges were unjustified, but was often more concerned about seemingly unrelated matters.

When told of the seriousness of the charges he faced, involving a maximum of four to seven years imprisonment, he explained that external things did not matter—only the truth mattered—and they could not touch him inside. He said that he loved the officers, wished them no harm, and only regretted that they did not respect him as a man.

When Mr. Watson appeared in court after three weeks' hospital care for the shotgun wounds, his speech and gestures were so strange that the judge committed him for mental observation. He was diagnosed as paranoid schizophrenic, found incompetent to understand the nature of the proceedings against him or to participate in his own defense, and committed to a state mental hospital for treatment until found competent to stand trial.

The doctors confirmed the diagnosis and prescribed chlorpromazine, a major antipsychotic agent, for his treatment. He refused the medication. A week later he had shown no improvement and was described as agitated, confused, abusive, and threatening, although not assaultive. The doctors believed his mental condition to be deteriorating and saw little hope for improvement without medication.

On the subject of medication, Mr. Watson was able to carry on a responsive discourse and was unusually clear and adamant in what he had to say. He acknowledged that the doctors believed he needed medication, but he thought them wrong and did not want it under any circumstances. Among other reasons, he said that medication would alter his brain and that he could handle things for himself. When told that medication might be the only way to gain his release from the hospital, he replied that he still did not want the medication and should be released without it.

Under the law of the state, it was possible for Mr. Watson's hospital commitment to continue as long as two-thirds of the maximum prison sentence he could receive if convicted, or four years, eight months. The doctor in charge thought that the patient was unlikely ever to agree to take the medication voluntarily but that forced medication would improve the situation. Five male attendants would be required to force the medication.

Mr. Watson's lawyer believed that, given the circumstances of the case and the fact that Mr. Watson had no prior record, it was likely that he would receive a very short prison term at most if convicted. There appeared to be no established rule of law on whether, or when, forced medication is permissible.

These two cases raise all the questions of consent found in the cases dealing with adults whose ability to consent is not questioned. The object may be to benefit the patient or to facilitate self-determination. In the case of the mentally ill patient, however, the goal of getting any kind of consent for whatever reason becomes much more problematic. The conflict is a basic one, between the desire to grant the mental patient the dignity that comes from assuming his ability to make at least some judgments, and the desire to determine what will really benefit the patient and what the patient really wants. In a discussion of this case, Jack Himmelstein, an attorney for the NAACP Legal Defense Fund, argues for the right of the patient to refuse psychiatric treatment even if the alternative is involuntary confinement:

> We give "normal" individuals the right to make innumerable decisions about their lives which by many standards may be against their self-interest. They are free to lead unhealthy lives, to refuse medical treatment, to be self-destructive and to have widely disparate views about the world . . . The psychiatric finding of a "mental illness" alone simply does not create a justifiable basis for forced administration of psychoactive drugs to anyone who refuses to take them voluntarily since we would deplore the use of such techniques absent a finding of mental illness.
>
> Posted in that position is admittedly the notion that some form of "choice" is exercised by those who "refuse" psychoactive drugs, and I would grant that the rule might be otherwise if the mentally ill person resisted medication without having any comprehension whatever, so that his resistance was a totally meaningless act. This exception is certainly imprecise and requires a difficult drawing of lines, but it would not include the case of Robert Watson who said he understood that the doctors wanted to medicate him and said he did not want it, regardless of the doctors' arguing that the decision was wrong, ill-informed, deleterious or a mask for the wish to be medicated.
>
> Robert Watson is a black youth who has been shot, charged with serious crimes (probably the more serious because of the need of the police to justify the severe injuries they inflicted), imprisoned, "hospitalized as incompetent" and now threatened with the forced administration of drugs as well as imprisonment upon recovery. He not only receives no protection from the presumption of innocence, he is given no opportunity to establish his innocence. He may be kept in such pretrial detention for years, without the right to bail, on the implicit assumption that his illness makes him dangerous, although on the explicit rationale that it is in the defendant's interest to be treated. This confinement, without a hearing, is unjustifiable and therefore presents no justifiable basis for forced administration of drugs.
>
> Taking this reality into account in balancing the interests of the state and the individual, it is clear that because of the likelihood of abuse and misuse of forced medication and the doubts about the drug's effects, some check is needed on the state hospital's power to force medication. A rule that would allow forced medication when it is determined by doctors to be in the medical interest of the patient— trusting to the goodwill, competence and self-discipline of the hospital staff—is insufficient. Relying on the authority of the courts to act as

more than a rubber stamp where the issue is "medical interest" is
unrealistic. Since the individual has most at stake, it does not appear
unreasonable to put the onus on the hospital staff to inform individuals of the effects of the drug, and to let the decision rest with the
individual.

I would think that having a rule that put the onus on trust and
discourse rather than force and the threat of force would also not be
anti-therapeutic. But let us assume that there are circumstances where
forced medication is the only acceptable alternative to justifiable
longterm confinement. I put to one side the issue of whether or when
such confinement is justified. At some point, the cost to society and to
the individual of indefinite, longterm confinement argues for allowing
forced medication. However, that point could not reasonably come in
the first week, as in the case of Robert Watson. Assuming a situation
where the individual is equally adamant against both confinement and
forced medication, I admit to a prejudice in favor of confinement
against medication.[13]

Robert Michels of the Cornell University Medical College offers
different arguments from the perspective of a psychiatrist, stressing the
difficulty of getting some people to understand the choices they are
making and emphasizing the right of those people to be protected by
society:

One of the most striking features of many emotionally disturbed
individuals is that they say one thing and mean another, or they say
things which at first seem meaningless, but with skill, patience and
experience their meaning can often be deciphered. We must recognize,
however, that there is a marked difference between the public verifia-
bility of meaning in most social transactions, and in the communications of a mentally disturbed person to his caretakers . . .

Once in the hospital, we are told that Robert Watson "refused
medication," but that is an interpretation—not a description of the
phenomenon. Did he understand what it was, why it was being given,
what its likely effects would be, what his life would be like with it,
without it? Does "refuse" mean the same thing when it refers to a
reasonable man who understands what he is refusing as to a man
whose thinking is deranged, whose mind is gripped by thoughts and
emotions which stem from the experiences of his past rather than the
realities of the present? For such a man to "refuse" medication may
have much more to do with childhood experiences of being injured by
adults than with his interest or disinterest in treatment today.

The report goes on to assure us that Robert Watson was "unusually
clear and adamant" on the subject of medicine. My own experiences
with people similar to him makes that seem highly unlikely. It is
certainly an exceptionally rare individual whose mind is deranged but
who retains an island of clarity which centers on his passionate desire
not to be treated. More likely, we are dealing with the pseudo-clarity
of the paranoid person who has a social facade of logical thinking with

the underlying substrate of an emotionally disturbed mind. If so, then the "unusual clarity" refers only to the surface appearance, and the word "refusal" is a misnomer, a term which has its origins in the discourse of reasonable men and is not appropriately transferred to the verbal productions of the mentally ill.

However, the dilemma which this creates is obvious. If anyone's "clear and adamant refusal" can be labeled by a psychiatrist as the symptom of mental illness, and not to be taken at face value, then who has any rights and how can they be safeguarded? A civil libertarian might argue that the psychiatrist's interpretations, whether valid or not, represent a step in the erosion of personal liberties which will eventually lead to an elitist group having the authority to tell all of us what we *really* think. The conclusion is that it is preferable to let some sick people go without treatment, even if their apparent refusal of it is really spurious, in order to protect the rights of the rest of us . . .

The problem can be formulated as a conflict of rights. One right is to health and the expectation that society will protect one from the vicissitudes of childish, deranged, or otherwise severely maladaptive behavior which would seriously impair one's health. The other is the right to liberty, to "do one's thing," no matter how different or unconventional, as long as it harms no others. The mentally healthy majority, with lawyers and politicians as their spokesmen, place liberty first, and are suspicious of the psychiatrist's arcane knowledge which could, if abused, give him the ultimate power to determine who shall be free and who shall not. The minority who suffer from psychiatric illness, with their caretakers as their ombudsmen, will suffer if a liberty they cannot enjoy is made superior to a health that must sometimes be forced upon them. For their lives, the preservation of individual liberty rather than the right to treatment is another of the tyrannies of the majority to which they might be subjected.

The only solution to this dilemma is the professional competence and ethical standards of the expert—in this case the psychiatrist, guided by judicial safeguards and review. Treatment should be available to all who might profit from it. If the individual's "refusal" is the product of disease or defect, if his illness is serious, if the treatment is relatively effective and relatively safe, then the individual's right to receive treatment should take precedence over his incompatible right to refuse it. Whether drugs or hospitalization or both is a technical question, but certainly in general, involuntary institutionalization is far more of an assault on a person's liberties than involuntary medication. Robert Watson "wanted" to be released, and wanted not to receive medication. The closest possible compromise might have been forced medication which could lead to earlier release.[14]

The two perspectives are radically different. They both recognize, however, that consent for psychiatric patients is problematic. The courts and laws have begun to recognize this also. Judgments about who is capable of giving consent and for what must become more sophisticated. If even the normal, healthy, middle-class adult has subtle pressures on him influencing his consent decision, residence in a psychiatric institution, even when commitment is involuntary, surely does not mean it is impossible to consent or withhold consent for any possible medical procedure. The state of New York in the 1973 Mental Hygiene Law revisions provides explicitly that mental patients may withhold consent for "surgery, shock treatment, major medical treatment in the nature of surgery, or the use of experimental drugs or procedures."[15] This does not imply, however, that consent for more routine medical procedures, such as an eye examination or a physical exam, are not required.

A 1972 New York court case supports the view that commitment to a mental institution does not necessarily imply that the patient is incompetent to make certain judgments about medical treatment. The case involved electroshock treatments for Paula Stein, whom the court had ordered retained at Bellevue Hospital for psychiatric care and treatment. After she protested the electroshock treatments, the court found: "she is sufficiently mentally ill to require further retention. However, that determination does not imply that she lacks the mental capacity to knowingly consent or withhold her consent to electroshock therapy . . . she does have the mental capacity to know and understand whether she wishes to consent to electroshock therapy. It does not matter whether this Court would agree with her judgment; it is enough that she is capable of making a decision, however unfortunate that decision may prove to be."[16]

A similar decision was reached in 1973 in the case of Maida Yetter, a 60-year-old at Allentown State Hospital who had been committed two years previously suffering from schizophrenia. She wanted to refuse a biopsy for diagnosis of a possible breast cancer. The judge supported her refusal, arguing that commitment is not necessarily evidence of incompetency.[17]

Consent for Treatment of Children

The decision that one is not competent to refuse treatment is even more complex than it is normally thought to be. In cases where the individual is judged incompetent to make the decision for himself whether to consent or to refuse consent for medical treatment, as with the child, the role of the guardian becomes critical. The question is one of when the guardian's consent or refusal of consent is sufficiently reasonable that it can be accepted as being in the interests of the person not capable of making the decision himself.

101 PARENTAL REFUSAL OF TREATMENT FOR A CHILD

Jim Powley, a 14-year-old, was on a summer vacation with his parents, two older brothers, and a younger sister. They were driving to a cabin they had rented in the country. On the way they were involved in a head-on automobile accident, killing the father and two older brothers. Jim Powley's leg was pinned in the wreckage, breaking the femur in two places and crushing some of the thigh muscle and hip. His mother and sister were cut severely but escaped permanent injury.

Jim spent several months hospitalized while the leg began to heal. For the past month he had been at home, with his mother providing the nursing care. The orthopedist was now recommending corrective surgery.

Mrs. Powley had not recovered from the trauma of losing her husband and two children. She had developed a pattern of praying every morning and evening for Jim's recovery and had visited him daily during the months he was hospitalized. When the orthopedist asked Mrs. Powley for permission to perform the operation, he explained that the risk was minimal. With the operation Jim would have an excellent chance of complete recovery of the function of the leg, perhaps walking with a slight limp. Without it, there was a 90 percent chance he would lose the use of his leg for life. The greatest risk was from the general anesthesia which, according to the physician, had a risk of about one death in two thousand cases.

After reflection, Mrs. Powley said that even though the risk was small, the thought of endangering his life was horrifying. She refused permission to operate, sayng, "God's will be done." Jim said he agreed with his mother.

----

1. Is the child completely at the mercy of the parent's wishes for medical consent? When a situation does not involve emergency or lifesaving treatment, under what circumstances might parental wishes be overridden?
2. Some cases involve parental refusal of blood transfusion for their children because of religious conviction. How do such cases compare with this one?
3. What steps should be taken by a physician or other concerned party if there is doubt about the parental refusal to consent for medical treatment?
4. If Jim Powley had disagreed with his mother, of what significance would it be? At what age should a minor be allowed to consent to medical treatment without the parent's consent or despite the parent's explicit refusal of consent?
5. Do state laws for birth control and venereal disease treatment for minors without parental consent imply that those youths are old enough to consent or withhold consent for medical treatment?

CHAPTER 13

Death
and Dying

The Bible says that the first shall be last, the last, first. While dying and death are the last stages in the life cycle and the last in many systematic discussions of medical ethics, the problems of death and dying are often the first encountered by the medical student, clinician, or student of medical ethics. It is often forgetten that the dying patient is first of all a person. He too faces the moral problems faced by any other patient who does not yet happen to be dying. Therefore many other cases are also relevant to the dying patient. Ethical problems of who should make decisions sometimes involve dying patients. Agonizing controversies over what the patient should be told often involve dying patients. Abortion cases in reality involve issues of death and dying of a special kind, as do decisions to stop hemodialysis treatment. The issue of informed consent for experimental and especially nonexperimental medical treatment is directly related to the issues of death and dying. One way of discussing euthanasia, or the stopping of treatment on the dying patient, is in terms of the refusal of consent for treatment by the dying patient or his agent. Ethical problems that are unique, however, to the dying patient are the definition of death and decisions about the medical treatment of the dying. Sometimes in fact there is confusion between the two.

102 HIS BRAIN IS GONE BUT IS HE DEAD?

Late one evening a 33-year-old man in jeans and workshirt was deposited at the door of the emergency room by three anonymous friends who made a swift departure. There was no sign of life. A nurse who was the first to see the patient initiated mouth-to-mouth resuscitation until the respirator team could attach the appropriate mechanical devices. A laboratory analysis confirmed the rapid visual diagnosis of the resident in charge for the evening: heroin overdose. The lack of oxygen to the brain had left the patient in a deep coma, but the next morning the heart was functioning normally while respiration was being maintained by machinery.

After an extensive examination, the neurologist announced that the patient showed no signs of any brain activity. He met the criteria of irreversible coma proposed by the Harvard Medical School Ad Hoc Committee To Examine the Definition of Brain Death. As called for by that report, the tests had been repeated after the heroin had clearly been metabolized and again twenty-four hours later. At this point there was complete agreement among the medical staff about the patient's medical condition. All evidence indicated, and the evidence was convincing, that the patient would never again recover consciousness. They agreed that the respirator, combined with appropriate intravenous feeding and careful monitoring, could keep the patient's cells and organs functioning for an indefinite period, perhaps years.

The neurologist claimed that the patient was dead; the criteria had been met. They should therefore go ahead and remove the kidneys. There was not a moment to spare if the young girl on the nephrology service was to get the organs in good condition. At this point, a major dispute broke out among the medical staff. Three identifiable camps emerged. The first group, representing about 40 percent of the staff, sided with the neurologist. The patient was dead. A second group, maybe another 40 percent of the staff, said, "No, the patient's heart is still beating. How can you possibly call the patient dead when he has a functioning heart? True, he is in an irreversible coma and will never regain consciousness. In fact he has reached a point where he should be allowed to die with dignity, but he is still living." A third and smaller group took the traditional position of medical ethics that the medical professional's duty is to preserve life when it can be preserved. They agreed with the second group that a patient with a beating heart is still alive, but they differed in saying that treatment, by whatever means available, should be continued.[1]

The position of the first group may seem similar to that of the second. In either case the patient will soon be dead. There are serious practical as well as theoretical differences, however. If the patient is taken to be dying and the decision is made to turn off the respirator so he can die "all the way," there well may be some damage to the organs needed for transplant. It is at least an unnecessary and foolish risk to take if one considers

that the patient is already dead. Even if there were no practical difference, the debate between the first and second groups is theoretically
fascinating. Since they disagree on whether the individual is dead or
alive, they must have a different understanding of what it means to be
alive. Since they both agree that the brain is irreversibly damaged, one
group must believe that brain function is not an essential part of what it
means for a human being to be living, while the other presumably
considers brain function to be part of the essence of human nature.

The debate between the second and third groups, often called the
euthanasia debate, focuses on a quite different issue. They both believe
that the patient is alive, albeit dying. One group, however, believes that
sometimes it is morally appropriate to allow the dying patient to die. The
other rejects this view as inconsistent with the moral duty of the medical
profession.

The Definition of Death

103 BRAIN DEATH: WELCOME DEFINITION OR DANGEROUS JUDGMENT

On May 25, 1968, at the beginning of the era of transplantation, Bruce
Tucker was brought to the operating room of the hospital of the Medical
College of Virginia. Mr. Tucker, a 56-year-old black laborer, had suffered a massive brain injury in a fall. He sustained a lateral basilar skull
fracture on the right side, subdural hematoma on the left, and brain stem
contusion.

The following timetable was included in the summary of the case by
Judge A. Christian Compton:

6:05 P.M. Admitted to the hospital.

11:00 P.M. Emergency right temporopatietal craniotomy and right
parietal burr hole.

2:05 A.M. Operation complete; patient fed intravenously and received
"medication" each hour.

11:30 A.M. Placed on respirator, which kept him "mechanically alive."

11:45 A.M. Treating physician noted "prognosis for recovery is nil and
death imminent."

1.00 P.M. Neurologist called to obtain an EEG [electroencephalo-
gram] with the results showing "flat lines with occasional artifact.
He found no clinical evidence of viability and no evidence of cortical
activity."

2:45 P.M. Mr. Tucker taken to the operating room. From this time
until 4:30 P.M. "he maintained vital signs of life, that is, he maintained, for the most part, normal body temperature, normal pulse,
normal blood pressure and normal rate of respiration."

3:30 P.M. Respirator cut off.
3:33 P.M. Incision made in Joseph Klett, heart recipient.
3:35 P.M. Patient pronounced dead.
4:25 P.M. Incision made to remove Tucker's heart.
4:42 P.M. Heart taken out.
4:33 P.M. Incision made to remove decedent's kidneys.

Tucker's heart and kidneys were then removed by the surgical team. The heart was transplanted to Joseph G. Klett, who died about one week later.

William E. Tucker, brother of the dead man, sued for $100,000 damages, charging the transplant team was engaged in a "systematic and nefarious scheme to use Bruce Tucker's heart and had hastened his death by shutting off the mechanical means of support." According to the judge's summary, "a close friend of the deceased was searching for him and made an inquiry at three of the hospital information desks, all without success." Tucker's brother, William, was "at his place of business, located within 15 city blocks of the hospital, all day on May 25th until he left his business to go find his brother in the afternoon when he heard he had been injured. Among the personal effects turned over to the brother later was a business card which the decedent had in his wallet which showed the plaintiff's (brother's) name, business address and telephone number thereon." The suit charged that the removal of organs was carried out with only minimal attempts to notify the victim's family and obtain permission for use of his organs.[2]

Whether this case should in fact be treated as a "brain death," that is the way the principals and the press handled it. The surgeons who removed Tucker's heart evidently also interpreted it as a case of deciding when a patient is dead. Dr. David M. Hume, chief of surgery at the Medical College of Virginia Hospital and the one who operated on Mr. Tucker, remarked that the court's decision, in favor of the physicians, "brings the law up to date with what medicine has known all along—that the only death is brain death."[3] Asked to decide whether the physicians were guilty of causing the death of the heart donor, the jury in the Tucker case were in effect being asked to make a public policy judgment about whether the irreversible loss of brain function is to be equated for moral, legal, and public policy purposes with the death of an individual.

The task of defining death is not a trivial exercise in terminology. Rather, it involves an attempt to understand the philosophical nature of man and what is essential to man which is lost at the time of death. When a person is said to have died, there are appropriate behavioral changes: people cease certain kinds of medical treatment, go into mourning, initiate a funeral ritual, read a will, or if the individual happens to be president of an organization, elevate the vice-president to his presidency role. According to many, including those who focus on the definition of death as crucial for the transplant debate, it is appropriate to remove vital, unpaired organs after, but not before, death. So there is a great deal at stake at the policy level in the definition of death.

There are four plausible candidates for the concept of death. All attempt to determine what is so significant to man that its loss constitutes a change in the moral and legal status of the individual. The traditional religious and philosophical view in Western culture is that a person dies at the time when the soul leaves the body. This separation of body and soul is difficult to verify experimentally and scientifically and is best left to the religious traditions, which in some cases still focus on the soul-departure concept of death.

Traditional secular thought has focused on the cessation of the flow of the vital body fluids, blood and breath. When the circulatory and respiratory functions cease, the individual is dead. This view of the nature of man identifies his essence with the flowing of fluids in the animal species.

The other two candidates for the concept of death are new. One is the complete loss of the body's integrating capacities, as signified by the activity of the central nervous system. This popular concept is frequently though inaccurately given the name "brain death." More recently some have begun to question the adequacy of the notion of brain death, claiming that it has already become old-fashioned. They ask why it is that one must identify loss of the entire brain with death, and whether it should only be the loss of consciousness, of ability to think, reason, feel, experience, interact with others, and control body functions. This distinction is crucial in the rare cases where the lower brain function remains intact while the cortex, which controls consciousness, is utterly destroyed.

The public policy debate about the meaning of death involves a choice among these several candidates. The Harvard Medical School Ad Hoc Committee To Examine the Definition of Brain Death established operational criteria for what it calls irreversible coma, based on sound scientific evidence. The four criteria are: unreceptivity and unresponsivity, no movement or breathing, no reflexes, and a flat electroencephalogram ("of great confirmatory value").[4]

What the committee did not do, however, and what it was not capable of doing, was to establish that a patient in irreversible coma is "dead," that is, should be treated as if he were no longer a living human being who is the possessor of the same moral rights and obligations as other human beings. While a patient in irreversible coma, according to the Harvard criteria, may have shifted to a status where he can no longer be considered living, the decision that he is "dead" cannot be derived from any amount of scientific investigation and demonstration. The choice among the many candidates for what is essential to the nature of man, and therefore the loss of which is to be called death, is essentially a philosophical or moral question, not a medical or scientific one.

This being so, it is troubling that a physician could cite the Virginia legal decision in favor of the physicians' actions as confirming "what medicine has known all along—that the only death is brain death." If some physicians believe this—and certainly there is no consensus among medical professionals—they know it from their general belief system about what is valuable in life and not from their training as medical scientists. It is also distressing that "expert" witnesses, including William Sweet of the Harvard Medical School, were called by the defense to testify before the jury. Dr. Sweet testified: "Death is a state in which the brain is dead. The rest of the body exists in order to support the brain. The brain is the individual." This may or may not be a sound moral philosophical argument. It is certainly not a medical argument. And to ask a chief of neurosurgery at Massachusetts General Hospital to make the moral argument is a kind of special pleading on the part of legal counsel for the defense. The New York *Times* nevertheless concurred with the argument in a report of the verdict: "A medical opinion that death occurs when the brain dies, even if the heart and other organs continue to function, has been reinforced by a jury here in a landmark heart transplant suit."[5] The claim that death occurs when the brain dies is opinion, to be sure, but it is not, and by the very nature of the case cannot be, medical opinion. To leave such decision-making in the hands of scientifically trained professionals would be a dangerous move.

Especially in such a fundamental matter as life and death itself, it is difficult to see how the rest of society can shirk its responsibility in defining the concept of death. To be sure, the scientific community can and should be asked to establish the criteria for measuring such things as irreversible coma, if the public, acting through its policy-making agencies in the legislature, ever does determine that irreversible coma is to be equated with death.

The confusion between social and medical responsibilities was highlighted in the Tucker trial. In the state of Virginia, according to the judge, a definition of death was operative, and that definition was specifically "the cessation of life; the ceasing to exist; a total stoppage of the circulation of the blood, and a cessation of the animal and vital functions consequent thereto such as respiration and pulsation." On a motion for summary judgment for the defendants, the judge ruled that the law-book definition of death must take precedence over medical opinion. He directed that the court was bound by the legal definition of death in Virginia until it was changed by the state legislature. Three days later, however, after considerable debate, Judge Compton appeared to backtrack on his commitment to the publicly established concept of death when he instructed the jury: "In determining the time of death, as aforesaid . . . you may consider the following elements none of which should necessarily be considered controlling, although you may feel under the evidence that one or more of these conditions are controlling: the time of the total stoppage of the circulation of the blood; the time of the total cessation of the other vital functions consequent thereto, such as respiration and pulsation; the time of complete and irreversible loss of all functions of the brain; and whether or not the aforesaid functions were spontaneous or were being maintained artificially or mechanically."

This instruction is ambiguous, to say the least. Judge Compton may have meant no innovation here. He could have meant merely that the "complete and irreversible loss of all function of the brain" was the "cause" of death as traditionally defined, in the sense of "a cessation of the animal and vital functions." Presumably if the head injury to Tucker led to the cessation of all brain function and thereby to the cessation of all other vital functions, death could have occurred in the traditional sense without or prior to the intervention of the surgeons. This almost certainly would have been the case if Mr. Tucker had received no medical attention. Traditional death would then have occurred, and the "complete and irreversible loss of all function of the brain" would have been simply a relevant factor.

But it is also possible to interpret the judge's instructions as authorizing the jury to use a new concept of death, one based directly on brain function, in determining the time of the patient's death. If this was the judge's intent, it would have been a complete reversal of his previous position and a major change in public policy. It would have contradicted the judge's earlier conclusion that "if such a radical change is to be made in the law of Virginia, the application should be made therefore not to the courts but to the legislature wherein the basic concept of our society relating to the preservation and extension of life could be examined and, if necessary, reevaluated." It is to be hoped that in the judge's later instruction to the jury he was not backing down from this important principle.

The other candidates for decision-maker in this case are the relatives of the patient. While it is the state's obligation to establish fundamental policy in this area, it would seem both reasonable and in the interest of the state to stipulate that no organs may be removed from an individual after death unless there is some authorization by the individual patient or the patient's relatives, such as is now called for under the Uniform Anatomical Gift Act. If it is true that in this case the relatives of the patient were not consulted and sufficient time was not taken to establish that relatives were available, this would seem to have been a most serious infringement upon the rights of the patient and the patient's family.

The removal of organs in the rare situations where relatives cannot be found raises a serious, if unusual, problem for transplant surgeons. It might be wiser to avoid the risk of abuse in these cases, which frequently involve indigent and lonely patients, by simply forbidding the use of organs. Certainly four hours—from the time Mr. Tucker was placed on a respirator until the respirator was turned off—was not sufficient time to seek permission from the next of kin.

The defense, the prosecution, and the press all interpreted this case as focusing on the meaning and concept of death. Yet the case record, as presented to the court, leaves open some serious questions. The medical team was operating with a definition of death that concentrated on the brain. Medical witnesses for the defense claimed that Mr. Tucker was "neurologically dead" several hours before the transplant operation. Yet according to the records presented in court, at 11:45 A.M. Mr. Tucker's physician said that the prognosis was nil and death imminent. At 1:00 P.M. the neurologist took an EEG reading that showed "flat lines with occasional artifact," and he reported "no evidence of viability and no signs of cortical activity." Presumably, according to the brain-oriented concept of death, Mr. Tucker was thought to be dead at that time by the surgeons. Yet the surgeons noted that at 3:30 P.M. they turned off the respirator. One must ask what possible moral principle would justify turning off a respirator on a dead patient. Presumably if the physician is dealing with a corpse, the moral imperative would be to preserve the organs for the benefit of the living in the best possible condition, that is, by continuing the respiration process until the heart can be removed. There would be no moral problem with such behavior; in fact, it would be morally irresponsible to run the risk of damaging the tissue. Yet the respirator was turned off, from which one can only surmise that it must have been done in order to permit the heart and lungs to stop function-ing. The only plausible reason would be that there was some lingering doubt about whether or not Mr. Tucker was dead. Of course, to intro-duce this dimension is to place doubt on the claim that the patient was dead at 1:00 P.M. when the EEG showed a flat tracing "with occasional artifact."

If, however, the purpose was to turn the respirator off in order to allow the patient to die all the way, the case is not one of a new definition of death at all; instead, it is the common situation of morally and pos-sibly legally deciding to continue treatment no longer on an irreversibly terminal patient. The morality of ceasing treatment on such a terminal patient has been widely accepted in medical ethics. The jury never announced that the brain-oriented concept of death was appropriate or that they themselves used such a concept. They were not asked or permitted to do so. They merely concluded that they found the defen-dants not guilty of wrongful death of the decedent. At least some of them may well have reasoned that the physicians indeed hastened the dying process by turning off the respirator, but that given the patient's condition, this was an acceptable way to behave; that is, they may have considered that the physician justifiably decided to withdraw the mechanical means of support as "extraordinary for a patient in Tucker's irreversibly dying condition." Whether they reasoned thus is not known, nor is it known whether the jury accepted a brain-oriented concept of death.

The proceedings raise some doubt as to whether the patient was dead even according to the concept of death that focuses on the brain. The Harvard criteria call for the use of irreversible coma. But the Harvard report appeared in the *Journal of the American Medical Association* of August 5, 1968, and the surgeons at the Medical College of Virginia had to make their decision two months earlier, on May 25. Nor was Mr. Tucker declared dead according to Harvard's minimal tests for establishing irreversible coma. At the very least, the tests were not repeated twenty-four hours later. The patient was pronounced dead less than two hours and thirty-five minutes after the EEG reading.

In order to accept the jury's decision in this case as demonstrating that the physicians were justified in the use of brain evidence of death, one would have to accept four debatable premises. The first is that the jury indeed based its decision on a brain-oriented concept of death. Second, a man is really dead when he no longer has any capacity for brain activity. Third, it was reasonable under 1968 conditions to conclude that the patient had irreversibly lost the capacity for any brain activity based on one EEG reading without repetition. And fourth, one would have to accept that individual medical professionals should be vested with the authority to change public policy in an area as fundamental as life and death.

The Dying Adult

Once it has been determined that the individual is not really dead, according to some definition of death, but a living human being who is suffering from a condition from which he might die, the most often asked ethical question is when, if ever, it is morally appropriate to let the dying take its course, or indeed to help it along with an action that hastens death. The debate over euthanasia is an ethical thicket, a tangled swamp overgrown with extraneous moral distinctions which entrap those who try to reflect on the moral dilemmas in the care of the dying. It can engulf the well-meaning in a morass of distinctions, leaving the patient to fend for himself. The term *euthanasia* means to some "a good and appropriate death" while to others a "morally outrageous death." When one term can mean both things simultaneously, it had best be dropped from the vocabulary.

The situation of the dying adult introduces real moral dilemmas for the patient, his family, his physician, and others near to him. These issues are most apparent when dealing with competent, conscious adults for whom death is seen variously as an immediate and inevitable fate or a welcome release. A moral distinction is often made between taking an action that will hasten the death of a terminally ill person, on the one hand, and omitting an intervention that will prolong the life of the person, on the other. These two kinds of response are sometimes called active and passive euthanasia, but since some traditions reject the view that omitting intervention is euthanasia at all, they are probably more appropriately called simply actions and omissions. In cases where omitting intervention is a possibility, another morally significant distinction is that between a terminally ill elderly person whose death is certain to be soon and for whom medical treatment will simply prolong the dying, and a person whose death may be rapid but for whom simple medical treatment may provide years of healthy living. The distinction is between prolonging the dying and prolonging the living.

104   TECHNOLOGY'S ASSAULT ON DEATH

The patient, a 21-year-old, left the hospital in November after treatment for leukemia and came back on New Year's Eve of the same year. At that time she was not expected to live through the night. When the psychiatrist went to visit her parents in the waiting room outside of the intensive treatment unit, she found the father to be in so much agony and pain that he could not relate. He sat numb and immobilized, unable to enter into the conversation between her and the patient's mother. The mother told the psychiatrist about two of the family's experiences. From the moment there had been any publicity about her daughter's illness, the tenants in their apartment house had stopped paying the rent, claiming that she must have made a lot of money because of all the publicity. Also, after receiving the emergency call from the hospital, they had tried to use the car, only to discover that the battery had been stolen.

The psychiatrist wondered for awhile why the mother had related these two strange incidents to her at a time when her daughter was dying. After she explored her own emotional reaction to the two incidents, however, it suddenly occurred to her that both of them concerned people who were insensitive, imperceptive, and cruel. She asked the mother if something cruel and insensitive had happened right now to her daughter. At this moment the father lifted his head and started to cry, and the mother pointed with her hands in the direction of her daughter's room.

When the psychiatrist visited the patient, she realized what the parents had been trying to say. The woman lay half-naked on the bed, hooked up on tubes, a tracheostomy, and a respirator, staring desperately around the room. The psychiatrist's first impulse was to cover her with a bed-sheet, but a nurse appeared and said, "Don't bother—she will push it off again in a minute." The psychiatrist approached the patient, who took her hand and pointed to the ceiling. The psychiatrist looked up and asked if the light was bothering her. The patient grabbed her hands and kissed them, communicating that her impression was correct. When the psychiatrist asked for the light to be switched off, however, the nurse reminded her of the rules and regulations of the intensive treatment unit, which required that the light stay on. Then the psychiatrist asked for a chair for the mother to sit with her daughter. She was told that they could not give her a chair anymore because during the previous visit the mother had stayed more than five minutes. The woman died eight hours after the physicians had informed the parents of her imminent death—she died with the room light in her eyes, the tubes in her mouth and veins, and the parents sitting outside in the waiting room. [6]

105   WHOSOEVER LOSES HIS LIFE SHALL GAIN IT

Charles Osborne was admitted to Cafritz Memorial Hospital with injuries and internal bleeding caused when a tree fell on him. He needed whole blood for a transfusion, but refused to give the necessary consent. His wife also refused. Both were Jehovah's Witnesses, holding religious beliefs that forbid the infusion of whole blood into the body. They believe that transfusion would violate the Biblical injunctions against "eating blood." [7]

The hospital brought a petition to the home of Judge Bacon on the night of the accident. Mr. Osborne's wife, brother, and grandfather were also present. They stated his views, explaining that they were based on strong religious convictions. The grandfather said that the patient "wants to live very much . . . He wants to live in the Bible's promised new world where life will never end. A few hours here would nowhere compare to everlasting life." His wife added, "He told me he did not want blood—he did not care if he had to die."

Judge Bacon was concerned with the patient's capacity to make such a decision in light of his serious condition. She also recognized the possibility that the use of drugs might have impaired his judgment and ability for choice. The lawyer for the hospital replied that Mr. Osborne was receiving fluid by vein but no drugs which could impair his judgment. He was conscious, knew what the doctor was saying, was aware of the consequences of his decision, and had with full understanding executed a statement refusing the recommended transfusion and releasing the hospital from liability.

The judge, afraid of relying solely on hearsay evidence, went to Mr.

Osborne's bedside. She asked him whether he believed that he would be deprived of the opportunity for "everlasting life" if transfusion were ordered by the court. His response was: "Yes. In other words, it is between me and Jehovah; not the courts . . . I'm willing to take my chances. My faith is that strong . . . I wish to live, but with no blood transfusions. Now get that straight."

Judge Bacon was concerned about Mr. Osborne's two young children, whom the state might have an overriding interest in protecting. She brought up the matter with his wife, who replied: "My husband has a business and it will be turned over to me. And his brothers work for him, so it will be carried on. That is no problem. In fact, they are working on it right now. Business goes on. As far as money is concerned, everybody is all right. We have money saved up. Everything will be all right. If anything ever happens, I have a big enough family, and the family is prepared to care for the children."[8]

106 TO END THE AGONY

Skin cancer had riddled the tortured body of Matthew Donnelly. A physicist, he had done research for the past thirty years on the use of X-rays. He had lost part of his jaw, his upper lip, his nose, and his left hand. Growths had been removed from his right arm and two fingers from his right hand. He was left blind, slowly deteriorating, and in agony of body and soul. The pain was constant; at its worst, he could be seen lying in bed with teeth clenched and beads of perspiration standing out on his forehead. Nothing could be done except continued surgery and analgesia. The physicians estimated that he had about a year to live.

Mr. Donnelly had three younger brothers ranging in age from 52 to 36. The youngest, Harold, was the one to whom he had always felt closest. When he pleaded for relief, the other brothers put him off, saying the doctors were doing all they could. To Harold the pleas were more explicit. For the past two months they had been repeated and unmistakable. Mr. Donnelly wanted to die.

Harold removed a .30-caliber pistol from his dresser drawer. He wandered through the town the rest of the afternoon and early evening, having drinks at local bars. He walked toward the hospital, arriving during the evening visiting hours. He claimed that he could remember nothing else, including how his brother was shot and killed. The brothers testified against him in the trial.

———————

These three cases presumably involve competent adults who are dying either necessarily or because of a choice they feel they must make. Yet the cases raise very different issues. Taken together, they force one to examine the relevance of the ethical distinctions that are sometimes made. Some see at least five significant distinctions.

The first is the distinction between actions and omissions in the case of the dying. Matthew Donnelly is dying in agony when he pleads with his brother Harold to put him out of his misery. The firing of a .30-caliber pistol into the dying brother's head would be an action causing death in any court of law as well as in common sense. Charles Osborne, on the contrary, asks no one to do anything. He simply demands that no blood transfusion be given to replace his own blood lost when the tree fell on him. Actions and omissions that produce death, also termed active and passive euthanasia, are traditionally seen as morally very different. The argument is complex, however, for in either case the result is normally the same—the patient dies. In both cases someone makes a decision that results in a death which is different from and probably sooner than the death that would otherwise have occurred. It would be dangerous to argue that one is never morally or legally responsible when he omits actions. The parent who maliciously lets his child starve to death must be as culpable as the one who actively hastens the child's death through battering. Yet several arguments have been made for the importance of maintaining the difference.

First, at least for most people, acting to hasten death is psychologically different from simply letting the death occur. But if the psychological difference is a product of the traditional view that action and omission are morally different, it cannot be used to prove the moral difference. Such an argument is circular.

Second, some argue that the physician has a moral duty to preserve life, because of the moral code of his profession. Although this argument might apply to both active killing and letting the patient die, it is particularly significant for direct action to hasten death. But argument of the medical profession's unique moral duty ignores certain cases. It certainly does not apply to the case of Mr. Donnelly whose brother, a medical layman, is the one asked to do the killing. Even if a physician were asked, the fact that a professional group has agreed, without any public sanction, that its members have a special moral duty to preserve life does not necessarily mean that the duty is binding on a member of the profession who does not accept it. A good case can be made that the public should hold the practitioners of medicine to the unique duty to preserve life, which might be a reason to exclude physicians from the role of euthanizer, but this would require an additional and independent argument, such as that physicians should be adversaries for life, much as lawyers are adversaries for their clients.

Third, some argue that to legitimate the active killing of suffering and dying patients might serve as a wedge to legitimate other forms of killing, as of mentally ill, useless, or undesirable persons, according to some-one's individual judgment. Leo Alexander, a physician who played a significant role in the Nuremberg trials, has observed about the Nazi holocaust: "It started with the acceptance of the attitude, basic in the euthanasia movement, that there is such a thing as life not worthy to be lived. This attitude in its early stages concerned itself merely with the severely and chronically sick. Gradually the sphere of those to be in-cluded in this category enlarged to encompass the socially unproductive, the ideologically unwanted, the racially unwanted and finally all non-Germans. But it is important to realize that the infinitely small wedge-in lever from which this entire trend of mind received its impetus was the attitude toward the non-rehabilitable sick."[9]

A fourth argument for maintaining a moral distinction between active killing and allowing the dying patient to die is that the cause of death in the two cases is different.[10] In active killing the cause of death will be the gunshot wound, the air bubble in the vein, or the potassium chloride injection. In the withdrawal of medical intervention it will be the disease process itself which causes death. Of course, in either case the human agent may be responsible.

The distinction is also made in the law. If a person acts to cause a harm, he is responsible in American law no matter what the motive. If, however, he omits an action and thereby permits a harm to take place, whether or not he is responsible for that harm will depend on the relation between the one who omits the action and the one who is harmed. If there is a clearly established obligation to act, as in the case of the parents' obligation to care for their children, then even an omission that permits harm there probably carries responsibility. In the case of Mr. Osborne, if a physician-patient relationship has been established, there might be some obligation on the part of the physician to bring the matter before the court. If the court supports Mr. Osborne's refusal, as it did in this case, then it can hardly be argued that the physician has an obliga-tion to act. On the contrary, he appears to have an obligation not to act.

There are some practical distinctions between actions causing the death of a patient thought to be terminally ill and suffering and simply omitting treatment so that death can take its course. First, the number of cases where pain cannot be relieved by adequate analgesic medication is small. If pain and suffering, which would appear to be the primary moral justification for actively hastening the death of the patient, can be controlled, then active killing may not be needed. Mr. Donnelly's pain, for instance, might succumb to higher levels of morphine. An argument could be made, however, that actively hastening death would be more humane, more "dignified," for the patient than maintaining him in his final hours with high levels of analgesia and sedation.

A second practical distinction is that the active hastening of death does not always have the same outcome as withdrawing heroic medical interventions. There are rare cases, either because of an error in judgment about the prognosis or because of a malicious desire to dispose of an unattractive patient, where actively hastening death will certainly lead to death, but withdrawal of heroic interventions will not.

The arguments about the distinctions between active killing and simple omission of intervention are complex. Even if one were to conclude that the theoretical and practical differences between the two are minimal, the question remains whether, for practical purposes, they should be treated in the law as equivalent.

The second ethical distinction raised by the three cases is that of dying versus lifesaving procedures. In this sense Mr. Osborne, the man who refuses a blood transfusion, differs from the young woman with leukemia and Mr. Donnelly. While the leukemia victim and Mr. Donnelly are both in the last stages of an inevitable dying process, Mr. Osborne, if he were to receive blood, would presumably recover completely and could look forward to a long period of healthy living. The question is whether there is any moral significance to the distinction between prolonging the living of a living patient and prolonging the dying of one who is in the last stages of inevitable death. Deciding that they are morally different, however, does not imply that the rejection of lifesaving treatment is always morally unacceptable while the cessation of treatment on the inevitably dying is always acceptable.

The third significant ethical distinction that characterizes the cases is between voluntary and nonvoluntary decisions. Mr. Osborne, although the blood would save his life, is vigorously refusing the treatment. He signs a release form expressing his refusal. Even the physicians do not claim he is incompetent to make the judgment. The judges confirm that judgment. Likewise, Mr. Donnelly is actively pleading for an end to his suffering. He is the source of the idea planted in his brother to take the gun and put him out of his misery. In Mr. Donnelly's case there is no judicial determination that the decision of the patient was competent and voluntary, as in Mr. Osborne's case. Even if the voluntary choice on the part of the patient himself is critical, there must be some method of ensuring that the patient has indeed expressed himself without undue pressure from others and that he understands what he is saying. In cases of the active killing of suffering and terminally ill patients, it is often necessary to rely on the word of the one who does the killing, on his own evaluation of the patient's plea.

In contrast with the Osborne and Donnelly cases, the woman with leukemia presents a more ordinary and troublesome situation. Certainly no one has requested that anything be done differently. The choice could have been made to ignore some of the last desperate measures to keep her alive. The parents could have been permitted into the room of their dying daughter. The tragedy of the case, however, is that no one appears to have considered any alternatives. To have stopped her treatment without consultation with her, assuming that she were competent to understand the alternatives, would have been a frighteningly bold decision. All too often the care of the terminally ill patient is discussed as if he were an object to be "managed" rather than as if he, or his agent, were a person with individual wishes.

The fourth important ethical distinction shown by these cases is between direct and indirect killing. Mr. Donnelly's agony in his last minutes, which led to his plea to his brother to put him out of his misery, raises the question of why he was not given an analgesia sufficient to relieve his pain, which might have obviated at least some of the grounds for the request. The terms *direct* and *indirect* as applied to the effect of an action come from Catholic moral theology but are grasped intuitively by many non-Catholics as well. The "Ethical and Religious Directives for Catholic Health Facilities" as revised in 1971 state the principal clearly: "It is not euthanasia to give a dying person sedatives and analgesics for the alleviation of pain, when such a measure is judged necessary, even though they may deprive the patient of the use of reason, or shorten his life."[11] But the situation would be different if one were to give morphine or to leave a bottle of phenobarbital at the bedside with the statement, "Don't take all of these or they will kill you," when the real intention was to hasten the death of the patient rather than to relieve the pain or insomnia. That action would not necessarily be morally different from giving potassium chloride. Whether or not the distinction between omission and commission or between direct and indirect effect is plausible, the distinction must at least be considered in reaching a moral conclusion, and some patients in some medical settings hold it to be a significant distinction.

One final distinction among these three cases has to do with the significance of the children of patients. The young woman with leukemia has no dependents; her parents remain her closest and most significant relatives. Mr. Donnelly has no dependent children. Mr. Osborne, however, has two young children. Even if one grants the right of any competent patient to refuse medical treatment for any reason whatsoever, it is possible that the state has a real concern in protecting the interests of those minor children. The judge in the Osborne case was concerned that they be provided for, and a persuasive argument was made that they would be. It would have posed a different problem if they might have suffered irreparable damage. In a related case in Washington, D.C., a 25-year-old mother who was a Jehovah's Witness with a seven-month-old child tried to refuse a lifesaving blood transfusion. The court considered the harm to the child to be a critical factor in ordering the transfusion.

The Dying Child

The fact that the state has a strong interest in protecting the welfare of children and others who are not competent to make reasoned decisions about their own care raises another series of cases, those involving children who themselves are dying. Many of the same problems that are raised for the dying adult—the difference between active killing and omission of medical intervention, the difference between treating a person who can live and one who is inevitably dying—are also important for the dying child. An added problem is determining who does and does not have the proper authority to make life and death decisions for children who cannot make the choices themselves.

When a child is dying, the tragedy, the emotion, the drama are often excruciating. At times the psychological and other needs of the parents, the physicians, the nurses, and others come to dominate the decision-making. This complex interaction of potential decision-makers can have a critical impact on the ethical dilemma. In cases involving dying children, some parents may want the struggle against death to continue even though hope seems virtually nonexistent, whereas other parents may feel that the child's suffering should not be prolonged. Another issue is the role of older children, who may understand something of their condition but should probably not have complete authority to make decisions about their case. A final problem is whether to preserve life when someone decides that the life is not going to be of sufficient quality.

107 PARENTS WHO REFUSE TO SAY "DIE"

A 32-year-old gave premature birth during the thirty-second week of pregnancy to a 1600-gram boy. The baby showed evidence of hyaline membrane disease and was placed on a respirator the second day after birth. Vital signs were present, although there was some difficulty in respiration. At the time that the decision was made to place the infant on a respirator, the father was consulted. He said that he wanted everything possible done to save the child.

The infant was on the respirator for forty-five days, after which time he showed no evidence of O_2 toxicity and was taken off the respirator. At that point PO_2 levels were within the normal range, all neurological signs were normal, and there was a normal EEG, but continued evidence of respiratory difficulty resulted in the decision to return the infant to the respirator. Approximately a week later the infant was taken off the respirator once again and maintained in the hospital. At two-and-a-half months there was evidence of congestive heart failure, which was treated with digitalis. There were noticeable changes in the neurological picture, including definite evidence of deterioration. At three months the physi-. cian, in consultation with other medical staff, decided that no resuscita- tion would be attempted in the event of a respiratory arrest. At four-and- a-half months the baby was doing poorly. His weight was ten pounds, two ounces.

During the following month several episodes of hypoxia, or lack of oxygen, were treated by nurses in the hospital ward, who felt motivated to carry out a lifesaving procedure on the infant. There were definite signs of brain damage and no hope for improvement in respiration.

The social case worker reported on the condition of the family during the period. She said that the events had wrecked the family, producing marital problems and causing the father to beat his young daughter who was residing at home. A third child, a nine-year-old girl, was in a military school and was not directly affected by the events. The case worker re- ported that the family had immigrated to the United States from an East- ern European country at the time of the communist takeover. The father came from a long line of distinguished military leaders, each of whom had borne the same first name. It was revealed that the infant son had been given this name by the father, and that the father had spent many of his hours in the hospital ward telling the nursing staff and other hospital personnel of the great military career anticipated for the infant when he overcame his present illness. He had further revealed that if the child died, this name could never again be used in the family.

During the course of discussing the case, several questions of a social and ethical nature were raised. An attending physician argued, "The intensive care unit is our livelihood. We get a lot of fun out of it. But does this mean that we have a right to put a patient in it who is going to die anyway, just so that we can train physicians who haven't seen a case like this before?" Another physician observed: "The parents really don't make the decision. You let them think they are making it." A medical student remarked: "If we insist that the parents become involved in the decision, we're copping out on our responsibility." Other questions were raised, such as the point at which the decision should be made to provide no further therapy for this child, or whether a decision to provide no fur- ther resuscitation should be made at all. Was the use of the respirator resorting to extraordinary means of medical care? What were the criteria for extraordinary care? Did the notion of extraordinary care refer to the type of instrument involved or to the condition of the patient? What should be the role of the parents in deciding therapeutic procedures? Did the physician have an obligation to consult with the parents? What should be the role of the other hospital personnel—the nurses, hospital administration, and administration of the pediatrics department—in reaching a decision?

108 PARENTS WHO SAY "LET HIM DIE"

The patient, an 11-year-old boy with cystic fibrosis, a disease of genetic origin, was going to die. Probably a few months were left, but barring a miracle, the medical staff knew that not much more could be hoped for. Now the boy's mother was in the hallway of the pediatrics ward of the hospital, a major center for the treatment of cystic fibrosis. She was creating a scene, demanding that the staff provide no special care for the boy. "Just maintain him," she said, "and let him die in peace."

The boy had been brought to the hospital by his mother two weeks previously. He was in an acute respiratory crisis. This had been the fifth attack in the last six months. He had been in and out of the hospital regularly for the last two years. This time it appeared that the mother may have been slow in bringing the boy to the hospital. Bronchial infection was well developed. There were lung abscesses and cor pulmonale.

Penicillin therapy was initiated immediately to supplement the prophylactic tetracycline regimen which the boy had been receiving regularly. A "sweat test" revealed chlorides at dangerous levels. Massive salt depletion indicated urgent intravenous saline, which was ordered. After two weeks further X-rays indicated generalized obstructive emphysema. Bilateral bronchopneumonia contributed to a rapidly deteriorating condition.

The staff agreed that if the boy's life was to be saved, bronchoscopy was essential. The procedure was of only occasional assistance, even to older patients, and was difficult in children. But the physician in charge felt it was their only chance.

At this point she encountered the boy's mother in the hall, who insisted that she stop the treatment. To make matters worse, the mother herself had a history of mental illness, having undergone three hospitalizations since the death of her husband seven years ago. This made some of the medical staff question her ability to think clearly in the life-and-death matter of her son's care.

The medical staff went into an emergency meeting. A resident who had cared for the boy on one previous admission argued: "We have to grant the wishes of the mother. It is only human to let him die peacefully." Others replied: "The fundamental task of medicine is to preserve the life and health of the patient. We just cannot refuse to provide the well-established procedures which will possibly save his life, even if for only a few days or weeks."

109 THE DYING TEENAGER

On November 22 a 13-year-old girl was admitted to a hospital in her community complaining of a lower abdominal pain of approximately one week's duration. She had a low-grade fever (102-104°), tender abdomen, and slight suprapubic distention. Examination revealed a large ovarian cyst.

On April 4 of the following year the patient was admitted to another hospital complaining of a lumbosacral pain of two weeks' duration. A left upper quadrant mass, both cystic and hemorrhagic, 16 cm. in length and 6-8 cm. in width, was removed surgically on May 1. A nodular lesion of the left fallopian tube was also found. A pathological analysis of the tube lesion was negative, but analysis of the mass showed that there were new, apparently malignant tissues. From this point the patient's course rapidly deteriorated. Postoperatively the hematocrit, which declined to below 30, was buoyed by packed red blood cells. The patient continued to complain of abdominal and back pain, especially on the left side. On May 11 there was a severe nosebleed. The first chemotherapy regimen was given on May 15. This was followed by a decline in platelet count from 750,000 to 224,000, a weight loss from 105 to 96 pounds, and a persistent low-grade fever.

On May 23 the second regimen of chemotherapy was given, followed by isolated episodic hematemesis and undulating fever. In the course of the following week the chart recorded incidents of liver toxicity, stomatitis, dermatitis of the thigh, and pharyngitis, and by June 1 the patient's hair had fallen out. On June 4 there was clear evidence of the extension of the mass, blotches on the face and forearm, and extensive rash. Fever persisted.

The white cell count increased progressively over the next three weeks. On June 14 she was allowed to return home for a short period after pleading from her and her parents so that she could attend a family birthday celebration for a brother who was particularly close to her. She took with her iron for anemia, a nonnarcotic pain reliever (propoxyphene), and multivitamins. Upon readmission to the hospital on June 26, her weight had dropped to 81-1/2 pounds. She continued to complain of pain in the upper left quadrant where distention indicated an increase in the size of the mass.

On July 1 a massive hemorrhage required her transfer to the intensive care unit. Two thousand cc's of whole blood were administered. She complained of intense pain, and a great extension of the epigastrium was evident. Her blood pressure fell to 74/30 by 5:30 P.M., and she suffered a cardiac syncope. By July 3 the hemorrhaging was under control but the patient's condition was deteriorating. Blood pressure dropped to 60/40, pulse was 152, respiration was labored. There were additional cardiac arhythmias. The hematocrit dropped again to 30 following a transient rise after transfusion. The patient was being maintained on nasal oxygen and was receiving diazepam, prochlorperazine, meperidine, and codeine.

At this point the patient experienced transient periods of delirium but for the most part was stuporous and occasionally communicative.

The patient was expected to live no more than two weeks. A final surgical procedure was under consideration to "clean the area out." The patient was being encouraged to continue her therapy in preparation for a return to school in the fall. Her parents visited daily. They were first-generation Armenian-Americans, which created a considerable language barrier between them and the physicians. They were now in the visitors' waiting room. Two medical students were discussing the case in the hall outside her room. Among the questions they asked each other were, When should treatment be stopped on the patient? Should the narcotic dosage be increased even if it would run a serious risk of respiratory depression and possibly hasten death? Should the contemplated surgery be performed, and why? And who should make these decisions—the resident, the attending physician, the medical staff meeting jointly, the parents, or the girl herself? The patient heard them as they discussed her minimal life expectancy.

110   REFUSING SURGERY FOR A BABY
WITH DOWN'S SYNDROME

The children's hospital transport team responsible for bringing seriously ill infants to a major medical center received a call from a distant city. A six-day-old baby with Down's syndrome, a bowel obstruction, and jaundice was being referred for treatment. Upon transfer, the baby underwent tests which confirmed the mongolism, identified the obstruction as duodenal stenosis with possible atresia lower in the tract, and a bilirubin of 17.

The parents of the child were young—the father 21, the mother 18—and the father's position as an hourly worker suggested modest means. This had been the woman's first pregnancy. Operative permission was sought from the parents both for an exchange transfusion in the event that the baby's hematologic status did not stabilize and for surgery to correct the bowel obstruction.

The parents had discussed the prognosis for the child with both their local physician and their clergyman. At their request, the baby had been baptized. When asked for permission to operate, they refused to grant it.

It was the opinion of the attending physician on the transport team that the future for this child as pictured by the local doctor had been unduly pessimistic. The tenor of the conversation with the clergyman was not known.

The hematologic condition did in fact stabilize overnight, forestalling the need for a transfusion. At a meeting of a wider consulting group the next morning, sentiments of varying degrees were expressed both for and against the decision of the parents.

Parents in that state were financially responsible, according to their means, up to an amount of $3000 or more per year, for the upkeep of a child in the state hospital. The responsibility lasted until the child was 15 years of age.

It may be that the competent adult who is dying has the right and the duty to decide when to continue or stop treatment, but in these four cases involving dying children that cannot be. Someone must act on behalf of the child. The question is whether the parents, the physician, or the state should have this awesome responsibility. In contrast with the case of the adult who apparently has the legal right, and many would say the moral right, to refuse treatment for any grounds whatsoever no matter how foolish they may seem, the parent or guardian of an incompetent patient clearly cannot have that same right.

While Jehovah's Witnesses are permitted to refuse blood for themselves even if it would return them to a normal and healthy life, they cannot refuse for their children, even if they argue on grounds of religious freedom. Three-year-old Kenneth Clark, for example, suffered from second- and third-degree burns over 40 percent of his body. When his parents, who were both Jehovah's Witnesses, refused a blood transfusion, the court ordered it.[12] An eight-day-old child suffering from erythroblastosis fetalis had a transfusion ordered by the Illinois Supreme Court over the parents' objections.[13] In a case in New Jersey the parents tried to refuse blood for their infant who would die or be mentally retarded without it. The Supreme Court opinion in that case reflects the principle that the interest of the state is so strong that it can override the religious freedom of the parents: "Thus the [first] amendment embraces two concepts—freedom to believe and freedom to act. The first is absolute but, in the nature of things, the second cannot be. The right to practice religion freely does not include the liberty to expose—a child—to ill health or death. Parents may be free to become martyrs themselves. But it does not follow they are free, in identical circumstances, to make martyrs of their children before they have reached the age of full and legal discretion when they can make that choice for themselves."[14]

If the parents do not have the right to refuse treatments when by doing so they unreasonably jeopardize the life of their children, the question arises whether it is reasonable to distinguish between preserving the life of the child and merely prolonging the dying? Is the baby with hyaline membrane disease who continues to deteriorate after four months and begins to show signs of brain damage having his life saved or merely having his dying prolonged? Is the 11-year-old with cystic fibrosis or the

13-year-old with the malignancy dying? Real differences in the prognoses exist in these cases, but there are also real differences in the attitudes of the parents and physicians. The question is what would constitute a reasonable refusal and who should have the authority to decide.

The father who desperately wants to have his name perpetuated in military honor and the mother whose competency is doubtful may not be in a good position to be the decision-makers. But physicians may be in no better position, for they have their own interests. One physician suggests that the intensive care unit is his livelihood and "a lot of fun." Continued intervention is also valuable for the training of students and young physicians, as in this case and that of the girl with the malignancy. Physicians may have unique attitudes in the face of death; they may feel unique moral commitments, such as that it is the physician's special duty to preserve life. Conflict between parents and professionals can be anticipated. Some would argue that the present presumption that the parent is in the best position to protect the welfare of the child is justified if the family relationship is to continue as an essential institution. As in the cases of parents offering religious objections to clearly lifesaving treatment, such as blood transfusion, legal mechanisms exist to intervene on behalf of the child. The courts are prepared for that intervention. Defenders of the parental role in treatment refusal argue that the courts should continue to be relied on for that purpose.

The older child who is dying raises a second problem. In the cases of the 11-year-old boy and the 13-year-old girl there is no evidence of consultation with the child or even consideration of the child's attitudes. The 13-year-old with the malignancy is in fact being told to prepare for school for the following year when she overhears two medical students talking in the hall outside her room about her minimal life expectancy. It is unrealistic to assume that 21 must continue to be the age when a "child" is capable of having some understanding of his medical condition. What should be the course of the parents and the physicians in these two cases if the probably dying children indicate that they want the treatment stopped? What if the boy with cystic fibrosis says he wants it to continue in the face of his mother's demand that it be stopped? Most important, what should be done to bring the older child into the decision-making process?

The case of the mongoloid infant raises a third problem. If parents cannot make what society interprets as a unreasonable refusal of blood for a child in need of a transfusion but may reasonably refuse heroic death-prolonging efforts on a child when he is clearly dying, it still leaves the possibility of a condition where it would be reasonable to refuse a lifesaving treatment, that is, one which would lead to a life so unacceptable that parents are justified in rejecting it. That is the claim of the parents of the mongoloid child. Certainly if the treatment is ordered for the child against the parents' wishes, there will be problems. The parents may well reject the child. The child may suffer psychologically. The parents, if forced to provide economically for the child, may neglect it. A case can be made that the child's life would be less than ideal even independent of the mongolism. This might be an argument for the position that the state should be responsible for providing for the child once it orders lifesaving treatment against the parents' wishes. This solution could be defended as an obligation to the parents, but more important as being in the best interests of the child.

But the parents' moral position is that it is in the best interests of the child, and perhaps other members of the family as well, that his life not continue at all even though it could continue. In an adult, such a decision may be understood and tolerated. Some medical treatments may be "extraordinary" or "heroic" or unreasonable even though they might save a life. Many would grant this to be the case in face of the psychic torture of continual hemodialysis on a kidney machine. Some would even grant that an older minor might morally make such a reasoned choice. Parents now do make such choices in the case of fetuses with major genetic defects, and some consider the choice to be morally acceptable. The question is whether such a decision by parents for their mongoloid infant can ever be considered reasonable or morally acceptable. This may be an ethically unique question to be argued independent of the other precedents.

The Incompetent Dying Adult

The case of the dying child is much more difficult than that of the dying competent adult who has the authority and responsibility to make some decisions about his own care. Unfortunately even for adults, however, in many cases dying is a debilitating process. Not all adults do their dying while fully in possession of the rational faculties. In some ways the dying adult who is not competent is like the child. Someone must exercise the decision-making authority for him as his guardian and protector. In other ways, however, he is very different from the child. For one thing, he was once competent. The formerly competent adult is in a morally unique status. One problem is what significance to attach to the person's wishes expressed while competent. Added to the tragedy of such cases is the fact that the dying have often been abandoned by the humanity of which they were once a part.

111 INSTRUCTIONS FROM THE FORMERLY COMPETENT

Constance Emerson had lived a long and full life. At age 92 she was in one of the most competent nursing homes in the county. Three years ago she had slipped on the pavement, striking her head. She suffered a severe cerebral hemorrhage and never fully recovered her mental faculties. Earlier in life she had been active in community activities and was president of the Women's Club. She had worked as a volunteer and later as a part-time paid worker at Homer House, a noted settlement house, where she had been a leading force in the development of an educational program for children of working mothers.

After the fall she had been cared for at home by her husband until his own health deteriorated to the point where this was no longer possible. For many years Mrs. Emerson had suffered from diabetes, for which she required a special diet and medical care. She could eat only soft foods, such as baby foods or liquids. She was completely bedridden, blind, and largely deaf. Occasionally she suffered from respiratory infection but was well cared for by the medical staff. Her heart was strong. Although she was bothered by her arthritis, she was not otherwise in pain. She sometimes recognized her husband when he came to visit. When she tried to talk to him, her speech was often unintelligible.

Six years ago Mrs. Emerson had given a talk on the miseries of prolonging the life of the dying elderly. Having seen the agony of deterioration in her relatives, she had made an eloquent plea for a "dignified and simple way to choose death." She had shown the manuscript of the talk to her husband and had mentioned publishing it, but no action was ever taken. Mr. Emerson was now afraid to bring up the subject with her, fearing she might infer that he wanted her to die. Their son, who visited Mrs. Emerson about once a week, felt that they should do nothing to disturb the care she was getting in the nursing home.

Mrs. Emerson's problem is a relatively new one in the care of the dying. She desperately wanted to avoid the indignity of bedridden helplessness. But she now lies in the nursing home with her family and her professional attendants utterly confused. One problem in the case is the lack of precision in her instructions. She gave a lecture some years earlier, but no one knows exactly when she would have considered herself to be so far deteriorated that the time for the hemlock had come. No one knows whether she would have changed her mind.

The Euthanasia Educational Council of New York has drafted a model letter which can be used by individuals as informal instructions to their family, physician, lawyer, or clergyman:

> If the time comes when I can no longer take part in decisions for my own future, let this statement stand as the testament of my wishes:
>
> If there is no reasonable expectation of my recovery from physical or mental disability, I, _____, request that I be allowed to die and not be kept alive by artificial means or heroic measures. Death is as much a reality as birth, growth, maturity and old age—it is the one certainty.

I do not fear death as much as I fear the indignity of deterioration, dependence and hopeless pain. I ask that drugs be mercifully administered to me for terminal suffering even if they hasten the moment of death.

This request is made after careful consideration. Although this document is not legally binding, you who care for me will, I hope, feel morally bound to follow its mandate. I recognize that it places a heavy burden of responsibility upon you, and it is with the intention of sharing that responsibility and of mitigating any feelings of guilt that this statement is made. [15]

This letter is clearly not meant to be legally binding. Others have suggested that legally binding forms be developed, perhaps by authorizing a power of attorney for someone, such as a spouse, to refuse medical treatment when in his or her judgment there is no reasonable expectation for recovery, or by passing other laws to facilitate treatment refusals. [16] All these proposals raise the question of the role of the family, particularly the next of kin, in deciding about the medical care of the family member who, like the child, is no longer able to make reasoned decisions for himself. The disputes that arise among family members can be agonizing.

112 ALONE, DYING, AND OUT OF CONTROL

The siren of the fire department ambulance screeched ominously as it approached the emergency room. In it a man, apparently in his sixties, seemed lifeless. They had found him in the charred remains of a third-floor apartment. The call for the burn team sounded on the hospital's paging system.

By the next day life had been pumped back into his internal organs. Burned over 70 percent of his body, he was headed for endless rounds of painful skin grafting even if by some miracle the medical staff should pull him through the immediate crisis and the subsequent period of high risk of infection.

Identification of the patient was difficult. The landlord was not located for two days. He was able to give the man's name but knew nothing else about him and seemed to care less. Others in the building knew little more. He had lived alone in the room for the last three months. No one had ever seen any visitors. One neighbor claimed that he had complained of being alone in the world. Apparently he had no family and had never married. He lived on a small pension.

After a week the patient was sufficiently conscious to moan in pain from the burns when he was not sedated. The medical staff purposely withheld the sedation for periods to see if he would more completely regain consciousness. He did not. He remained semi-comatose but

writhed in agony each time the pain returned. He retained brain function, but the neurologist could not predict when, if ever, he would regain
anything resembling normal consciousness.

Two nurses on the burn unit agonized with the patient during the
week. They knew, as did the physicians, that there was little hope. Even
if they could pull him through, he would require months, perhaps years,
of medical care. One nurse remarked that if it were he, he hoped the
medical staff or his family would simply let him go in peace. They approached one of the physicians, asking if treatment really had to continue. He did not respond with the traditional view that the physician's
duty is to preserve life. He was in fact quite willing to follow the instructions of the patient or the family. He agreed that he himself would never
want to have such treatment continue. But there was no family—no one
who could speak for the patient. Certainly he could not speak for himself. As a matter of principle, the physician wanted to give all benefit of
the doubt to continuing the best possible care. All too often he had seen
lower-class, lonely patients abandoned in the wards of this and similar
big city hospitals—abandoned not only by family and friends, if they had
any, but also by the medical personnel. "Who," he asked the nurses,
"should have the authority to decide to give up on someone who is alone,
dying, and out of control?"

Most tragic of all is the dilemma of decision-making for an incompetent
and dying person who has no family available or willing to play a role. To
be alone, dying, and out of control is, according to one understanding of
human nature, to have lost some of the most important human qualities.
The situation eliminates one of the most obvious solutions to the question asked over and over in medical ethics: Who should decide what to
do? The question in these circumstances does not lend itself to easy
resolution.

To establish a working policy for such decisions about the dying
incompetent in general, one must make certain assumptions. First,
sufficient reasons do exist to stop certain treatments in certain cases.
Some may hold to the view that those aiding the dying patient—the
family, friends, and medical professionals—must strive to sustain life to
the last gasp, but this view is not held by any major social group,
religious or professional. It cannot in practical terms be the basis for care
of patients, because there is always something that people can do which
they choose not to do because it is inappropriate. Another necessary
assumption, which many but not all would endorse, is that if the patient
were conscious and competent, he would have the right, morally and
legally, to decide when the treatment ought to be stopped. The final
assumption required for decisions about the dying incompetent is that

when a family member or guardian is available, as in the case of the dying child, the ultimate decision ought to rest with that person. These views would resolve many cases of the treatment of the dying, but they would not help in this particular case.

The question posed by this case is what the policy out to be when critical decisions have to be made about the care of patients and there are no family or friends to serve as agent for the patient to represent his interests. Should the physician plan the guardian role? Should a committee be appointed at the hospital to be the "God squad"? Should the nurses, the chaplain, the hospital administration, or the courts have a role? What ought to be the decision?

In order to resolve the issues posed in this case, one must first decide which of the three basic principles is to guide the choice. Perhaps the most obvious principle is that of doing the thing that will produce the greatest good for the greatest number of people. The task is to do what will benefit society. The principle of classical utilitarianism has some shocking and unacceptable implications, especially in the medical context. A defender of this principle would ask what action is the most beneficial to society. It is hard to see how continued expenditures of time and money for the treatment of this helpless and lonely old man could add to the greatest good. In this particular case the utilitarian calculus might lead to a resolution that many would find acceptable, namely, to let him die in peace.

Even though the principle of doing what will benefit society leads to this possibly acceptable solution, it is not necessarily the proper solution because of this principle. The decision could be made that, on balance, it would be more beneficial to society to keep him alive in order to try out a new and exotic burn treatment. Or the decision could be made that medical students would learn from him in practicing their burn intervention techniques. If the overriding principle is to do what will benefit society, and it is decided that society will benefit more by keeping him alive, then it will be correct to keep him alive and suffering to serve the greater good.

There might also be more acceptable social benefits in keeping him alive. For instance, crassly to abandon this patient who is alone might start a social momentum of abandoning the lonely suffering. If people think ahead to a time when they themselves might be lonely and suffering, they will be troubled. They might conclude that a practice of treating the lonely and suffering produces the greater good after all, because it relieves everyone from worrying about one day being in that same condition. Thus it is conceivable that this patient might either be treated or allowed to die for the greater good of society.

The second principle that might govern the choice is the traditional Hippocratic ethic: the physician's duty is to do what he thinks will benefit the patient. This perspective sets aside the greater good of the greater number as morally irrelevant. It is still not clear what the physician should decide, but the things considered relevant to the decision will be quite different. Excluded would be a long list of now extraneous social impacts: the usefulness of the treatment for research and medical education, the cost to society in terms of time and money, and even the precedent established and the fears generated in those who are now well. The physician, if he were to follow the Hippocratic maxim, would decide what in his opinion is in the patient's best interest. This ethic also, however, leads to serious and probably insurmountable problems. Decisions cannot really be made with complete disregard for such social factors as cost. Nor can the physician make a patient-centered decision with complete disregard for others, including other patients of his who may be competing for the physician's time or the burn unit bed. The hospital cannot accept a total commitment to present patients to the disregard of those who are not now patients because they are too poor or are in some other way excluded from the health care system. Finally, and probably most critically for the Hippocratic patient-benefiting ethic, a situation in which the physician's guess about what is in the patient's interest incorporates all of his own biases, his own feelings about death, and his own religious, ethical, or other values cannot be tolerated. The Hippocratic patient-benefiting ethic is ultimately very individualistic and paternalistic as well as consequential. There is no particular reason that the physician's determination will be in the patient's interest according to his own system of beliefs and values. This is the great moral danger of Golden Rule ethics. To do unto others as you would have them do unto you may be interpreted to mean that you will impose your peculiar biases and values on someone who does not and perhaps ought not to share them. A physician who believes that the physician's role is to treat until the last gasp might take the view that, if he were a patient suffering from burns to the extent that he was out of control and presumably dying, he would want his physician to continue the treatment. On the contrary, if he were among the minority of physicians who believe that the "useless" and suffering ought to be hastened out of their misery by an air bubble injection, he might concede that if he were in that condition, he would want the physician quickly to find the vein for the injection. The fact that physicians might hold either of these views cannot make it right for this patient.

This leads to the third approach to the decision. It steps back from a consideration of consequences, either to society or to the patient, and asks whether there are certain characteristics of actions that make them right independent of the consequentialist considerations. There is a long tradition in ethical theory which says there are. It dates from the Ten Commandments and the Stoic natural law theorists and has its modern expression in Kant, Hobbes, Locke, Rousseau, and those who talk about inalienable rights. These right-making characteristics include the principles of justice, reparation, truth-telling, liberty, and promise- or contract-keeping. For medicine the primary competitor to the Hippocratic patient-benefiting ethic is the ethic of the contract. The question in this case is whether any basic rights and wrongs are important in making a decision independent of the question of benefits and harms either to the patient or to society.

There do seem to be such considerations, and they may lead in either direction. The consideration that seems most relevant to a decision to keep on treating is the claim of a right to life. One who believes monisticly in the right to life and is willing to subordinate all other moral claims to this fundamental right may think that it concedes too much to grant that some treatments are expendable and may want to reopen the debate at this point. Others may concede that the right to life is important but that other right-making characteristics are important as well. In this particular case it might be argued that there comes a time when continued treatment on one who is suffering and dying is such an assault on the dignity and humanity of the patient that the humane course is to stop the treatment. Some treatments are so incompatible with the nature of the human being that they are unnatural, unacceptable, or inappropriate. The contract between the patient and the physician and between the society and the physician may set limits as well as obligations on the treatments that can be offered. As with the other basic principles, the approach based on right-making characteristics can lead to either the continuation or the cessation of the treatment in this case. The basis of the decision, however, will be very different.

Even after the question of the principle for making the decision is resolved, there is still the physician's question: Who should have the authority to decide to give up on someone who is alone, dying, and out of control? For one who has no family and is alone, there are three basic choices: the physician or some other medical professional can decide, a particular patient's interests might be, these two requirements tend to retreat to the fiction of treating to the end.

In this particular case there is no reason to suspect the concern and compassion of the physician. He seems thoroughly committed to the protection of the patient. He himself, however, makes the case against the physician having the authority to decide to stop the treatment. There are two kinds of problems with giving the physician this authority. First, there is danger in inserting the physician's judgment about the patient's interest into the decision. Second, such lonely and abandoned patients run a great risk of being deserted by the medical team as well. While this particular physician seems committed to his patient's welfare, at times his colleagues are not. Paradoxically, patients may be better served in general by a rule that treatment ought not to be stopped when they cannot make the decision for themselves and have no guardian to make it for them. This is the physician's argument. Even if this particular patient's interests and the right will be served by stopping the treatment, in general the interests of this group of patients and the right will be better served if there is a policy of continuing to treat, of bending over backward to make sure the patient is not abandoned prematurely.

If, however, the physician cannot be the ultimate authority and it seems intolerably inhumane to follow the rule of always trying to treat to the end, the remaining choice seems to be to designate someone as an agent for the patient. He or she should be either one who is capable of representing the patient's interests or one who is capable of determining what is reasonable or right on balance. When there is no idea what the particular patient's interests might be, these two requirements tend to merge. A court-appointed guardian has been proposed as the agent for this purpose. He would serve as a second agent, as a check against the physician. Either would have the right to appeal if he thought the right choices were not being made.

The use of an agent for the patient appointed by the court or some other public body is an inadequate alternative. But this is a tragic case where the normal human decision-making mechanisms are not available. Some may find the alternative of a patient agent so inadequate that they prefer some other resolution, such as a policy of always trying to treat to the end when there is no instruction from the patient or his natural agent. The human person is a remarkable creature, normally endowed with a will and a reason to make choices, including the infinitely complex ethical choices in the medical area. When that will and reason are compromised, medicine as well as humanity suffer.

APPENDIXES
BIBIOGRAPHY
NOTES
INDEX

Codes of Medical Ethics

HIPPOCRATIC OATH

I swear by Apollo Physician and Asclepius and Hygieia and Panaceia and all the gods and goddesses, making them my witness, that I will fulfil according to my ability and judgment this oath and this covenant:

To hold him who has taught me this art as equal to my parents and to live my life in partnership with him, and if he is in need of money to give him a share of mine, and to regard his offspring as equal to my brothers in male lineage and to teach them this art—if they desire to learn it—without fee and covenant; to give a share of precepts and oral instruction and all the other learning to my sons and to the sons of him who has instructed me and to pupils who have signed the covenant and have taken an oath according to the medical law, but to no one else.

I will apply dietetic measures for the benefit of the sick according to my ability and judgment; I will keep them from harm and injustice.

I will neither give a deadly drug to anybody if asked for it, nor will I make a suggestion to this effect. Similarly I will not give to a woman an abortive remedy. In purity and holiness I will guard my life and my art.

I will not use the knife, not even on sufferers from stone, but will withdraw in favor of such men as are engaged in this work.

Whatever houses I may visit, I will come for the benefit of the sick, remaining free of all intentional injustice, of all mischief and in particular of sexual relations with both female and male persons, be they free or slaves.

What I may see or hear in the course of the treatment or even outside of the treatment in regard to the life of men, which on no account one must spread abroad, I will keep to myself holding such things shameful to be spoken about.

If I fulfil this oath and do not violate it, may it be granted to me to enjoy life and art, being honored with fame among all men for all time to come; if I transgress it and swear falsely, may the opposite of all this be my lot.[1]

PATIENT'S BILL OF RIGHTS

The American Hospital Association presents a Patient's Bill of Rights with the expectation that observance of these rights will contribute to more effective patient care and greater satisfaction for the patient, his physician, and the hospital organization. Further, the Association presents these rights in the expectation that they will be supported by the hospital on behalf of its patients, as an integral part of the healing process. It is recognized that a personal relationship between the physician and the patient is essential for the provision of proper medical care. The traditional physician-patient relationship takes on a new dimension when care is rendered within an organizational structure. Legal precedent has established that the institution itself also has a responsibility to the patient. It is in recognition of these factors that these rights are affirmed.

1. The patient has the right to considerate and respectful care.

2. The patient has the right to obtain from his physician complete current information concerning his diagnosis, treatment, and prognosis in terms the patient can be reasonably expected to understand. When it is not medically advisable to give such information to the patient, the information should be made available to an appropriate person in his behalf. He has the right to know by name, the physician responsible for coordinating his care.

3. The patient has the right to receive from his physician information necessary to give informed consent prior to the start of any procedure and/or treatment. Except in emergencies, such information for informed consent, should include but not necessarily be limited to the specific procedure and/or treatment, the medically significant risks involved, and the probable duration of incapacitation. Where medically significant alternatives for care or treatment exist, or when the patient requests information concerning medical alternatives, the patient has the right to such information. The patient also has the right to know the name of the person responsible for the procedures and/or treatment.

4. The patient has the right to refuse treatment to the extent permitted by law, and to be informed of the medical consequences of his action.

5. The patient has the right to every consideration of his privacy concerning his own medical care program. Case discussion, consultation, examination, and treatment are confidential and should be conducted discreetly. Those not directly involved in his care must have the permission of the patient to be present.

6. The patient has the right to expect that all communications and records pertaining to his care should be treated as confidential.

7. The patient has the right to expect that within its capacity a hospital must make reasonable response to the request of a patient for services. The hospital must provide evaluation, service and/or referral as indicated by the urgency of the case. When medically permissible a patient may be transferred to another facility only after he has received complete information and explanation concerning the needs for and alternatives to such a transfer. The institution to which the patient is to be transferred must first have accepted the patient for transfer.

8. The patient has the right to obtain information as to any relationship of his hospital to other health care and educational institutions insofar as his care is concerned. The patient has the right to obtain information as to the existence of any professional relationships among individuals, by name, who are treating him.

9. The patient has the right to be advised if the hospital proposes to engage in or perform human experimentation affecting his care or treatment. The patient has the right to refuse to participate in such research projects.

10. The patient has the right to expect reasonable continuity of care. He has the right to know in advance what appointment times and physicians are available and where. The patient has the right to expect that the hospital will provide a mechanism whereby he is informed by his physician or a delegate of the physician of the patient's continuing health care requirements following discharge.

11. The patient has the right to examine and receive an explanation of his bill regardless of source of payment.

12. The patient has the right to know what hospital rules and regulations apply to his conduct as a patient.

No catalogue of rights can guarantee for the patient the kind of treatment he has a right to expect. A hospital has many functions to perform, including the prevention and treatment of disease, the education of both health professionals and patients, and the conduct of clinical research. All these activities must be conducted with an overriding concern for the patient, and, above all, the recognition of his dignity as a human being. Success in achieving this recognition assures success in the defense of the rights of the patient.[2]

AMERICAN MEDICAL ASSOCIATION
PRINCIPLES OF MEDICAL ETHICS

Preamble. These principles are intended to aid physicians individually and collectively in maintaining a high level of ethical conduct. They are not laws but standards by which a physician may determine the propriety of his conduct in his relationship with patients, with colleagues, with members of allied professions, and with the public.

Section 1. The principal objective of the medical profession is to render service to humanity with full respect for the dignity of man. Physicians should merit the confidence of patients entrusted to their care, rendering to each a full measure of service and devotion.

Section 2. Physicians should strive continually to improve medical knowledge and skill, and should make available to their patients and colleagues the benefits of their professional attainments.

Section 3. A physician should practice a method of healing founded on a scientific basis; and he should not voluntarily associate professionally with anyone who violates this principle.

Section 4. The medical profession should safeguard the public and itself against physicians deficient in moral character or professional competence. Physicians should observe all laws, uphold the dignity and honor of the profession and accept its self-imposed disciplines. They should expose, without hesitation, illegal or unethical conduct of fellow members of the profession.

Section 5. A physician may choose whom he will serve. In an emergency, however, he should render service to the best of his ability. Having undertaken the care of a patient, he may not neglect him; and unless he has been discharged he may discontinue his services only after giving adequate notice. He should not solicit patients.

Section 6. A physician should not dispose of his services under terms or conditions which tend to interfere with or impair the free and complete exercise of his medical judgment and skill or tend to cause a deterioration of the quality of medical care.

Section 7. In the practice of medicine a physician should limit the source of his professional income to medical services actually rendered by him, or under his supervision, to his patients. His fee should be commensurate with the services rendered and the patient's ability to pay. He should neither pay nor receive a commission for referral of patients. Drugs, remedies or appliances may be dispensed or supplied by the physician provided it is in the best interests of the patient.

Section 8. A physician should seek consultation upon request; in doubtful or difficult cases; or whenever it appears that the quality of medical service may be enhanced thereby.

Section 9. A physician may not reveal the confidences entrusted to him in the course of medical attendance, or the deficiencies he may observe in the character of patients, unless he is required to do so by law or unless it becomes necessary in order to protect the welfare of the individual or of the community.

Section 10. The honored ideals of the medical profession imply that the responsibilities of the physician extend not only to the individual, but also to society where these responsibilities deserve his interest and participation in activities which have the purpose of improving both the health and the well-being of the individual and the community.[3]

INTERNATIONAL CODE OF MEDICAL ETHICS

Adopted by the Third General Assembly of The World Medical Association, London, England, October 1949.

Duties of Doctors in General

A doctor must always maintain the highest standards of professional conduct.

A doctor must practice his profession uninfluenced by motives of profit.

The following practices are deemed unethical:

a) Any self advertisement except such as is expressly authorized by the national code of medical ethics.

b) Collaborate in any form of medical service in which the doctor does not have professional independence.

c) Receiving any money in connection with services rendered to a patient other than a proper professional fee, even with the knowledge of the patient.

Any act, or advice which could weaken physical or mental resistance of a human being may be used only in his interest.

A doctor is advised to use great caution in divulging discoveries or new techniques of treatment.

A doctor should certify or testify only to that which he has personally verified.

Duties of Doctors to the Sick

A doctor must always bear in mind the obligation of preserving human life.

A doctor owes to his patient complete loyalty and all the resources of his science. Whenever an examination or treatment is beyond his capacity he should summon another doctor who has the necessary ability.

A doctor shall preserve absolute secrecy on all he knows about his patient because of the confidence entrusted in him.

A doctor must give emergency care as a humanitarian duty unless he is assured that others are willing and able to give such care.

Duties of Doctors to Each Other

A doctor ought to behave to his colleagues as he would have them behave to him.

A doctor must not entice patients from his colleagues.

A doctor must observe the principles of "The Declaration of Geneva" approved by The World Medical Association.[4]

DECLARATION OF GENEVA

Medical vow adopted by the General Assembly of The World Medical Association at Geneva, Switzerland, September 1948, and amended by the 22nd World Medical Assembly, Sydney, Australia, August 1968.

At the Time of Being Admitted as a Member of the Medical Profession:

I solemnly pledge myself to consecrate my life to the service of humanity.

I will give to my teachers the respect and gratitude which is their due;

I will practice my profession with conscience and dignity;

The health of my patient will be my first consideration;

I will respect the secrets which are confided in me; even after the patient has died.

I will maintain by all the means in my power, the honor and the noble traditions of the medical profession;

My colleagues will be my brothers;

I will not permit considerations of religion, nationality, race, party politics or social standing to intervene between my duty and my patient;

I will maintain the utmost respect for human life, from the time of conception; even under threat, I will not use my medical knowledge contrary to the laws of humanity.

I make these promises solemnly, freely and upon my honor.[5]

Guidelines for
Human Experimentation

THE NUREMBERG CODE

1. The voluntary consent of the human subject is absolutely essential.

This means that the person involved should have legal capacity to give consent; should be so situated as to be able to exercise free power of choice, without the intervention of any element of force, fraud, deceit, duress, over-reaching, or other ulterior form of constraint or coercion; and should have sufficient knowledge and comprehension of the elements of the subject matter involved as to enable him to make an understanding and enlightened decision. This latter element requires that before the acceptance of an affirmative decision by the experimental subject there should be made known to him the nature, duration, and purpose of the experiment; the method and means by which it is to be conducted; all inconveniences and hazards reasonably to be expected; and the effects upon his health or person which may possibly come from his participation in the experiment.

The duty and responsibility for ascertaining the quality of the consent rests upon each individual who initiates, directs, or engages in the experiment. It is a personal duty and responsibility which may not be delegated to another with impunity.

2. The experiment should be such as to yield fruitful results for the good of society, unprocurable by other methods or means of study, and not random and unnecessary in nature.

3. The experiment should be so designed and based on the results of animal experimentation and a knowledge of the natural history of the disease or other problem under study that the anticipated results will justify the performance of the experiment.

4. The experiment should be so conducted as to avoid all unnecessary physical and mental suffering and injury.

5. No experiment should be conducted where there is an *a priori* reason to believe that death or disabling injury will occur; except, perhaps, in those experiments where the experimental physicians also serve as subjects.

6. The degree of risk to be taken should never exceed that determined by the humanitarian importance of the problem to be solved by the experiment.

7. Proper preparations should be made and adequate facilities provided to protect the experimental subject against even remote possibilities of injury, disability, or death.

8. The experiment should be conducted only by scientifically qualified persons. The highest degree of skill and care should be required through all stages of the experiment of those who conduct or engage in the experiment.

9. During the course of the experiment the human subject should be at liberty to bring the experiment to an end if he has reached the physical or mental state where continuation of the experiment seems to him to be impossible.

10. During the course of the experiment the scientist in charge must be prepared to terminate the experiment at any stage, if he has probable cause to believe, in the exercise of the good faith, superior skill, and careful judgment required of him that a continuation of the experiment is likely to result in injury, disability, or death to the experimental subject.[6]

DECLARATION OF HELSINKI

Recommendations guiding medical doctors in biomedical research involving human subjects, adopted by the 18th World Medical Assembly, Helsinki, Finland, 1964, and revised by the 29th World Medical Assembly, Tokyo, Japan, 1975.

Introduction

It is the mission of the medical doctor to safeguard the health of the people. His or her knowledge and conscience are dedicated to the fulfillment of this mission.

The Declaration of Geneva of the World Medical Association binds the doctor with the world, "The health of my patient will be my first consideration," and the International Code of Medical Ethics declares that, "Any act or advice which could weaken physical or mental resistance of a human being may be used only in his interest."

The purpose of biomedical research involving human subjects must be to improve diagnostic, therapeutic and prophylactic procedures and the understanding of the aetiology and pathogenesis of disease.

In current medical practice most diagnostic, therapeutic or prophylactic procedures involve hazards. This applies *a fortiori* to biomedical research.

Medical progress is based on research which ultimately must rest in part on experimentation involving human subjects.

In the field of biomedical research a fundamental distinction must be recognized between medical research in which the aim is essentially diagnostic or therapeutic for a patient, and medical research, the essential object of which is purely scientific and without direct diagnostic or therapeutic value to the person subjected to the research.

Special caution must be exercised in the conduct of research which may affect the environment, and the welfare of animals used for research must be respected.

Because it is essential that the results of laboratory experiments be applied to human beings to further scientific knowledge and to help suffering humanity, The World Medical Association has prepared the following recommendations as a guide to every doctor in biomedical research involving human subjects. They should be kept under review in the future. It must be stressed that the standards as drafted are only a guide to physicians all over the world. Doctors are not relieved from criminal, civil and ethical responsibilities under the laws of their own countries.

I. Basic Principles

1. Biomedical research involving human subjects must conform to generally accepted scientific principles and should be based on adequately performed laboratory and animal experimentation and on a thorough knowledge of the scientific literature.

2. The design and performance of each experimental procedure involving human subjects should be clearly formulated in an experimental protocol which should be transmitted to a specially appointed independent committee for consideration, comment and guidance.

3. Biomedical research involving human subjects should be conducted only by scientifically qualified persons and under the supervision of a clinically competent medical person. The responsibility for the human subject must always rest with a medically qualified person and never rest on the subject of the research, even though the subject has given his or her consent.

4. Biomedical research involving human subjects cannot legitimately be carried out unless the importance of the objective is in proportion to the inherent risk to the subject.

5. Every biomedical research project involving human subjects should be preceded by careful assessment of predictable risks in comparison with forseeable benefits to the subject or to others. Concern for the interests of the subject must always prevail over the interest of science and society.

6. The right of the research subject to safeguard his or her integrity must always be respected. Every precaution should be taken to respect the privacy of the subject and to minimize the impact of the study on the subject's physical and mental integrity and on the personality of the subject.

7. Doctors should abstain from engaging in research projects involving human subjects unless they are satisfied that the hazards involved are believed to be predictable. Doctors should cease any investigation if the hazards are found to outweigh the potential benefits.

8. In publication of the results of his or her research, the doctor is obliged to preserve the accuracy of the results. Reports of experimentation not in accordance with the principles laid down in this Declaration should not be accepted for publication.

9. In any research on human beings, each potential subject must be adequately informed of the aims, methods, anticipated benefits and potential hazards of the study and the discomfort it may entail. He or she should be informed that he or she is at liberty to abstain from participation in the study and that he or she is free to withdraw his or her consent to participation at any time. The doctor should then obtain the subject's freely given informed consent, preferably in writing.

10. When obtaining informed consent for the research project the doctor should be particularly cautious if the subject is in a dependent relationship to him or her or may consent under duress. In that case the informed consent should be obtained by a doctor who is not engaged in the investigation and who is completely independent of this official relationship.

11. In case of legal incompetence, informed consent should be obtained from the legal guardian in accordance with national legislation. Where physical or mental incapacity makes it impossible to obtain informed consent, or when the subject is a minor, permission from the responsible relative replaces that of the subject in accordance with national legislation.

12. The research protocol should always contain a statement of the ethical considerations involved and should indicate that the principles enunciated in the present Declaration are complied with.

II. Medical Research Combined with Professional Care (Clinical Research)

1. In the treatment of the sick person, the doctor must be free to use a new diagnostic and therapeutic measure, if in his or her judgment it offers hope of saving life, reestablishing health or alleviating suffering.

2. The potential benefits, hazards and discomfort of a new method should be weighed against the advantages of the best current diagnostic and therapeutic methods.

3. In any medical study, every patient—including those of a control group, if any—should be assured of the best proven diagnostic and therapeutic method.

4. The refusal of the patient to participate in a study must never interfere with the doctor-patient relationship.

5. If the doctor considers it essential not to obtain informed consent, the specific reasons for this proposal should be stated in the experimental protocol for transmission to the independent committee (I,2).

6. The doctor can combine medical research with professional care, the objective being the acquisition of new medical knowledge, only to the extent that medical research is justified by its potential diagnostic or therapeutic value for the patient.

III. Non-therapeutic Biomedical Research Involving Human Subjects (Non-clinical Biomedical Research)

1. In the purely scientific application of medical research carried out on a human being, it is the duty of the doctor to remain the protector of the life and health of that person on whom biomedical research is being carried out.

2. The subjects should be volunteers—either healthy persons or patients for whom the experimental design is not related to the patient's illness.

3. The investigator or the investigating team should discontinue the research if in his/her or their judgment it may, if continued, be harmful to the individual.

4. In research on man, the interest of science and society should never take precedence over considerations related to the wellbeing of the subject.[7]

AMERICAN MEDICAL ASSOCIATION
ETHICAL GUIDELINES FOR CLINICAL INVESTIGATION

The following guidelines are intended to aid physicians in fulfilling their ethical responsibilities when they engage in the clinical investigation of new drugs and procedures.

(1) A physician may participate in clinical investigation only to the extent that his activities are a part of a systematic program competently designed, under accepted standards of scientific research, to produce data which is scientifically valid and significant.

(2) In conducting clinical investigation, the investigator should demonstrate the same concern and caution for the welfare, safety and comfort of the person involved as is required of a physician who is furnishing medical care to a patient independent of any clinical investigation.

(3) In clinical investigation *primarily for treatment*—

A. The physician must recognize that the physician-patient relationship exists and that he is expected to exercise his professional judgment and skill in the best interest of the patient.

B. Voluntary consent must be obtained from the patient, or from his legally authorized representative if the patient lacks the capacity to consent, following: (a) disclosure that the physician intends to use an investigational drug or experimental procedure, (b) a reasonable explanation of the nature of the drug or procedure to be used, risks to be expected, and possible therapeutic benefits, (c) an offer to answer any inquiries concerning the drug or procedure, and (d) a disclosure of alternative drugs or procedures that may be available.

   i. In exceptional circumstances and to the extent that disclosure of information concerning the nature of the drug or experimental procedure or risks would be expected to materially affect the health of the patient and would be detrimental to his best interests, such information may be withheld from the patient. In such circumstances such information shall be disclosed to a responsible relative or friend of the patient where possible.

   ii. Ordinarily, consent should be in writing, except where the physician deems it necessary to rely upon consent in other than written form because of the physical or emotional state of the patient.

   iii. Where emergency treatment is necessary and the patient is incapable of giving consent and no one is available who has authority to act on his behalf, consent is assumed.

(4) In clinical investigation *primarily for the accumulation of scientific knowledge*—

A. Adequate safeguards must be provided for the welfare, safety and comfort of the subject.

B. Consent, in writing, should be obtained from the subject, or from his legally authorized representative if the subject lacks the capacity to consent, following: (a) a disclosure of the fact that an investigational drug or procedure is to be used, (b) a reasonable explanation of the nature of the procedure to be used and risks to be expected, and (c) an offer to answer any inquiries concerning the drug or procedure.

C. Minors or mentally incompetent persons may be used as subjects only if:

i. The nature of the investigation is such that mentally competent adults would not be suitable subjects.

ii. Consent, in writing, is given by a legally authorized representative of the subject under circumstances in which an informed and prudent adult would reasonably be expected to volunteer himself or his child as a subject.

D. No person may be used as a subject against his will.[8]

EXCERPTS FROM DEPARTMENT OF HEALTH, EDUCATION, AND WELFARE REGULATIONS ON THE PROTECTION OF HUMAN SUBJECTS

46.2 Policy

(a) Safeguarding the rights and welfare of subjects at risk in activities supported under grants and contracts from DHEW is primarily the responsibility of the organization which receives or is accountable to DHEW for the funds awarded for the support of the activity. In order to provide for the adequate discharge of this organizational responsibility, it is the policy of DHEW that no activity involving human subjects to be supported by DHEW grants or contracts shall be undertaken unless a committee of the organization has reviewed and approved such activity, and the organization has submitted to DHEW a certification of such review and approval, in accordance with the requirements of this part.

(b) This review shall determine whether these subjects will be placed at risk, and, if risk is involved, whether:

(1) The risks to the subject are so outweighed by the sum of the benefit to the subject and the importance of the knowledge to be gained as to warrant a decision to allow the subject to accept these risks;

(2) the rights and welfare of any such subjects will be adequately protected;

(3) legally effective informed consent will be obtained by adequate and appropriate methods in accordance with the provisions of this part; and

(4) the conduct of the activity will be reviewed at timely intervals . . .

(c) No grant or contract involving human subjects at risk shall be made to an individual unless he is affiliated with or sponsored by an organization which can and does assume responsibility for the subjects involved.

46.3 Definitions

(a) "Organization" means any public or private institution or agency (including Federal, State, and local government agencies).

(b) "Subject at risk" means any individual who may be exposed to the possibility of injury, including physical, psychological, or social injury, as a consequence of participation as a subject in any research, development, or related activity which departs from the application of those established and accepted methods necessary to meet his needs, or which increases the ordinary risks of daily life, including the recognized risks inherent in a chosen occupation or field of service.

(c) "Informed consent" means the knowing consent of an individual or his legally authorized representative, so situated as to be able to exercise free power of choice without undue inducement or any element of force, fraud, deceit, duress, or other form of constraint or coercion. The basic elements of information necessary to such consent include:

(1) A fair explanation of the procedures to be followed, and their purposes, including identification of any procedures which are experimental;

(2) a description of any attendant discomforts and risks reasonably to be expected;

(3) a description of any benefits reasonably to be expected;

(4) a disclosure of any appropriate alternative procedures that might be advantageous for the subject;

(5) an offer to answer any inquiries concerning the procedures; and

(6) an instruction that the person is free to withdraw his consent and to discontinue participation in the project or activity at any time without prejudice to the subject.

(d) "Secretary" means the Secretary of Health, Education, and Welfare or any other officer or employee of the Department of Health, Education, and Welfare to whom authority has been delegated.

(e) "DHEW" means the Department of Health, Education, and Welfare.

(f) "Approved assurance" means a document that fullfills the requirements of this part and is approved by the Secretary.

(g) "Certification" means the official organizational notification to DHEW in accordance with the requirements of this part that a project or activity involving human subjects at risk has been reviewed and approved by the organization in accordance with the "approved assurance" on file at DHEW.

(h) "Legally authorized representative" means an individual or judicial or other body authorized under applicable law to consent on behalf of a prospective subject to such subject's participation in the particular activity or procedure.

46.6 Minimum Requirements for General Assurances

. . .(b) A committee or committee structure which will conduct initial and continuing reviews in accordance with the policy outlines in 46.2. Such committee structure or committee shall meet the following requirements:

(1) The committee must be composed of not less than five persons with varying backgrounds to assure complete and adequate review of activities commonly conducted by the organization. The committee must be sufficiently qualified through the maturity, experience, and expertise of its members and diversity of its membership to insure respect for its advice and counsel for safeguarding the rights and welfare of human subjects. In addition to possessing the professional competence necessary to review specific activities, the committee must be able to ascertain the acceptability of proposals in terms of organizational commitments and regulations, applicable law, standards of professional conduct and practice, and community attitudes. The committee must therefore include persons whose concerns are in these areas.

(2) The committee members shall be identified to DHEW by name; earned degrees, if any; position or occupation; representative capacity; and by other pertinent indications of experience such as board certification, licenses, etc., sufficient to describe each member's chief anticipated contributions to committee deliberations. Any employment or other relationship between each member and the organization shall be identified, i.e., full-time employee, part-time employee, member of governing panel or board, paid consultant, unpaid consultant. Changes in committee membership shall be reported to DHEW in such form and at such times as the Secretary may require.

(3) No member of a committee shall be involved in either the initial or continuing review of an activity in which he has a conflicting interest, except to provide information requested by the committee.

(4) No committee shall consist entirely of persons who are officers, employees, or agents of, or are otherwise associated with the organization, apart from their membership on the committee.

(5) No committee shall consist entirely of members of a single professional group.

(6) The quorum of the committee shall be defined, but may in no event be less than a majority of the total membership duly convened to carry out the committee's responsibilities under the terms of the assurance . . .

(c) Procedures which the organization will follow in its initial and continuing review of proposals and activities.

(d) Procedures which the committee will follow (1) to provide advice and counsel to activity directors and investigators with regard to the committee's actions, (2) to insure prompt reporting to the committee of proposed changes in an activity and of unanticipated problems involving risk to subjects or others and (3) to insure that any such problems, including adverse reactions to biologicals, drugs, radioisotope labelled drugs, or to medical devices, are promptly reported to the DHEW.

(e) Procedures which the organization will follow to maintain an active and effective committee and to implement its recommendations.

46.9 Obligation To Obtain Informed Consent; Prohibition of Exculpatory Clauses

Any organization proposing to place any subject at risk is obligated to obtain and document legally effective informed consent. No such informed consent, oral or written, obtained under an assurance provided pursuant to this part shall include any exculpatory language through which the subject is made to waive, or to appear to waive, any of his legal rights, including any release of the organization or its agents from liability for negligence.

46.10 Documentation of Informed Consent

The actual procedure utilized in obtaining legally effective informed consent and the basis for committee determinations that the procedures are adequate and appropriate shall be fully documented. The documentation of consent will employ one of the following three forms:

(a) Provision of a written consent document embodying all of the basic elements of informed consent. This may be read to the subject or to his legally authorized representative, but in any event he or his legally authorized representative must be given adequate opportunity to read it. This document is to be signed by the subject or his legally authorized representative. Sample copies of the consent form as approved by the committee are to be retained in its records.

(b) Provision of a "short form" written consent document indicating that the basic elements of informed consent have been presented orally to the subject or his legally authorized representative. Written summaries of what is to be said to the patient are to be approved by the committee. The short form is to be signed by the subject or his legally authorized representative and by an auditor witness to the oral presentation and to the subject's signature. A copy of the approved summary, annotated to show any additions, is to be signed by the persons officially obtaining the consent and by the auditor witness. Sample copies of the consent form and of the summaries as approved by the committee are to be retained in its records.

(c) Modification of either of the primary procedures outlined in paragraphs (a) and (b) of this section. Granting of permission to use modified procedures imposes additional responsibility upon the review committee and the organization to establish: (1) that the risk to any subject is minimal, (2) that use of either of the primary procedures for obtaining informed consent would surely invalidate objectives of considerable immediate importance, and (3) that any reasonable alternative means for attaining these objective would be less advantageous to the subjects. The committee's reasons for permitting the use of modified procedures must be individually and specifically documented in the minutes and in reports of committee actions to the files of the organization. All such modifications should be regularly reconsidered as a function of continuing review and as required for annual review, with documentation of reaffirmation, revision, or discontinuation, as appropriate.[9]

BASIC WORKS ON MEDICAL ETHICS

Cadbury, Henry J., et al. *Who Shall Live? Man's Control over Birth and Death: A Report Prepared for the American Friends Service Committee.* New York: Hill & Wang, 1970.

Callahan, Daniel. "Bioethics as a Discipline." *Hastings Center Studies* 1, no. 1 (1973): 66-73.

Campbell, A. V. *Moral Dilemmas in Medicine.* Baltimore: Williams & Wilkins, 1972.

Clouser, K. Danner. "What is Medical Ethics?" *Annals of Internal Medicine 80* (May 1974): 657-660.

Curran, Charles E. *Politics, Medicine and Christian Ethics.* Philadelphia: Fortress Press, 1973.

Cutler, Donald R., ed. *Updating Life and Death: Essays in Ethics and Medicine.* Boston: Beacon Press, 1969.

Engelhardt, H. Tristram, Jr., and Callahan, Daniel, eds. *Science, Ethics and Medicine.* Hastings-on-Hudson, N.Y.: Institute of Society, Ethics and the Life Sciences, 1976.

Fletcher, Joseph. *Morals and Medicine.* Boston: Beacon Press, 1954.

Golding, Martin. "Ethical Issues in Biological Engineering." *U.C.L.A. Law Review* 15 (February 1968): 443-479.

Gorovitz, Samuel, et al. *Moral Problems in Medicine.* Englewood Cliffs, N.J.: Prentice-Hall, 1976.

Gustafson, James. "Basic Ethical Issues in the Bio-Medical Fields." *Soundings* 53 (Summer 1970): 151-180.

_____. *The Contributions of Theology to Medical Ethics.* 1975 Pere Marquette Theology Lecture. Milwaukee: Marquette University Theology Department, 1975.

Haring, Bernard. *Medical Ethics*. Notre Dame, Ind.: Fides Publishers, 1973.

Jakobovits, Immanuel. *Jewish Medical Ethics*. New York: Bloch, 1959.

Kelly, Gerald. *Medico-Moral Problems*. St. Louis: Catholic Hospital Association, 1958.

Leach, Gerald. *The Biocrats*. Baltimore: Penguin Books, 1972.

McFadden, Charles J. *Medical Ethics*. 6th ed. Philadelphia: F. A. Davis Company, 1967.

Nelson, James B. *Human Medicine: Ethical Perspectives on New Medical Issues*. Minneapolis: Augsburg, 1973.

O'Donnell, Thomas J. *Morals in Medicine*. 2nd ed. Westminster, Md.: Newman Press, 1960.

Ramsey, Paul. *The Patient as Person*. New Haven: Yale University Press, 1970.

Smith, Harmon. *Ethics and the New Medicine*. Nashville: Abingdon Press, 1970.

Torrey, E. Fuller, ed. *Ethical Issues in Medicine*. Boston: Little, Brown, 1968.

Vaux, Kenneth. *Biomedical Ethics: Morality for the New Medicine*. New York: Harper & Row, 1974.

Veatch, Robert M. "Medical Ethics: Professional or Universal?" *Harvard Theological Review* 65 (1972): 531-559.

Walters, LeRoy, ed. *Bibliography of Bioethics*. Vol. 1. Detroit: Gale Research, 1975.

Wertz, Richard W., ed. *Readings on Ethical and Social Issues in Biomedicine*. Englewood Cliffs, N.J.: Prentice-Hall, 1973.

Williams, Robert H., ed. *To Live and To Die: When, Why, and How*. New York: Springer-Verlag, 1973.

BASIC WORKS ON ETHICAL THEORY

Baier, Kurt. *The Moral Point of View: A Rational Basis of Ethics*. New York: Random House, 1968.

Bayles, Michael D., ed. *Contemporary Utilitarianism*. New York: Doubleday, 1968.

Beach, Waldo, and Neibuhr, H. Richard, eds. *Christian Ethics*. New York: Ronald Press, 1955.

Bentham, Jeremy. *An Introduction to the Principles of Morals and Legislation*. Ed. J. Lafleur. New York: Hafner Press, 1948. (Originally published 1789.)

Bernfield, Simon. *The Foundations of Jewish Ethics*. New York: KTAV, 1968.

Brandt, Richard B. *Ethical Theory*. Englewood Cliffs, N.J.: Prentice-Hall, 1959.

_____. *Value and Obligation*. New York: Harcourt, Brace & World, 1961.

Broad, Charlie Dunbar. *Ethics and the History of Philosophy*. New York: Humanities Press, 1952.

_____. *Five Types of Ethical Theory*. New York: Humanities Press, 1962.

Ewing, A. C. *Ethics*. New York: Free Press, 1965.

Foot, Philippa, ed. *Theories of Ethics*. New York: Oxford University Press, 1967.

Fox, Marvin, ed. *Modern Jewish Ethics: Theory and Practice*. Columbus: Ohio State University Press, 1975.

Frankena, William K. *Ethics*. 2nd ed. Englewood Cliffs, N.J.: Prentice-Hall, 1973.

Fried, Charles. *An Anatomy of Values: Problems of Personal and Social Choice.* Cambridge: Harvard University Press, 1970.

Gert, Bernard. *The Moral Rules.* New York: Harper & Row, 1970.

Gustafson, James M. *Can Ethics Be Christian?* Chicago: University of Chicago Press, 1975.

Hare, R. M. *Applications of Moral Philosophy.* Berkeley: University of California Press, 1973.

————. *Freedom and Reason.* New York: Oxford University Press, 1965.

————. *The Language of Morals.* New York: Oxford University Press, 1962.

Hudson, William Donald. *The Is/Ought Question: A Collection of Papers on the Central Problems in Moral Philosophy.* London: Macmillan, 1969.

Kant, Immanuel. *Foundations of the Metaphysics of Morals: Text and Critical Essays.* Ed. Robert P. Wolff. New York: Bobbs-Merrill, 1969. (Originally published 1785.)

————. *Lectures on Ethics.* New York: Harper & Row, 1963. (Ed. P. Menzer from a student's notes taken in 1780 and first published in Berlin, 1924.)

Ladd, John. *Ethical Relativism.* Belmont, Cal.: Wadsworth, 1973.

Lehmann, Paul L. *Ethics in a Christian Context.* New York: Harper & Row, 1963.

Long, Edward Leroy. *A Survey of Christian Ethics.* New York: Oxford University Press, 1967.

Lyons, David. *Forms and Limits of Utilitarianism.* New York: Oxford University Press, 1965.

MacIntyre, Alasdair. *A Short History of Ethics.* New York: Macmillan, 1966.

McClosky, Henry John. *Meta-Ethics and Normative Ethics.* The Hague: Martinus Nijhoff, 1969.

Melden, A. I., ed. *Ethical Theories.* 2nd ed. Englewood Cliffs, N.J.: Prentice-Hall, 1967.

Mill, John Stuart. *Utilitarianism and Other Writings.* Cleveland: Meridian, 1962. (Originally published 1863.)

Moore, G. E. *Ethics.* London: Williams and Norgate, 1912.

————. *Principia Ethica.* London: Cambridge University Press, 1903.

Neibuhr, Reinhold. *An Interpretation of Christian Ethics.* Cleveland: World, 1956.

Niebuhr, H. Richard. *The Responsible Self.* New York: Harper & Row, 1963.

Nowell-Smith, P. H. *Ethics.* Baltimore: Penguin Books, 1954.

Outka, Gene H. *Agape: An Ethical Analysis.* New Haven: Yale University Press, 1972.

Perry, Ralph Barton. *General Theory of Value: Its Meaning and Basic Principles Construed in Terms of Interest.* Cambridge: Harvard University Press, 1926.

Rachels, James, ed. *Moral Problems: A Collection of Philosophical Essays.* New York: Harper & Row, 1971.

Ramsey, Paul. *Basic Christian Ethics.* New York: Charles Scribner's Sons, 1950.

Ross, W. David. *Foundations of Ethics.* New York: Oxford University Press, 1939.

————. *The Right and the Good.* New York: Oxford University Press, 1930.

Sellars, James. *Theological Ethics.* New York: Macmillan, 1966.

Sellars, W. S., and Hospers, John, eds. *Readings in Ethical Theory.* 2nd ed. New York: Appleton-Century-Crofts, 1970.

Sidgwick, Henry. *The Methods of Ethics*. 7th ed. London: Macmillan, 1907.

Smart, J. J. C., and Williams, Bernard. *Utilitarianism: For and Against*. New York: Cambridge University Press, 1973.

Stevenson, Charles L. *Ethics and Language*. New Haven: Yale University Press, 1944.

_____. *Facts and Values: Studies in Ethical Analysis*. New Haven: Yale University Press, 1963.

Thielicke, Helmut. *Theological Ethics*. 2 vols. Philadelphia: Fortress Press, 1966.

Williams, Bernard. *Morality: An Introduction to Ethics*. New York: Harper & Row, 1972.

1. VALUES IN HEALTH AND ILLNESS
2. RESPONSIBILITY FOR THE DECISION

Identifying Values

Boorse, Christopher. "On the Distinction Between Disease and Illness." *Philosophy and Public Affairs* 5 (Fall 1975): 49-68.

Callahan, Daniel. "The WHO Definition of Health." *Hastings Center Studies* 1, no. 3 (1973): 77-87.

Freidson, Eliot. *Professional Dominance: The Social Structure of Medical Care*. Chicago: Aldine, 1970.

Goffman, Erving. *Asylums: Essays on the Social Situation of Mental Patients and Other Inmates*. New York: Doubleday Anchor, 1961.

Kluckhohn, Florence, and Strodtbeck, Fred L. *Variations in Value Orientations*. Westport, Conn.: Greenwood Press, 1973. Originally published 1961.

Laski, Harold J. *The Limitations of the Expert*. Fabian Tract No. 235. London: Fabian Society, 1931.

Macklin, Ruth. "Mental Health and Mental Illness: Some Problems of Definition and Concept Formation." *Philosophy of Science* 39 (September 1972): 341-365. Reprinted in *Biomedical Ethics and the Law,* ed. James M. Humber and Robert F. Almeder. New York: Plenum, 1976.

Mechanic, David. "Health and Illness in Technological Societies." *Hastings Center Studies* 1, no. 3 (1973): 7-18.

Parsons, Talcott. "Social Structure and Dynamic Process: The Case of Modern Medical Practice." *The Social System*. New York: Macmillan, 1951.

Rieff, Philip. *Triumph of the Therapeutic: Uses of Faith after Freud*. New York: Harper & Row, 1968.

Sedgwick, Peter. "Illness—Mental and Otherwise." *Hastings Center Studies* 1, no. 3 (1973): 19-40.

Siegler, Miriam, and Osmond, Humphrey. *Models of Madness, Models of Medicine*. New York: Macmillan, 1974.

Swyhart, Barbara Ann DeMartino. *Bioethical Decision-Making: Releasing Religion from the Spiritual*. Philadelphia: Fortress Press, 1975.

Szasz, Thomas S. *The Myth of Mental Illness*. New York: Dell, 1961.

Veatch, Robert M. "Generalization of Expertise: Scientific Expertise and Value Judgments." *Hastings Center Studies* 1, no. 2 (1973): 29-40.

_____. "The Medical Model: Its Nature & Problems." *Hastings Center Studies* 1, no. 3 (1973): 59-76.

_____. *Value-Freedom in Science and Technology: A Study of the Importance of Religious, Ethical, and Other Socio-Cultural Factors in Selected Medical Decisions Regarding Birth Control*. Missoula, Mont.: Scholars Press, 1976.

Mastectomy

Cope, Oliver. *Man, Mind and Medicine: The Doctor's Education,* pp. 32-36. Philadelphia: J. B. Lippincott, 1968.

Crile, George. "Results of Conservative Treatment of Breast Cancer at Ten and Fifteen Years." *Annals of Surgery* 181, no. 1 (January 1975): 26-30.

_____, and Angelm, Thomas J. "Debates in Medicine: Management of Breast Cancer." *Journal of the American Medical Association* 230 (Oct. 7, 1974): 95-109.

Cutler, S. J., and Heise, H. W. "Efficacy of Current Treatment Methods— Cancer of the Breast." *Cancer* 24 (1969): 1117.

Fisher, Bernard. "Cooperative Clinical Trials in Primary Breast Cancer: A Critical Appraisal." *Cancer* 31 (May 1973): 1271-1286.

Roberts, M. Maureen, et al. "Simple Versus Radical Mastectomy." *The Lancet,* May 19, 1973, pp. 1073-1076.

Drugs, Values, and Society

Brecher, Edward M., and the Editors of Consumer Reports. *Licit and Illicit Drugs*. Boston: Little, Brown, 1972.

Kunnes, Richard. *The American Heroin Empire: Power, Profits, and Politics*. New York: Dodd, Mead, 1972.

Musto, David. *The American Disease: Origins of Narcotic Control*. New Haven: Yale University Press, 1973.

Nelkin, Dorothy. *Methadone Maintenance: A Technological Fix*. New York: George Braziller, 1973.

Osmond, Humphrey, and Aaronson, Bernard, eds. *Psychedelics: The Uses and Implications of Psychedelic Drugs*. Garden City, N.Y.: Doubleday Anchor, 1970.

Szasz, Thomas S. *Ceremonial Chemistry: The Ritual Persecution of Drugs, Addicts and Pushers*. Garden City, N.Y.: Doubleday Anchor, 1974.

_____. "The Ethics of Addiction." *American Journal of Psychiatry* 128 (November 1971): 541-546.

Zinberg, Norman E., and Robertson, John A. *Drugs and the Public*. New York: Simon & Schuster, 1972.

Sterilization

Holder, Angela Roddy. "Voluntary Sterilization." *Journal of the American Medical Association* 225 (Sept. 24, 1973): 1743-1744.

McKenzie, James F. "Contraceptive Sterilization: The Doctor, the Patient, and the United States Constitution." *University of Florida Law Review* 25 (Winter 1973): 327-347.

Presser, Harriet B. "Voluntary Sterilization: A World View." *Reports on Population/Family Planning*, no. 5 (July 1970): 1-36.

Schima, Marilyn E., et al., eds. *Advances in Voluntary Sterilization: Proceedings of the Second International Conference.* Princeton: Excerpta Medica, 1974.

Generic Name Prescriptions

Chewning, J. B. "Legal Implications of Generic Drug Substitution." *Ohio State Medical Journal* 71, no. 5 (May 1975): 323-336.
Kemp, Bernard A., and Moyer, Paul R. "Equivalent Therapy at Lower Cost: The Oral Penicillins." *Journal of the American Medical Association* 228 (May 20, 1974): 1009-1014.
"Limitations on Payment or Reimbursement for Drugs." *Federal Register* 40, no. 148 (July 31, 1975): 32284.
Lowy, Douglas R.; Lowy, Lyndia; and Warner, R. Stephen. "A Survey of Physicians' Awareness of Drug Costs." *Journal of Medical Education* 47 (May 1972): 349-351.
Manninen, Vesa, and Korhonen, Aila. "Inequal Digoxin Tablets." *The Lancet,* Dec. 1, 1973, p. 1268.

Trisomy-18

Hecht, Frederick. "Chromosome Eighteen Trisomy Syndrome." In *Birth Defects Atlas and Compendium,* ed. Daniel Bergsma. Baltimore: Williams and Wilkins, for National Foundation-March of Dimes, 1973.
Smith, D. W., et al. "The No. 18 Trisomy Syndrome." *The Journal of Pediatrics* 60 (1962): 513-527.
Valentine, G. H. *The Chromosome Disorders: An Introduction for Clinicians.* 2nd ed. Philadelphia: J. B. Lippincott, 1969.

Hospital Committees

"Optimum Care for Hopelessly Ill Patients: A Report of the Clinical Care Committee of the Massachusetts General Hospital." *New England Journal of Medicine* 295 (Aug. 12, 1976): 362-364.
Rabkin, Mitchell T.; Gillerman, Gerald; and Rice, Nancy R. "Orders Not To Resuscitate." *New England Journal of Medicine* 295 (Aug. 12, 1976): 364-366.
Veatch, Robert M. "Human Experimentation Committees: Professional or Representative?" *Hastings Center Report* 5 (October 1975): 31-40.
Waldman, A. Martin. "Medical Ethics and the Hopelessly Ill Child." *The Journal of Pediatrics* 88 (May 1976): 890-892.

3. DUTY TO THE PATIENT AND SOCIETY
4. HEALTH CARE DELIVERY

Relationship of Individual and Society

Bentham, Jeremy. *Introduction to the Principles of Morals and Legislation,* ed. J. Lafleur. New York: Hafner Press, 1948.
Feinberg, Joel. *Social Philosophy.* Englewood Cliffs, N.J.: Prentice-Hall, 1973.

Locke, John. *Second Treatise of Government,* ed. Thomas P. Peardon. New York: Bobbs-Merrill, 1952.

Lukes, Steven. *Individualism.* New York: Harper & Row, 1973.

McWilliams, Wilson C. *The Idea of Fraternity in America.* Berkeley: University of California Press, 1973.

Mill, John Stuart. *On Liberty.* New York: Oxford University Press, 1912. Originally published 1859.

———. *Utilitarianism,* ed. Samuel Gorovitz. New York: Bobbs-Merrill, 1971.

Olafson, Frederick A. *Society, Law, and Morality.* Englewood Cliffs, N.J.: Prentice-Hall, 1961.

Sedgwick, Peter. "Medical Individualism." *Hastings Center Studies* 2 (September 1974): 69-80.

Sidel, Victor W., and Sidel, Ruth. "Medicine in China: Individual and Society." *Hastings Center Studies* 2 (September 1974): 23-36.

Ward, John William. "Individualism: Ideology or Utopia?" *Hastings Center Studies* 2 (September 1974): 11-22.

Wasserstrom, Richard A. *Morality and the Law.* Belmont, Cal.: Wadsworth, 1911.

Theories of Justice

Barry, Brian. "John Rawls and the Priority of Liberty." *Philosophy and Public Affairs* 2 (Spring 1973): 274-290.

———. *The Liberal Theory of Justice.* New York: Oxford University Press, 1974.

Bedau, Hugo A. *Justice and Equality.* Englewood Cliffs, N.J.: Prentice-Hall, 1971.

Brandt, Richard. *Social Justice.* Englewood Cliffs, N.J.: Prentice-Hall, 1962.

Brunner, Emil. *Justice and the Social Order.* New York: Harpers, 1945.

Daniels, Norman, ed. *Reading Rawls: Critical Studies on Rawls' A Theory of Justice.* New York: Basic Books, 1975.

McBride, William Leon. "The Concept of Justice in Marx, Engels, and Others." *Ethics* 85 (April 1975): 204-218.

Nagel, Thomas. "Equal Treatment and Compensatory Discrimination." *Philosophy and Public Affairs* 2 (Summer 1973): 348-363.

Nozick, Robert. *Anarchy, State, and Utopia.* New York: Basic Books, 1975.

Olafson, Frederick A., ed. *Justice and Social Policy.* Englewood Cliffs, N.J.: Prentice-Hall, 1961.

Rawls, John. "Justice as Fairness." *The Philosophical Review* 67 (April 1958).

———. *A Theory of Justice.* Cambridge: Harvard University Press, 1971.

Rescher, Nicholas. *Distributive Justice.* Indianapolis: Bobbs-Merrill, 1966.

Equity, Rights, and Health Care Delivery

Alford, Robert R. *Health Care Politics: Ideological and Interest Group Barriers to Reform.* Chicago: University of Chicago Press, 1975.

Annas, George J. "The Hospital: A Human Rights Wasteland." *The Civil Liberties Law Review,* Fall 1974, pp. 9-27.

_____. "Medical Remedies and Human Rights." *Human Rights* 2 (Fall 1972): 151-167.

_____. *The Rights of Hospital Patients: The Basic ACLU Guide to a Hospital Patient's Rights.* New York: Avon Books, 1975.

_____, and Healy, Joseph M., Jr. "The Patient Rights Advocate: Redefining the Doctor-Patient Relationship in the Hospital Context." *Vanderbilt Law Review* 27 (March 1974): 243-269.

Bermant, Gordon; Brown, Peter; and Dwokin, Gerald. "Of Morals, Markets, and Medicine." *Hastings Center Report* 5 (February 1975): 14-16.

Childress, James F. "Who Shall Live When Not All Can Live?" *Soundings* 53 (Winter 1970): 339-354.

Committee on Ways and Means. *National Health Insurance Resource Book.* Washington, D.C.: U.S. Government Printing Office, 1974.

Ehrenreich, Barbara, and Ehrenreich, John. *The American Health Empire: Power, Profits and Politics.* New York: Random House, 1970.

Fein, Rashi. "On Measuring Economic Benefits of Health Programmes." In *Medical History and Medical Care,* ed. Gordon McLachlan and Thomas McKeown. London: Oxford University Press, 1971.

Foucault, Michel. *The Birth of the Clinic.* New York: Pantheon, 1973.

Fried, Charles. "Equality and Rights in Medical Care." *Hastings Center Report* 6 (February 1976): 29-34.

_____. *Medical Experimentation: Personal Integrity and Social Policy.* New York: American Elsevier, 1974.

_____. "Rights and Health Care—Beyond Equity and Efficiency." *New England Journal of Medicine* 293 (July 31, 1975): 241-245.

Fuchs, Victor R. *Who Shall Live? Health, Economics, and Social Change.* New York: Basic Books, 1974.

Galdston, Iago. "Humanism and Public Health." *Bulletin of the History of Medicine* 8 (1940): 1032-1039.

Garfield, Sidney. "The Delivery of Medical Care." *Scientific American* 222 (1970): 15-23.

Halberstam, Michael. "Liberal Thought, Radical Theory and Medical Practice." *New England Journal of Medicine* 284 (May 27, 1971): 1180-1185.

Havighurst, Clark C., and Blumstein, James F. "Coping with Quality/Cost Trade-offs in Medical Care: The Role of PSROs." *Northwestern University Law Review* 70 (March-April 1975): 6-68.

Hiatt, Howard H. "Protecting the Medical Commons: Who Is Responsible?" *New England Journal of Medicine* 293 (July 31, 1975): 235-241.

Illich, Ivan. *Medical Nemesis.* New York: Random House, 1976.

Kass, Leon R. "Regarding the End of Medicine and the Pursuit of Health." *The Public Interest* 40 (Summer 1975): 11-42.

Krizay, John, and Wilson, Andrew. *The Patient as Consumer: Health Care Financing in the United States.* Lexington, Mass.: D. C. Heath, 1974.

Leys, Duncan. "A Doctor's Thoughts on Justice." *The Lancet,* Nov. 6, 1971, pp. 1026-1028.

Outka, Gene. "Social Justice and Equal Access to Health Care." *The Journal of Religious Ethics* 2 (Spring 1974): 11-32.

Pauker, Stephen G., and Kassierer, Jerome P. "Therapeutic Decision Making:

A Cost-Benefit Analysis." *New England Journal of Medicine* 293 (July 31, 1975): 229-234.

Pilpel, Harriet, "Minors' Rights to Medical Care." *Albany Law Review* 36 (1972): 462-487.

Sade, Robert M. "Medical Care as a Right: A Refutation." *New England Journal of Medicine* 285 (Dec. 2, 1971): 1288-1292.

Sidel, Victor, and Sidel, Ruth. *Serve the People.* Boston: Beacon Press, 1973.

Strickland, Stephen P. *Politics, Science, and Dread Disease: A Short History of United States Medical Research Policy.* Cambridge: Harvard University Press, 1972.

Szasz, Thomas. *Psychiatric Justice.* New York: Macmillan, 1965.

Tancredi, Laurence, ed. *Ethics of Health Care.* Washington, D.C.: National Academy of Sciences, 1975.

Taylor, Vincent. "How Much Is Good Health Worth?" *Policy Sciences* 1 (1970): 49-72.

Veatch, Robert M., and Branson, Roy, eds. *Ethics and Health Policy.* Cambridge: Ballinger, 1976.

5. CONFIDENTIALITY

American Psychiatric Association. "Position Statement on the Need for Preserving Confidentiality of Medical Records in Any National Health Care System." *American Journal of Psychiatry* 128 (April 1972): 1349.

Beigler, Jerome S. "The 1971 Amendment of the Illinois Statute on Confidentiality: A New Development in Privilege Law." *American Journal of Psychiatry* 129 (September 1972): 311-314.

Carroll, James D. "A Report of the APSA Confidentiality in Social Science Research Data Project." *PS* 8 (Summer 1975): 258-261. (Available from American Political Science Association, 1527 New Hampshire Ave. N.W., Washington, D.C. 20036)

"The Confidentiality of Health Records." *Psychiatric Opinion* 12 (January 1975).

Curran, William J. "Law-Medicine Notes: Confidentiality and the Prediction of Dangerousness in Psychiatry." *New England Journal of Medicine* 293 (Aug. 7, 1975): 285-286.

———, et al. "Protection of Privacy and Confidentiality." *Science* 182 (Nov. 23, 1973): 797-802.

Daley, Dennis W. "*Tarasoff v. Regents of the University of California* (Cal 529 P 2nd 553) and the Psychotherapist's Duty To Warn." *San Diego Law Review* 12 (July 1975): 932-951.

Davidson, Henry A. "Professional Secrecy." In *Ethical Issues in Medicine,* ed. E. Fuller Torrey. Boston: Little, Brown, 1968.

Group for the Advancement of Psychiatry. "Confidentiality and Privileged Communication in the Practice of Psychiatry." Report No. 45, 1960. Rev. 1966. (Available from Publications Office, G. A. P., 419 Park Ave. South, New York, N.Y. 10016)

McFadden, Charles J. "Truthfulness and Professional Secrecy." In *Medical Ethics.* Philadelphia: F. A. Davis, 1967.

Medical Research Council. "Responsibility in the Use of Medical Information for Research." *British Medical Journal,* Jan. 27, 1973, pp. 213-216.

National Research Council. The Committee on Federal Agency Evaluation Research, Assembly of Behavioral and Social Sciences. *Protecting Individual Privacy in Evaluation Research.* Washington, D.C.: National Academy of Sciences, 1975.

"Public Access to Government Held Computerized Information." *Northwestern University Law Review* 68 (May/June 1973): 431-462.

Robitscher, Jonas B. "Public Life and Private Information." *Journal of the American Medical Association* 202 (Oct. 30, 1967), 398-400.

Schwitzgebel, R. B. "Confidentiality of Research Information in Public Health Studies." *Harvard Legal Commentary* 6 (1969): 187-197.

Solomon, Phillip, et al. "Confidentiality in Psychiatry Screening for Security Clearance." *American Journal of Psychiatry* 127 (May 1971): 1566-1568.

Thomson, Judith Jarvis. "The Right to Privacy." *Philosophy and Public Affairs* 4 (Summer 1975), 295-314.

U.S. Department of Health, Education and Welfare. Secretary's Advisory Committee on Automated Personal Data Systems. *Records, Computers and the Rights of Citizens.* Cambridge, Mass.: M.I.T. Press, 1973.

U.S. District Court of the District of Columbia. "Freedom of Information Act." Civil Action No. 1279-73 (1974).

Westin, Alan F., and Baker, Michael A., Project Directors. *Databanks in a Free Society: Computers, Record-Keeping and Privacy.* Report of the Project on Computer Databanks of the Computer Science and Engineering Board, National Academy of Sciences. New York: Quadrangle Books, 1972.

6. TRUTH-TELLING

Aitken-Swan, Jean, and Easson, E. C. "Reactions of Cancer Patients on Being Told Their Diagnosis." *British Medical Journal,* Mar. 21, 1959, pp. 779-783.

Branch, C. H. "Psychiatric Aspects of Malignant Disease." *CA: Bulletin of Cancer Progress* 6 (May 1956): 102-104.

Cramond, W. A. "Psychotherapy of the Dying Patient." *British Medical Journal,* Aug. 15, 1970, pp. 389-393.

Davies, Edmund. "The Patient's Right To Know the Truth." *Proceedings of the Royal Society of Medicine* 66 (June 1973): 533-536.

Dellinger, Anne M., and Warren, David G. "Frankness in the Doctor-Patient Relationship." *Popular Government,* June 1972, pp. 14-17.

Drillen, C. M., and Wilkinson, E. M. "Mongolism: When Should Parents Be Told?" *British Medical Journal* 2 (Nov. 21, 1964): 1306.

Eck, Marcel. *Lies and Truth.* New York: Macmillan, 1970. (See ch. 9.)

Fitts, Williams T., Jr., and Ravdin, I. S. "What Philadelphia Physicians Tell Patients with Cancer." *Journal of the American Medical Association* 153 (Nov. 7, 1953): 901-904.

Fletcher, Joseph. "Medical Diagnosis: Our Right To Know the Truth." In *Morals and Medicine.* Boston: Beacon Press, 1964.

Henderson, L. J. "Physician and Patient as a Social System." *New England*

Journal of Medicine 212 (May 2, 1935): 819-823.

Kaiser, B. L. "Patients' Rights of Access to Their Own Medical Records: The Need for a New Law." *Buffalo Law Review* 24 (Winter 1975): 317-330.

Kant, Immanuel. "On the Supposed Right To Lie from Altruistic Motives." In *Critique of Practical Reason,* trans. and ed. Lewis White Beck. Chicago: University of Chicago Press, 1949.

Kelly, W. D., and Friesen, S. R. "Do Cancer Patients Want To Be Told?" *Surgery* 27 (June 1950): 822-826.

Litin, E. M. "Should the Cancer Patient Be Told?" *Postgraduate Medicine* 28 (November 1960): 470-475.

Lund, Charles C. "The Doctor, the Patient and the Truth." *Annals of Internal Medicine* 24 (June 1946): 955.

Marmor, J. "What Shall We Tell the Cancer Patient?" *Bulletin of the Los Angeles County Medical Association* 84 (November 1954): 1324.

Meyer, B. C. "Truth and the Physician." *Bulletin of the New York Academy of Medicine* 45 (January 1969): 59-71.

National Association for Mental Health. "The Birth of an Abnormal Child: Telling the Parents." *The Lancet,* Nov. 13, 1971, pp. 1075-1077.

Oken, Donald. "What To Tell Cancer Patients." *Journal of the American Medical Association* 175 (Apr. 1, 1961): 1120-1128.

Peck, Arthur. "Emotional Reactions to Having Cancer." *CA—A Cancer Journal for Physicians* 22 (September-October 1972): 284-291.

Pemberton, L. B. "Diagnosis: Ca/Should We Tell the Truth?" *Bulletin of the American College of Surgeons,* May 1971, pp. 7-13.

Samp, Robert J., and Curreri, Anthony R. "A Questionnaire Survey on Public Cancer Education Obtained from Cancer Patients and Their Families." *Cancer* 10 (March-April 1957): 382-384.

Shenkin, Budd N., and Warner, David C. "Giving the Patient His Medical Record: A Proposal To Improve the System." *New England Journal of Medicine* 289 (Sept. 27, 1973): 688-692.

Siegler, Mark. "Pascal's Wager and the Hanging of Crepe." *New England Journal of Medicine* 293 (Oct. 23, 1975): 853-857.

Standard, Samuel, and Nathan, Helmuth, eds. *Should the Patient Know the Truth?* New York: Springer, 1955.

Vernick, J., and Karon, M. "Who's Afraid of Death on a Leukemia Ward?" *American Journal of Diseases of Children* 109 (1965): 393.

Wangensteen, O. H. "Should Patients Be Told They Have Cancer?" *Surgery* 27 (June 1950): 944-947.

7. ABORTION, STERILIZATION AND CONTRACEPTION

Abortion

Becker, Laurence C. "Human Being: The Boundaries of the Concept." *Philosophy and Public Affairs* 4 (Summer 1975): 334-359.

Bok, Sissela. "Ethical Problems of Abortion." *Hastings Center Studies* 2 (January 1974): 33-52.

Brandt, R. B. "The Morality of Abortion." *The Monist* 36 (October 1972): 503-526.

Brody, Baruch A. "Abortion and the Law." *Journal of Philosophy,* June 17, 1971, pp. 357-369.

―――. "Abortion and the Sanctity of Life." *American Philosophical Quarterly* 10 (April 1973): 133-140.

―――. "Thomson on Abortion." *Philosophy and Public Affairs* 1 (1972), 335-340.

Callahan, Daniel. *Abortion: Law, Choice and Morality.* New York: Macmillan, 1970.

Cohen, Marshall, et al., eds. *The Rights and Wrongs of Abortion.* Princeton: Princeton University Press, 1974.

Committee on Psychiatry and Law of the Group for the Advancement of Psychiatry. *The Right to Abortion: A Psychiatric View.* New York: Charles Scribner's Sons, 1970.

Diamond, James J. "Abortion, Animation, and Biological Hominization." *Theological Studies* 36 (June 1975): 305-324.

"*Doe v. Doe:* The Wife's Right to an Abortion over Her Husband's Objections." *New England Law Review* 11 (Fall 1975): 205-224.

Dyck, Arthur J. "Perplexities of the Would-be Liberal in Abortion." *Journal of Reproductive Medicine* 8 (June 1972): 351-354.

Engelhardt, H. Tristram, Jr. "Bioethics and the Process of Embodiment." *Perspectives in Biology and Medicine* 18 (Summer 1975): 486-500.

―――. "The Ontology of Abortion." *Ethics* 84 (April 1974): 217-234.

Fletcher, Joseph. "Indicators of Humanhood: A Tentative Profile of Man." *Hastings Center Report* 2 (November 1972): 1-4.

Foot, Philippa. "The Problem of Abortion and the Doctrine of the Double Effect." *Oxford Review* 5 (1967): 5-15.

Grisez, Germain G. *Abortion: The Myths, the Realities, and the Arguments.* New York: World, 1970.

Hall, Robert E., ed. *Abortion in a Changing World.* 2 vols. New York: Columbia University Press, 1970.

Hirsch, Harold L. "Legal Guidelines for the Performance of Abortions." *American Journal of Obstetrics and Gynecology* 122 (July 15, 1975): 679-682.

Nathanson, Bernard N. "Deeper into Abortion." *New England Journal of Medicine* 291 (Nov. 28, 1974): 1189-1190.

Noonan, John T., Jr., ed. *The Morality of Abortion: Legal and Historical Perspectives.* Cambridge: Harvard University Press, 1970.

Pilpel, Harriet F., and Patton, Dorothy E. "Abortion, Conscience, and the Constitution," *Columbia Human Rights Law Review* 6 (Fall-Winter 1974-75): 279-305.

Potter, Ralph. "The Abortion Debate." In *Updating Life and Death: Essays in Ethics and Medicine,* ed. Donald R. Cutler. Boston: Beacon Press, 1969.

Ramsey, Paul. "Abortion: A Review Article." *The Thomist* 37 (January 1973): 174-226.

"A Review of State Abortion Laws Enacted since January 1973." *Family Planning Population Reporter* 4 (December 1975): 108-113.

Roe v. Wade, 93 Supreme Court 705 (1973).

Rosner, Fred. "The Jewish Attitude Toward Abortion." *Tradition* 10 (1968): 48-71.

"A Statement on Abortion by One Hundred Professors of Obstetrics." *American Journal of Obstetrics and Gynecology* 112 (Apr. 1, 1972): 992-998.

Thomson, Judith. "A Defense of Abortion." *Philosophy and Public Affairs* 1 (Fall 1971): 47-66.

Tietze, Christopher. "The Effect of Legalization of Abortion on Population Growth and Public Health." *Family Planning Perspectives* 7 (May/June 1975): 123-127.

————, and Murstein, Marjorie Cooper. "Induced Abortion: 1975 Factbook." *Reports on Population/Family Planning* 14 (December 1975).

"Toward a Definition of Fetal Life: Ethical and Legal Options and Their Implications for Biologists and Physicians." *Clinical Research* 23 (October 1975).

Walbert, David F., and Butler, J. Douglas, eds. *Abortion, Society and the Law.* Cleveland: The Press of Case-Western Reserve University, 1973.

Wertheimer, Roger. "Understanding the Abortion Argument." *Philosophy and Public Affairs* 1 (Fall 1971): 67-95.

World Medical Assembly. "A Statement on Therapeutic Abortion." Declaration of Oslo. *World Medical Journal* 17 (1970): 125.

Sterilization

Bass, Medora S. "Attitudes of Parents of Retarded Children Toward Voluntary Sterilization." *Eugenics Quarterly* 14 (March 1967): 45-53.

Buck v. Bell 274 U.S. 200 (1927).

Bumpass, Larry L., and Presser, Harriet B. "Contraceptive Sterilization in the United States: 1965 and 1970." *Demography* 9 (November 1972): 531-548.

Davis, Morris E. "Involuntary Sterilization: A History of Social Control." *Journal of Black Health* 1 (August/September 1974).

Fletcher, Joseph. "Sterilization—Our Right To Foreclose Parenthood." In *Morals and Medicine.* Boston: Beacon Press, 1960.

McFadden, Charles. "Sterilization." In *Medical Ethics.* 6th ed. Philadelphia: F. A. Davis, 1967.

McKenzie, James F. "Contraceptive Sterilization: The Doctor, the Patient, and the United States Constitution." *University of Florida Law Review* 25 (Winter 1973): 327-347.

Meyers, David W. "Voluntary Sterilization" and "Compulsory Sterilization and Castration." In *The Human Body and the Law.* Chicago: Aldine Press, 1970.

Murdock, Charles W. "Sterilization of the Retarded: A Problem or a Solution?" *California Law Review* 62 (May 1974): 917-935.

Neuwirth, Gloria S.; Heisler, Phyllis A.; and Goldrich, Kenneth S. "Capacity, Competence, Consent: Voluntary Sterilization of the Mentally Retarded." *Columbia Human Rights Law Review* 6 (Fall-Winter 1974-75): 447-472.

Richart, R. M., and Prager, D. J. *Human Sterilization.* Springfield, Ill.: Charles C Thomas, 1972.

Robitscher, Jonas, ed. *Eugenic Sterilization.* Springfield, Ill.: Charles C Thomas, 1973.

Scrimshaw, Susan, and Pasquariella, Bernard. "Obstacles to Sterilization in One Community." *Family Planning Perspectives* 2 (1970): 40-42.

Veatch, Robert M. "Sterilization: Its Socio-cultural and Ethical Determinants." In *Advances in Voluntary Sterilization,* ed. Marilyn E. Schima, Ira Lubell, Joseph E. Davis, and Elizabeth Connell. New York: American Elsevier, 1974.

Contraception

Bumpass, Larry, and Westoff, Charles F. "The Perfect Contraceptive Population." *Science* 169 (Sept. 18, 1970): 1177-1182.

Callahan, Daniel, ed. *The Catholic Case for Contraception.* New York: Macmillan, 1969.

Feldman, David M. *Marital Relations, Birth Control and Abortion in Jewish Law.* New York: Schocken Books, 1974.

Grisez, Germain G. *Contraception and the Natural Law.* Milwaukee: Bruce, 1964.

Griswold v. Connecticut, 381 U.S. 479, 1965.

Hatcher, Robert A., et al. *Contraceptive Technology, 1976-77.* 8th edition. New York: Irvington, 1976.

Himes, Norman E. *Medical History of Contraception.* New York: Gamut Press, 1963.

Noonan, John T., Jr. *Contraception: A History of Its Treatment by the Catholic Theologians and Canonists.* Cambridge: Harvard University Press, 1966.

Paul VI. *Humanae Vitae: On the Regulation of Birth.* New York: Paulist Press, 1968.

Silver, Morton A. "Birth Control and the Private Physician." *Family Planning Perspectives* 4 (April 1972): 42-46.

Veatch, Robert M. "Experimental Pregnancy: The Ethical Complexities of Experimentation with Oral Contraceptives." *Hastings Center Report* 1 (June 1971): 2-3.

8. GENETICS, BIRTH AND THE BIOLOGICAL REVOLUTION

General Readings

Birch, Charles, and Abrecht, Paul, eds. *Genetics and the Quality of Life.* Elmsford, N.Y.: Pergamon Press, 1975.

Callahan, Daniel. "What Obligations Do We Have to Future Generations?" *American Ecclesiastical Review* 164 (April 1971): 265-280.

Cavelli-Sforza, L. L., and Bodmer, W. F. *The Genetics of Human Populations.* San Francisco: W. H. Freeman, 1971.

Dobzhansky, T. *Mankind Evolving.* New Haven: Yale University Press, 1962.

Fletcher, Joseph. *The Ethics of Genetic Control: Ending Reproductive Roulette.* New York: Doubleday, 1974.

Frankel, Mark S. "The Application of Genetic Technology: Ethics and Pitfalls." *Impact of Science on Society* 25 (March 1975): 85-90.

———. *Genetic Technology: Promises and Problems.* Program of Policy Studies in Science and Technology, Monograph No. 15. Washington, D.C.: George Washington University, March 1973.

"Genetic Science and Man." *Theological Studies* 33 (September 1972).

Golding, Martin. "Obligations to Future Generations." *The Monist* 56 (January 1972): 85-99.

Hamilton, Michael, ed. *The New Genetics and the Future of Man.* Grand Rapids, Mich.: Eerdmans, 1972.

Hilton, Bruce, et al., eds. *Ethical Issues in Human Genetics.* New York: Plenum Press, 1973.

Leach, Gerald. *The Biocrats.* New York: McGraw-Hill, 1970.

Levitan, Max, and Montagu, Ashley. *Textbook of Human Genetics.* New York: Oxford University Press, 1971.

Ludmerer, Kenneth M. *Genetics and American Society.* Baltimore: Johns Hopkins University Press, 1972.

McKusick, Victor. *Mendelian Inheritance in Man.* 4th ed. Baltimore: Johns Hopkins University Press, 1975.

Milunsky, Aubrey. *The Prevention of Genetic Disease and Mental Retardation.* Philadelphia: W. B. Saunders, 1975.

————, and Annas, G. J., eds. *Genetics and the Law.* New York: Plenum Press, 1976.

Motulsky, Arno G. "Brave New World?" *Science* 185 (Aug. 23, 1974): 653-663.

Paoletti, Robert A., ed. *Selected Readings: Genetic Engineering and Bioethics.* 2nd rev. ed. New York: MSS Information Corp., 1974. (Available from publisher, 655 Madison Ave., New York, N.Y. 10021.)

Ramsey, Paul. *Fabricated Man: The Ethics of Genetic Control.* New Haven: Yale University Press, 1970.

Roberts, J. Fraser. *Introduction to Medical Genetics.* 6th ed. New York: Oxford University Press, 1973.

Rosenfeld, Albert. *The Second Genesis: The Coming Control of Life.* New York: Random House, 1975.

Science Policy Research Division, Congressional Research Service, Library of Congress. *Genetic Engineering: Evolution of a Technological Issue.* Report prepared for the Subcommittee on Science, Research and Development of the Committee on Science and Astronautics, U.S. House of Representatives. Washington, D.C.: Government Printing Office, 1974.

Shinn, Roger L. "Perilous Progress in Genetics." *Social Research* 41 (Spring 1974): 83-103.

Sorenson, James R. "Social Aspects of Applied Human Genetics." New York: Russell Sage Foundation, 1971.

Veatch, Robert M. "Ethical Issues in Genetics." In *Progress in Medical Genetics,* vol. 10, ed. Arthur G. Steinberg and Alexander G. Bearn. New York: Grune & Stratton, 1974.

Vukovich, William T. "The Dawning of a Brave New World—Legal, Ethical, and Social Issues of Genetics." *University of Illinois Law Forum,* 1971, pp. 189-231.

Screening for Genetic Traits and Diseases

Beckwith, Jon, and King, Jonathan. "The XYY Syndrome: A Dangerous Myth." *New Scientist* 14 (November 1974): 474-476.

Borgaonkar, Digambers, and Shah, Saleem A. "The XYY Chromosome Male—
    or Syndrome?" *Progress in Medical Genetics* 10 (1974): 135-222.
Fletcher, Joseph. "Ethical Aspects of Genetic Controls." *New England Journal
    of Medicine* 285 (Sept. 20, 1971): 776-783.
Fort, A. T. "Counseling the Patient with Sickle Cell Disease about Reproduc-
    tion: Pregnancy Outcome Does Not Justify the Maternal Risk!" *American
    Journal of Obstetrics and Gynecology* 111 (1971): 324-327.
Hampton, Mary L., et al. "Sickle Cell 'Nondisease': A Potentially Serious Pub-
    lic Health Problem." *American Journal of Diseases of Childhood* 128 (July
    1974): 58-61.
Headings, Verle, and Fielding, Jon. "Guidelines for Counseling Young Adults
    with Sickle-Cell Trait." *American Journal of Public Health* 65 (August
    1975): 819-827.
Hook, Ernest B. "Behavioral Implications of the Human XYY Genotype."
    Science 179 (Jan. 12, 1973): 139-150.
Institute of Society, Ethics and the Life Sciences: Research Group on Ethical,
    Social and Legal Issues in Genetic Counseling and Genetic Engineering.
    "Ethical and Social Issues in Screening for Genetic Disease." *New England
    Journal of Medicine* 286 (May 25, 1972): 1129-1132.
Kellon, Dale B., et al. "Physicians' Attitudes about Sickle Cell Disease and
    Sickle Cell Trait." *Journal of the American Medical Association* 227 (Jan.
    7, 1974): 71-72.
Lappé, Marc. "Human Genetics." *Annals of the New York Academy of Sci-
    ences* 216 (May 18, 1973): 152-159.
———; Roblin, Richard O.; and Gustafson, James M. "Ethical, Social and
    Legal Dimensions of Screening for Human Genetic Disease." In *Birth De-
    fects Original Articles Series,* vol. 10, ed. Daniel Bergsma. Miami, Fla.:
    Symposia Specialists, 1974.
McQueen, David V. "Social Aspects of Genetic Screening for Tay-Sachs Dis-
    ease: The Pilot Community Screening Program in Baltimore and Washing-
    ton." *Social Biology* 22 (Summer 1975): 125-133.
"Screening for Disease." *Lancet,* Oct. 5, 1974, pp. 819-821.
Starfield, Barbara, and Holtzman, Neil A. "A Comparison of Effectiveness of
    Screening for Phenylketonuria in the United States, United Kingdom and
    Ireland." *New England Journal of Medicine* 293 (July 17, 1975): 118-121.
Waltz, Jon R., and Thigpen, Carol R. "Genetic Screening and Counseling: The
    Legal and Ethical Issues." *Northwestern University Law Review* 68 (Sep-
    tember/October 1973): 696-767.

Genetic Counseling

Bergsma, Daniel, ed. "Advances in Human Genetics and Their Impact on Soci-
    ety." *Birth Defects Original Article Series,* vol. 8, July 1972.
Fletcher, John. "Moral Problems in Genetic Counseling." *Pastoral Psychology*
    23 (April 1972): 47-60.
Fraser, F. C. "Genetic Counseling." *American Journal of Human Genetics* 26
    (September 1974): 636-659.

Lappé, Marc. "Allegiances of Human Geneticists: A Preliminary Typology." *Hastings Center Studies* 1, no. 1 (1973): 63-78.

Reisman, L. E., and Matheny, A. P., Jr. *Genetics and Counseling in Medical Practice.* St. Louis: C. V. Mosby, 1969.

Prenatal Diagnosis

Emery, Alan E. H., ed. *Antenatal Diagnosis of Genetic Disease.* New York: Longman, 1973.

Friedmann, Theodore. "Prenatal Diagnosis of Genetic Disease." *Scientific American* 225 (November 1971): 34-42.

Harris, Harry. *Prenatal Diagnosis and Selective Abortion.* London: Nuffield Provincial Hospitals Trust, 1974.

Harris, Maureen, ed. *Early Diagnosis of Human Genetic Defects: Scientific and Ethical Considerations.* Fogarty International Center Proceedings, No. 6, 1972.

Milunsky, Aubrey. *Prenatal Diagnosis of Hereditary Disorders.* Springfield, Ill.: Charles C Thomas, 1973.

Artificial Insemination and Sperm Banking

British Medical Association. Annual Report of the Council. "Appendix V: Report of Panel on Human Artificial Insemination." *British Medical Journal, Supplement,* Apr. 7, 1973, pp. 3-5.

Frankel, Mark S. *The Public Policy Dimensions of Artificial Insemination and Human Semen Cryobanking.* Program of Policy Studies in Science and Technology, Monograph No. 18. Washington, D.C.: George Washington University, December 1973.

Horne, Herbert W., Jr. "Artificial Insemination, Donor: An Issue of Ethical and Moral Values." *New England Journal of Medicine* 293 (Oct. 23, 1975): 873-874.

Law and Ethics of A.I.D. and Embryo Transfer. Ciba Foundation Symposium 17 (new series). New York: Associated Scientific Publishers, 1973.

Gene Therapy and Genetic Engineering

Berg, Paul, et al. "Letter to the Editor—Potential Biohazards of Recombinant DNA Molecules." *Science* 185 (July 26, 1974): 303.

_____; Baltimore, David; Brenner, Sydney; Roblin, Richard O.; and Singer, Maxine F. "Asilomar Conference on Recombinant DNA Molecules." *Science* 188 (June 6, 1975): 991-994.

Cohen, Stanley N. "The Manipulation of Genes." *Scientific American* 233 (July 1975): 25-33.

Friedmann, Theodore, and Roblin, Richard O. "Gene Therapy for Human Genetic Disease?" *Science* 175 (Mar. 3, 1972): 949-955.

Green, Harold P. "Genetic Technology: Law and Policy for the Brave New World." *Indiana Law Journal* 48 (Summer 1973): 559-580.

Hamilton, Michael, ed. *The New Genetics and the Future of Man.* Grand Rapids, Mich.: Eerdmans, 1972.

Hirschhorn, Kurt. "On Re-Doing Man." *Annals of the New York Academy of Sciences* 184 (June 1971): 103-112.

Hudock, George A. "Gene Therapy and Genetic Engineering: Frankenstein Is Still a Myth, But It Should Be Reread Periodically." *Indiana Law Journal* 48 (Summer 1973): 533-558.

Lappé, Marc. "Human Uses of Molecular Genetics." *Federation Proceedings* 34 (1975).

————, and Morison, Robert S., eds. "Ethical and Scientific Issues Posed by Human Uses of Molecular Genetics." *Annals of the New York Academy of Sciences* 265 (1976): 1-208.

In Vitro Fertilization and Cloning

Edwards, Robert G. "Fertilization of Human Eggs in Vitro: Morals, Ethics, and the Law." *Quarterly Review of Biology* 49 (March 1974): 3-26.

————. "Studies on Human Conception." *American Journal of Obstetrics and Gynecology* 117 (Nov. 1, 1973): 587-601.

————, and Fowler, Ruth E. "Human Embryos in the Laboratory." *Scientific American* 233 (October 1970): 45-54.

Francoeur, Robert T. *Utopian Motherhood.* New York: Doubleday, 1970.

Gaylin, Willard. "We Have the Awful Knowledge To Make Exact Copies of Human Beings." *New York Times Magazine,* Mar. 6, 1972, pp. 10ff.

Kass, Leon R. "Babies by Means of In Vitro Fertilization: Unethical Experiments on the Unborn?" *New England Journal of Medicine* 285 (Nov. 18, 1971): 1174-1179.

Pizzulli, Francis C. "Asexual Reproduction and Genetic Engineering: A Constitutional Assessment of the Technology of Cloning." *Southern California Law Review* 47 (February 1974): 476-484.

Ramsey, Paul. "Shall We 'Reproduce'?" *Journal of the American Medical Association* 220 (June 5, 1972): 1346-1350; (June 12, 1972): 1480-1485.

Tribe, Laurence H. *Channeling Technology Through Law.* San Francisco: Brackton Press, 1973. (See esp. "Biomedical Technology and Asexual Reproduction," pp. 155-303.)

Watson, James D. "Moving Toward Clonal Man: Is This What We Want?" *Atlantic Monthly* 227 (May 1971): 50-53.

9. TRANSPLANTATION, HEMODIALYSIS, AND THE ALLOCATION OF SCARCE RESOURCES

Transplantation

Advisory Committee to the Renal Transplant Registry. "The 12th Report of the Human Renal Transplant Registry." *Journal of the American Medical Association* 233 (Aug. 18, 1975): 787.

American Medical Association Judicial Council. "Ethical Guidelines for Organ Transplantation." *Journal of the American Medical Association* 205 (Aug. 5, 1968): 341-342.

British Medical Association. "Report of the Special Committee on Organ Transplantation." *British Medical Journal,* Mar. 21, 1970, pp. 750-751.

British Transplantation Society. "The Shortage of Organs for Clinical Transplantation: Document for Discussion." *British Medical Journal,* Feb. 1, 1975, pp. 251-256.

Christopherson, Lois K., and Gonda, Thomas A. "Patterns of Grief: End-Stage Renal Failure and Kidney Transplantation." *Journal of Thanatology* 3, no. 1 (1975): 49-58.

"Compulsory Removal of Cadaver Organs." *Columbia Law Review* 69 (April 1969): 693-705.

Curran, W. J. "Kidney Transplantation in Identical Twin Minors." *New England Journal of Medicine* 287 (July 6, 1972): 26-27.

_____. "A Problem of Consent: Kidney Transplantation in Minors." *New York University Law Review* 34 (1959): 891-898.

Dukeminier, J., Jr., and Sanders, D. "Organ Transplantation: A Proposal for Routine Salvaging of Cadaver Organs." *New England Journal of Medicine* 279 (Aug. 22, 1968): 413-419.

Eastwood, R. T., et al. *Cardiac Replacement: Medical, Ethical, Psychological and Economic Implications.* Report by Ad Hoc Task Force on Cardiac Replacement, National Heart Institute, National Institutes of Health. Washington, D.C.: U.S. Government Printing Office, 1969.

Fox, Renée C. "A Sociological Perspective on Organ Transplantation and Hemodialysis." *New Dimensions in Legal and Ethical Concepts for Human Research. Annals of the New York Academy of Sciences* 169 (January 1970): 406-428.

Leavell, Jerome F. "Legal Problems in Organ Transplantation." *Mississippi Law Journal* 44 (1973): 865-891.

Levine, Melvin D., et al. "The Medical Ethics of Bone Marrow Transplantation." *Journal of Pediatrics* 86 (January 1975): 145-150.

Lyons, Catherine. *Organ Transplants: The Moral Issues.* Philadelphia: Westminster Press, 1970.

McCormick, Richard A. "Transplantation of Organs: A Comment on Paul Ramsey." *Theological Studies* 36 (September 1975): 503-509.

Miller, George W. *Moral and Ethical Implications of Human Organ Transplants.* Springfield, Ill.: Charles C Thomas, 1971.

Ramsey, Paul. *The Patient as Person.* New Haven: Yale University Press, 1970. (See esp. chs. 4-6.)

Reemtsma, K. "Ethical Problems with Artificial and Transplanted Organs: An Approach by Experiential Ethics." In *Ethical Issues in Medicine,* ed. E. Fuller Torrey. Boston: Little, Brown, 1968.

Richardson, In re, 284 So. 2d 185 (La. App., 1973).

Sadler, Alfred M., Jr., and Sadler, Blair L. "Transplantation and the Law: Progress Toward Uniformity." *New England Journal of Medicine* 282 (Mar. 26, 1970): 717-723.

_____, and Stason, E. B. "The Uniform Anatomical Gift Act: A Model for Reform." *Journal of the American Medical Association* 206 (Dec. 9, 1968): 2501-2506.

Simmons, Roberta G., et al. "The Prospective Organ Transplant Donor: Problems and Prospects of Medical Innovation." *Omega* 3 (November 1972): 319-339.

Strunk v. Strunk, 445 S. W. 2d 145, 1969.

"The Totally Implantable Artificial Heart." Report by Artificial Heart Assessment Panel, National Heart and Lung Institute. June, 1973. Reprinted September 1973. (Available from National Heart and Lung Institute, National Institutes of Health, Bethesda, Md. 20014.)

Wolstenholme, E. W., and O'Connor, Maeve, eds. *Ethics in Medical Progress: With Special Reference to Transplantation.* Boston: Little, Brown, 1966.

Hemodialysis

Burton, Benjamin T., et al. "National Registry of Long-Term Dialysis Patients." *Journal of the American Medical Association* 218 (Nov. 1, 1971): 718-722.

Buxton, M. J., and West, R. R. "Cost-Benefit Analysis of Long-Term Hemodialysis for Chronic Renal Failure." *British Medical Journal,* May 17, 1975, pp. 376-379.

Levy, Norman B., and Wynbrandt, Gary D. "The Quality of Life on Maintenance Haemodialysis." *The Lancet* 1 (June 14, 1975): 1328-1330.

McKegney, F. P., and Lange, P. "The Decision To No Longer Live on Chronic Hemodialysis." *American Journal of Psychiatry* 128 (September 1971): 267.

Norton, Charles E. "Attitudes Toward Living and Dying in Patients on Chronic Hemodialysis." *Annals of the New York Academy of Sciences* 164 (Dec. 19, 1969): 720-732.

Allocation of Scarce Resources

American Heart Association Committee of Ethics. "Ethical Considerations of the Left Ventricular Assist Device." *Journal of the American Medical Association* 235 (Feb. 23, 1976): 823-824.

Beard, B. H. "Fear of Death and Fear of Life: The Dilemma in Chronic Renal Failures, Hemodialysis, and Kidney Transplantation." *Archives of General Psychiatry* 21 (1969): 373-380.

Bernstein, Dorothy M., and Simmons, Roberta G. "The Adolescent Kidney Donor: The Right To Give." *American Journal of Psychiatry* 131 (December 1974): 1338-1343.

Childress, James F. "Who Shall Live When Not All Can Live?" *Soundings* 53 (Winter 1970): 339-362. Reprinted in *Readings on Ethical and Social Issues in Biomedicine,* ed. Richard W. Wertz. Englewood Cliffs, N.J.: Prentice-Hall, 1973.

Daube, David. "Limitations of Self-Sacrifice in Jewish Law and Tradition." *Theology* 72 (July 1969): 291-304.

Fletcher, John C. "Dialogue Between Medicine and Theology: Death and Transplantation." In *Should Doctors Play God?* ed. Claude A. Frazier. Nashville: Broadman Press, 1971.

Fletcher, Joseph. "Our Shameful Waste of Human Tissue." In *Updating Life and Death,* ed. Donald Cutler. Boston: Beacon Press, 1969.

Fox, Renée C. "A Sociological Perspective on Organ Transplantation and Hemodialysis." *Annals of the New York Academy of Sciences* 169 (1970): 406-428.

――――, and Swazey, Judith P. *The Courage To Fail: A Social View of Organ*

Transplants and Dialysis. Chicago: University of Chicago Press, 1974.

Gaylin, Willard. "Harvesting the Dead: The Potential for Recycling Human Bodies." *Harper's* 249 (September 1974): 23ff.

Greenberg, Roger P., et al. "The Psychological Evaluation of Patients for a Kidney Transplant and Hemodialysis Program." *American Journal of Psychiatry* 130 (March 1973): 274-277.

Kaplan, Morris Bernard. "The Case of the Artificial Heart Panel." *Hastings Center Report* 5 (October 1975): 41-48.

Katz, Jay, and Capron, Alexander Morgan. *Catastrophic Diseases: Who Decides What? A Psychological and Legal Analysis of the Problems Posed by Hemodialysis and Organ Transplantation.* New York: Russell Sage Foundation, 1975.

Ramsey, Paul. "Choosing How To Choose: Patients and Sparse Medical Resources." In *The Patient as Person.* New Haven: Yale University Press, 1970.

Rescher, Nicholas. "The Allocation of Exotic Medical Life-saving Therapy." *Ethics* 79 (April 1969): 173-186.

"The Sale of Human Body Parts." *Michigan Law Review* 72 (May 1974): 1182-1264.

Sanders, David, and Dukeminier, Jesse, Jr. "Medical Advance and Legal Lag: Hemodialysis and Kidney Transplantation." *U.C.L.A. Law Review* 15 (February 1968): 357-413.

"Scarce Medical Resources." *Columbia Law Review* 69 (April 1969): 620-692.

Simmons, R. G. "Family Tension in the Search for a Kidney Donor." *Journal of the American Medical Association* 215 (Feb. 8, 1971): 909.

Smith, Harmon L. *Ethics and the New Medicine.* Nashville: Abingdon Press, 1970. (See esp. ch. 3.)

Titmuss, Richard. *The Gift Relationship: From Human Blood to Social Policy.* New York: Pantheon, 1971. Penguin Paperback, 1973.

10. PSYCHIATRY AND THE CONTROL OF HUMAN BEHAVIOR

General Readings

Ayd, Frank J., ed. *Medical, Moral and Legal Issues in Mental Health Care.* Baltimore: Williams & Wilkins, 1974.

Dworkin, Gerald. "Autonomy and Behavior Control." *Hastings Center Report* 6 (February 1976): 23-28.

Gaylin, Willard. "What's Normal?" *New York Times Magazine,* Apr. 1, 1973, pp. 14ff.

London, Perry. *Behavior Control.* New York: Harper & Row, 1969.

Neville, Robert. "Ethical and Philosophical Issues of Behavior Control." Paper presented at American Association for the Advancement of Science meeting, 1973.

Skinner, B. F. *Beyond Freedom and Dignity.* New York: Alfred A. Knopf, 1971.

Szasz, Thomas. *Manufacture of Madness: A Comparative Study of the Inquisition and the Mental Health Movement.* New York: Harper & Row, 1970.

Ulrich, Roger; Stachik, Thomas; and Mabry, John. *Control of Human Behavior.* Vol. 1, *Expanding the Behavioral Laboratory.* Vol. 2, *From Cure to Prevention.* Vol. 3, *Behavior Modification in Education.* Glenview, Ill.: Scott, Foresman, 1974.

U.S. Senate Subcommittee on Constitutional Rights of the Committee on the Judiciary. *Individual Rights and the Federal Role in Behavior Modification.* Washington, D.C.: Government Printing Office, 1974.

Physical Manipulation of the Brain

Andy, O. J. "Neurosurgical Treatment of Abnormal Behavior." *American Journal of Medical Science* 252 (August 1966): 232-238.

———. "Thalamotomy in Hyperactive and Aggressive Behavior." *Confinia Neurologica* 32 (1970): 322-325.

Breggin, Peter R. "The Return of Lobotomy and Psychosurgery." *Congressional Record* 118 (Feb. 24, 1972): E1602-E1612.

Burt, Robert A. "Why We Should Keep Prisoners from the Doctors." *Hastings Center Report* 5 (February 1975): 23-34.

Delgado, José M. R. *Physical Control of the Mind: Toward a Psychocivilized Society.* New York: Harper & Row, 1969.

Gaylin, Willard M.; Meister, Joel S.; and Neville, Robert C., eds. *Operating on the Mind.* New York: Basic Books, 1975.

Hitchcock, E. R.; Laitinen, L.; and Vaernet, K., eds. *Psychosurgery: Proceedings of the Second International Conference.* Springfield, Ill.: Charles C Thomas, 1972.

Kaimowitz v. *Department of Mental Health.* Michigan Circuit Court for Wayne County, Civil Action No. 73-19434-AW (July 10, 1973).

Mark, Vernon H., and Ervin, Frank R. *Violence and the Brain.* New York: Harper & Row, 1970.

———, and Neville, Robert. "Brain Surgery in Aggressive Epileptics." *Journal of the American Medical Association* 226 (Nov. 12, 1973): 765-772.

"Physical Manipulation of the Brain." *Hastings Center Report,* special supplement, May 1973.

Pribram, Karl H. *Languages of the Brain.* Englewood Cliffs, N.J.: Prentice-Hall, 1971.

Shapiro, Michael H. "Legislating the Control of Behavior Control: Autonomy and the Coercive Use of Organic Therapies." *Southern California Law Review* 47 (February 1974): 237-357.

Slovenko, Ralph. "Commentary: On Psychosurgery." *Hastings Center Report* 5 (October 1975): 19-22.

Spoonhour, J. M. "Psychosurgery and Informed Consent." *University of Florida Law Review* 26 (Spring 1974): 432-452.

"Symposium on Psychosurgery." *Boston University Law Review* 54 (March 1974): 215-353.

Tribe, Laurence H. "Electronic Monitoring and Neurological Manipulation." In *Channeling Technology Through Law.* San Francisco: Brackton Press, 1973.

Winter, Arthur. *Surgical Control of Behavior.* Springfield, Ill: Charles C. Thomas, 1971.

Drugs and Drug Therapy

Cantwell, Dennis P., ed. *The Hyperactive Child: Diagnosis, Management, Current Research.* New York: Spectrum, 1975.

Duster, Troy. *The Legislation of Morality: Law, Drugs and Moral Judgment.* New York: Free Press, 1970.

Evans, Wayne, and Kline, Nathan S. *Psychotropic Drugs in the Year 2000: Use by Normal Humans.* Springfield, Ill.: Charles C Thomas, 1971.

Fish, Barbara. "The 'One Child, One Drug' Myth of Stimulants in Hyperkinesis." *Archives of General Psychiatry* 25 (September 1971): 193-203.

———. "Treating the Hyperactive Child." *Journal of the American Medical Association* 218 (Nov. 29, 1971): 1427.

Grinspoon, Lester, and Hedblom, Peter. *The Speed Culture: Amphetamine Use and Abuse in America.* Cambridge: Harvard University Press, 1975.

———, and Singer, Susan. "Amphetamines in the Treatment of Hyperkinetic Children." *Harvard Educational Review* 43 (November 1973): 515-555.

Gross, Mortimer B., and Wilson, William C. *Minimal Brain Dysfunction.* New York: Brunner/Mazel, 1975.

"Minimal Brain Dysfunction." *Lancet* II (Sept. 1, 1973): 48-88.

Schrag, Peter, and Divoky, Diane. *The Myth of the Hyperactive Child: And Other Means of Child Control.* New York: Pantheon Books, 1975.

Szasz, Thomas. "The Ethics of Addiction." *American Journal of Psychiatry* 128 (November 1971): 541-546.

Valenstein, Eliot S. *Brain Control: A Critical Examination of Brain Stimulation and Psychosurgery.* New York: Wiley-Interscience, 1973.

Veatch, Robert M. "Drugs and Competing Drug Ethics." *Hastings Center Studies* 2 (January 1974): 68-80.

Wells, William W. "Drug Control of School Children: The Child's Right To Choose." *Southern California Law Review* 46 (March 1973): 585-616.

Wender, Paul H. "The Case of MBD." *Hastings Center Studies* 2 (January 1974): 94-102.

———. *The Hyperactive Child.* New York: Crown, 1973.

West, Louis Jolyon. "Hallucinogenic Drugs: Perils and Possibilities." *Hastings Center Studies* 2 (January 1974): 103-112.

World Medical Association. "The Use and Misuse of Psychotropic Drugs." Adopted by the 29th World Medical Assembly, Tokyo, Japan, October 1975. (Available from World Medical Association, 1841 Broadway, New York, N.Y. 10023.)

Psychotherapy and Psychology

Bandura, A. *Principles of Behavior Modification.* New York: Holt, Rinehart and Winston, 1969.

Birk, Lee, et al. *Behavior Therapy in Psychiatry: A Report of the American*

Psychiatric Association Task Force on Behavior Therapy. New York: Jason Aronson, 1974.

Birnbaum, Morton. "The Right to Treatment." *American Bar Association Journal* 46 (May 1960): 499-505.

Breggin, Peter R. "Psychotherapy as Applied Ethics." *Psychiatry* 34 (1971): 59-74.

Carrera, Frank, and Adams, P. L. "An Ethical Perspective on Operant Conditioning." *Journal of the American Academy of Child Psychiatry* 9 (1970): 607-623.

"Developments in the Law—Civil Commitment of the Mentally Ill." *Harvard Law Review* 87 (April 1974): 1190-1406.

Halleck, Seymour L. "Legal and Ethical Aspects of Behavioral Control." *American Journal of Psychiatry* 131 (April 1974): 381-385.

————. *The Politics of Therapy.* New York: Science House, 1971.

Hartmann, H. *Psychoanalysis and Moral Values.* New York: International Universities Press, 1960.

Lazare, Aaron. "Hidden Conceptual Models in Clinical Psychiatry." *New England Journal of Medicine* 288 (Feb. 15, 1973): 345-351.

London, Perry. *The Modes and Morals of Psychotherapy.* New York: Holt, Rinehart and Winston, 1964.

Mechanic, David. *Mental Health and Social Policy.* Englewood Cliffs, N.J.: Prentice-Hall, 1969.

Medvedev, Roy A., and Medvedev, Zhores A. *A Question of Madness.* New York: Alfred A. Knopf, 1971.

Rieff, Philip. *The Triumph of the Therapeutic: Uses of Faith after Freud.* New York: Harper Torchbooks, 1968.

Robitscher, Jonas. "Courts, State Hospitals and the Right to Treatment." *American Journal of Psychiatry* 129 (September 1972): 298-304.

Roman, Paul, and Trice, Harrison, eds. *The Sociology of Psychotherapy.* New York: Jason Aronson, 1974.

Siegler, Miriam, and Osmond, Humphrey. *Models of Madness, Models of Medicine.* New York: Macmillan, 1974.

Total Institutions, Incarceration, Commitment, and the Right to Treatment

Annas, George J. *The Rights of Hospital Patients.* An American Civil Liberties Union Handbook. New York: Avon Books, 1975.

Ennis, Bruce. *Prisoners of Psychiatry.* New York: Harcourt, Brace, Jovanovich, 1972.

————, and Siegel, Loren. *The Rights of Mental Patients.* New York: Avon Books, 1973.

Gaylin, Willard, and Blatte, Helen. "Behavior Modification in Prisons." *The American Criminal Law Review* 13 (Summer 1975): 11-35.

Goffman, Erving. *Asylums.* New York: Doubleday Anchor, 1961.

Harris, Robert W. "Implementing the Right to Treatment for Involuntarily Confined Mental Patients: Wyatt v. Stickney." *New Mexico Law Review* 3 (May 1973): 338-351.

Hoffman, P. Browning, and Dunn, Robert C. "Beyond *Rouse* and *Wyatt:* An Administrative-Law Model for Expanding and Implementing the Mental Patient's Right to Treatment." *Virginia Law Review* 61 (March 1975): 297-339.

Ingraham, Barton L., and Smith, Gerald W. "The Use of Electronics on the Observation and Control of Human Behavior and Its Possible Use in Rehabilitation and Parole." *Issues in Criminology* 7 (Fall 1972): 35-53.

Kittrie, Nicholas N. *The Right To Be Different: Deviance and Enforced Therapy.* Baltimore: Johns Hopkins University Press, 1971.

O'Connor v. *Donaldson,* 95 S. Ct. 2486 (U.S. Sup. Ct., June 26, 1975).

Robitscher, Jonas. "The Right to Psychiatric Treatment: A Social-Legal Approach to the Plight of the State Hospital Patient." *Villanova Law Review* 18 (November 1972): 11-36.

Rosenhan, D. L. "On Being Sane in Insane Places." *Science* 179 (Jan. 19, 1973): 250-258.

Rouse v. *Cameron,* 373 F. 2d 451 (1966).

Spece, Roy G., Jr. "Conditioning and Other Technologies Used To 'Treat?' 'Rehabilitate?' 'Demolish?' Prisoners and Mental Patients." *Southern California Law Review* 45 (Spring 1972): 616-684.

Stone, Alan. "Overview: The Right to Treatment—Comments on the Law and Its Impact." *American Journal of Psychiatry* 132 (November 1975): 1125-1134.

Tarasoff v. *Regents of the University of California,* 118 Cal. Rptr. 129, 529 P. 2d 553 (1974).

Wyatt v. *Aderholt,* 503 F. 2d 1305 (C.A.5, Ala., Nov. 8, 1974).

11. EXPERIMENTATION ON HUMAN BEINGS

12. CONSENT AND THE RIGHT TO REFUSE TREATMENT

Clinical Investigation

Alexander, Leo. "Medical Science under Dictatorship." *New England Journal of Medicine* 241 (July 14, 1949): 39-47.

Altman, Lawrence K. "Auto-Experimentation: An Unappreciated Tradition in Medical Science." *New England Journal of Medicine* 286 (Feb. 17, 1972): 346-352.

Barber, Bernard. "The Ethics of Experimentation with Human Subjects." *Scientific American* 234 (February 1976): 25-31.

———, et al. *Research on Human Subjects: Problems of Social Control in Medical Experimentation.* New York: Russell Sage Foundation, 1973.

Beecher, Henry K. "Ethics and Clinical Research." *New England Journal of Medicine* 274 (1966): 1354-1360.

———. *Experimentation in Man.* Springfield, Ill.: Charles C Thomas, 1959.

———. *Research and the Individual: Human Studies.* Boston: Little, Brown, 1970.

Bernard, Claude. *An Introduction to the Study of Experimental Medicine.* Trans. Henry Copley Green. New York: Dover, 1957.

Bok, Sissela. "The Ethics of Giving Placebos." *Scientific American* 231 (November 1974): 17-23.

Case Western Reserve Law Review 25 (Spring 1975).

Chalmers, Thomas, et al. "Controlled Studies in Clinical Cancer Research." *New England Journal of Medicine* 287 (July 13, 1972): 75-78.

Curran, W. J. "The Tuskegee Syphilis Study." *New England Journal of Medicine* 289 (Oct. 4, 1973): 730-731.

Freund, Paul A., ed. *Experimentation with Human Subjects.* New York: George Braziller, 1970.

Fried, Charles. *Medical Experimentation: Personal Integrity and Social Policy.* Vol. 5 of *Clinical Studies,* ed. A. G. Bearn, D. A. K. Black, and H. H. Hiatt, New York: American Elsevier, 1974.

Gray, Bradford H. *Human Subjects in Medical Experimentation.* New York: John Wiley & Sons, 1975.

Havighurst, C. C. "Compensating Persons Injured in Human Experimentation." *Science* 169 (July 10, 1969): 154.

Katz, Jay, with Alexander M. Capron and Eleanor Swift Glass. *Experimentation with Human Beings.* New York: Russell Sage Foundation, 1972.

Ladimer, Irving, and Newman, Roger W., eds. *Clinical Investigation in Medicine: Legal, Ethical and Moral Aspects.* Boston: Law-Medicine Research Institute, Boston University, 1963.

McCormick, Richard. "Proxy Consent in the Experimentation Situation." *Perspectives in Biology and Medicine* 18 (Autumn 1974): 2-20.

Mitscherlich, Alexander, and Mielke, Fred. *Doctors of Infamy: The Story of the Nazi Medical Crimes.* New York: Henry Schuman, 1949.

New York Academy of Sciences. *New Dimensions in Legal and Ethical Concepts of Human Research, Annals of the New York Academy of Sciences* 169, Art. 2 (Jan. 21, 1970): 293-593.

Pappworth, M. H. *Human Guinea Pigs: Experimentation on Man.* Boston: Beacon Press, 1968.

Rivlin, Alice M., and Timpane, P. Michael, eds. *Ethical and Legal Issues of Social Experimentation.* Washington, D.C.: Brookings Institution, 1975.

Rosenthal, Robert, and Rosnow, Ralph L. *The Volunteer Subject.* New York: Wiley-Interscience, 1975.

Informed Consent

Alfidi, Ralph J. "Informed Consent: A Study of Patient Reaction." *Journal of the American Medical Association* 216 (May 24, 1971): 1325-1329.

Beecher, Henry K. "Consent in Clinical Experimentation: Myth and Reality." *Journal of the American Medical Association* 195 (Jan. 3, 1966): 34-35.

Canterbury v. *Spence,* 464 F 2d 722, 791 (D.C. Cir. 1972).

Capron, Alexander Morgan. "Informed Consent in Catastrophic Disease Research and Treatment." *University of Pennsylvania Law Review* 123 (December 1974): 340-438.

Cassidy, Patrick Sean. "Cooper v. Roberts: A 'Reasonable Patient' Test for Informed Consent." *University of Pittsburgh Law Review* 34 (Spring 1973): 500-509.

Cobbs v. *Grant,* 8 Cal. 3d 229, 502P. 2d 1, 104 Cal. Rptr. 505 (1972).

Dickens, Bernard M. "Information for Consent in Human Experimentation." *University of Toronto Law Journal* 24 (1974): 381-410.

Fletcher, John. "Human Experimentation: Ethics in the Consent Situation." *Law and Contemporary Problems* 32 (1967): 620-649.

Fost, Norman C. "A Surrogate System for Informed Consent." *Journal of the American Medical Association* 233 (Aug. 18, 1975): 800-803.

McCormick, Richard A. "Proxy Consent in the Experimentation Situation." *Perspectives in Biology and Medicine* 18 (Autumn 1974): 2-20.

Morris, R. Curtis, et al. "Guidelines for Accepting Volunteers: Consent, Ethical Implications, and the Function of Peer Review." *Clinical Pharmacology and Therapeutics* 13 (September 1972): 782-802.

Riskin, Leonard L. "Informed Consent: Looking for the Action." *University of Illinois Law Forum,* no. 4 (1975): 580-611.

Wilkinson v. *Vesey,* 295 *Atlantic* 2nd, p. 676.

Institutional Guidelines for Human Research

American Medical Association. *Judicial Council: Opinions and Reports,* 1971, pp. 11-12.

Frankel, Mark S. "The Development of Policy Guidelines Governing Human Experimentation in the United States: A Case Study of Public Policy-Making for Science and Technology." *Ethics in Science and Medicine* 2 (May 1975): 43-59.

Gray, Bradford H. "An Assessment of Institutional Review Committees in Human Experimentation." *Medical Care* 13 (April 1975): 318-328.

Public Law 93-348 (formerly H.R. 7724). Title II, "Protection of Human Subjects of Biomedical and Behavioral Research." July 12, 1974.

U.S. Department of Health, Education, and Welfare. "Protection of Human Subjects: Fetuses, Pregnant Women, and In Vitro Fertilization." *Federal Register* 40 (Aug. 8, 1975): pt. III, pp. 33526-33552.

_____. National Institutes of Health. "Protection of Human Subjects." *Federal Register* 39 (May 30, 1974): pt. II.

Veatch, Robert M. "Human Experimentation Committees: Professional or Representative?" *Hastings Center Report* 5 (October 1975): 31-40.

Behavioral Research

American Psychological Association. "Ethical Principles in the Conduct of Research with Human Participants." *American Psychologist* 28 (January 1973): 79-80.

Baumrind, Diana. "Reactions to the May 1972 Draft Report of the Ad Hoc Committee on Ethical Standards in Psychological Research." *American Psychologist* 27 (November 1972): 1083-1086.

Brody, Eugene B. "Biomedical Innovation, Values and Anthropological Research." *Journal of Nervous and Mental Disease* 158 (February 1974): 85-87.

Kelman, Herbert C. *A Time To Speak: On Human Values and Social Research.* San Francisco: Jossey-Bass, 1968.

Milgram, Stanley. *Obedience to Authority.* New York: Harper & Row, 1974.

Reynolds, Paul D. "On the Protection of Human Subjects and Social Science." *International Social Science Journal* 24 (1972): 693-719.

Ruebhausen, Oscar M., and Brim, Orville G., Jr. "Privacy and Behavioral Research." *Columbia Law Review* 65 (1965): 1184-1211.

Sjoberg, Gideon, ed. *Ethics, Politics, and Social Research.* Cambridge: Schenkman, 1967.

Consent of Prisoners and Mental Patients

Adams, Aileen, and Cowan, Geoffrey. "The Human Guinea Pig: How We Test New Drugs." *World Magazine,* Dec. 5, 1972, pp. 20-24.

Ayd, Frank J. "Drug Studies in Prisoner Volunteers." *Southern Medical Journal* 65 (April 1972): 440-444.

Burt, Robert A. "Why We Should Keep Prisoners from the Doctors: Reflections on the Detroit Psychosurgery Case." *Hastings Center Report* 5 (February 1975): 25-34.

Capron, Alexander M. "Medical Research in Prisons." *Hastings Center Report* 3 (June 1973): 4-6.

Gold, Jay Alexander. "*Kaimowitz v. Department of Mental Health:* Involuntary Mental Patient Cannot Give Informed Consent to Experimental Psychosurgery." *New York University Review of Law and Social Change* 4 (Spring 1974): 207-227.

Hodges, Robert E., and Bean, William B. "The Use of Prisoners for Medical Research." *Journal of the American Medical Association* 202 (Nov. 6, 1967): 177-179.

McDonald, John C. "Why Prisoners Volunteer To Be Experimental Subjects." *Journal of the American Medical Association* 202 (Nov. 6, 1967): 175-176.

Slovenko, Ralph. "Commentary: On Psychosurgery." *Hastings Center Report* 5 (October 1975): 19-22.

Consent for Fetuses

American Academy of Pediatrics Task Force on Pediatric Research, Informed Consent and Medical Ethics. "AAP Code of Ethics for the Use of Fetuses and Fetal Material for Research." *Pediatrics* 56, no. 2 (August 1975): 304-305.

Ayd, Frank J., Jr., "Fetology: Medical and Ethical Implications of Intervention in the Prenatal Period." *Annals of the New York Academy of Sciences* 169 (1970): 376-381.

Hastings Center Report 5 (June 1975). Special issue on fetal research.

Kass, Leon. "Babies by Means of *In Vitro* Fertilization: Unethical Experiments on the Unborn?" *New England Journal of Medicine* 285 (Nov. 18, 1971): 1174-1178.

Martin, Michael M. "Ethical Standards for Fetal Experimentation." *Fordham Law Review* 43 (April 1975): 548-570.

Nathan, David G. "Ethical Problems in Fetal Research." *Journal of General Education* 27 (Fall 1975): 165-175.

Powledge, Tabitha M. "Fetal Experimentation: Sorting Out the Issues." *Hastings Center Report* 5 (April 1975): 8-10.

Ramsey, Paul. *The Ethics of Fetal Research.* New Haven: Yale University Press, 1975.

Reback, Gary L. "Fetal Experimentation: Moral, Legal and Medical Implications." *Stanford Law Review* 26 (May 1974): 1191-1207.

Tiefel, Hans O. "The Cost of Fetal Research: Ethical Considerations." *New England Journal of Medicine* 294 (Jan. 8, 1976): 85-90.

Consent of Children and Minors

Baker, James A. "Court Ordered Non-Emergency Medical Care for Infants." *Cleveland Marshall Law Review* 18 (1969): 296-307.

Campbell, A. G. M. "Infants, Children and Informed Consent." *British Medical Journal,* Aug. 3, 1974, pp. 334-338.

Capron, Alexander M. "Legal Considerations Affecting Clinical Pharmacological Studies in Children." *Clinical Research* 21 (February 1973): 141-150.

Curran, William J. "A Problem of Consent: Kidney Transplant in Minors." *New York University Law Review* 34 (1959): 891-898.

————, and Beecher, Henry K. "Experimentation in Children." *Journal of the American Medical Association* 210 (Oct. 6, 1969): 77-83.

Hofmann, Adele, and Pilpel, Harriet F. "The Legal Rights of Minors." *Pediatric Clinics of North America* 20 (November 1973): 989-1004.

Lower, Charles U., et al. "Nontherapeutic Research on Children: An Ethical Dilemma." *Journal of Pediatrics* 84 (April 1974): 468-473.

McCormick, Richard A. "Proxy Consent in the Experimentation Situation." *Perspectives in Biology and Medicine* 18 (Autumn 1974): 2-20.

Raitt, G. Emmett, Jr. "The Minor's Right To Consent to Medical Treatment: A Corollary of the Constitutional Right of Privacy." *Southern California Law Review* 48 (June 1975): 1417-1456.

Ramsey, Paul. *The Patient as Person.* New Haven: Yale University Press, 1970. (See pp. 1-58.)

Schwartz, A. Herbert. "Children's Concepts of Research Hospitalization." *New England Journal of Medicine* 287 (Sept. 21, 1972): 589-592.

13. DEATH AND DYING

General Readings

Ariès, Philippe. *Western Attitudes Toward Death: From the Middle Ages to the Present.* Trans. Patricia M. Ranum. Baltimore: Johns Hopkins University Press, 1974.

Becker, Ernest. *The Denial of Death.* New York: Free Press, 1973.

Choron, Jacques. *Death and Western Thought.* New York: Collier Books, 1973.

Cutler, Donald, ed. *Updating Life and Death.* Boston: Beacon Press, 1969.

Gatch, Milton McC. *Death: Meaning and Mortality in Christian Thought and Contemporary Culture.* New York: Seabury Press, 1969.

Goldberg, Ivan K.; Malitz, Sidney; and Kutscher, Austin H., eds. *Psychophar-*

macologic Agents for the Terminally Ill and Bereaved. New York: Columbia University Press, 1973.

Gorer, Geoffrey. *Death, Grief and Mourning.* New York: Doubleday, 1965.

Hendin, David. *Death as a Fact of Life.* New York: W. W. Norton, 1973.

Klufe, Eike-Henner W. *The Practice of Death.* New Haven: Yale University Press, 1975.

Kübler-Ross, Elisabeth. *On Death and Dying.* New York: Macmillan, 1969.

Mack, Arien, ed. *Death in the American Experience.* New York: Schocken Books, 1973.

May, William. "Attitudes Toward the Newly Dead." *Hastings Center Studies* 1, no. 1 (1973): 3-13.

————. "The Sacral Power of Death in Contemporary Experience." *Social Research* 39 (Autumn 1972): 463-488.

Morison, Robert S. "Dying." *Scientific American* 229 (September 1973): 55-62.

Neale, Robert E. *The Art of Dying.* New York: Harper & Row, 1973.

Ramsey, Paul. *The Patient as Person.* New Haven: Yale University Press, 1970. (See esp. chs. 2-3.)

Riemer, Jack, ed. *Jewish Reflections on Death.* New York: Schocken Books, 1975.

Shneidman, Edwin S. *Deaths of Man.* New York: Quadrangle Books, 1973.

Sophocles. *Antigone.*

Steinfels, Peter, and Veatch, Robert M., eds. *Death Inside Out.* New York: Harper & Row, 1975.

Tolstoy, Leo. *Death of Ivan Illyich.* New York: New American Library, Signet Books, 1960.

Toynbee, Arnold, et al. *Man's Concern with Death.* New York: McGraw-Hill, 1968.

Winter, Arthur, ed. *The Moment of Death: A Symposium.* Springfield, Ill: Charles C Thomas, 1965.

World Medical Association. "A Statement on Death." Declaration of Sydney. *World Medical Journal* 15 (1968): 133-134.

Care of the Dying Patient

Annas, George J. "Rights of the Terminally Ill Patient." *Journal of Nursing Administration* 4 (March/April 1974): 40-44.

Brim, Orville G., Jr., et al., eds. *The Dying Patient.* New York: Russell Sage Foundation, 1970.

Crane, Diana. *The Sanctity of Social Life: Physicians' Treatment of Critically Ill Patients.* New York: Russell Sage Foundation, 1975.

Feifel, Herman, et al. "Physicians Consider Death." *Proceedings, American Psychological Association Convention,* 1967, pp. 201-202.

Goldberg, Ivan K., et al., eds. *Psychopharmacologic Agents for the Terminally Ill and Bereaved.* New York: Columbia University Press, 1973.

Montange, Charles H. "Informed Consent and the Dying Patient." *Yale Law Journal* 83 (July 1974): 1632-1664.

Neale, Robert E. "Between the Nipple and the Everlasting Arms." *Archives of the Foundation of Thanatology* 3 (Spring 1971): 21-30.

Pearson, Leonard, ed. *Death and Dying: Current Issues in the Treatment of the Dying Person.* Cleveland: Case Western Reserve University Press, 1969.

Solzhenitsyn, A. *Cancer Ward.* New York: Bantam Books, 1969.

Sudnow, David. *Passing On: The Social Organization of Dying.* Englewood Cliffs, N.J.: Prentice-Hall, 1960.

White, Laurens P., ed. "Care of Patients with Fatal Illness." *Annals of the New York Academy of Sciences* 164 (December 1969): 635-896.

Worcester, Alfred. *The Care of the Aging, the Dying, and the Dead.* 2nd ed. Springfield, Ill.: Charles C Thomas, 1961.

Euthanasia and Lifesaving Treatment

Bard, B., and Fletcher, J. "The Right To Die." *Atlantic Monthly,* April 1968, pp. 59-64.

Baughman, William H., et al. "Euthanasia: Criminal Tort, Constitutional and Legislative Questions." *Notre Dame Lawyer* 48 (1973): 1202-1260.

Baylor Law Review 27 (Winter 1975). Symposium Issue on Euthanasia.

Behnke, John A., and Bok, Sissela. *The Dilemmas of Euthanasia.* New York: Doubleday Anchor, 1975.

Brill, Howard W. "Death with Dignity: A Recommendation for Statutory Change." *University of Florida Law Review* 12 (Winter 1970): 368-383.

Brown, Norman, et al. "The Preservation of Life." *Journal of the American Medical Association* 221 (Jan. 5, 1970): 76-82.

Byrn, Robert M. "Compulsory Life-Saving Treatment for the Competent Adult." *Fordham Law Review* 44 (1975): 1-36.

Cantor, Norman L. "A Patient's Decision To Decline Life-Saving Medical Treatment: Bodily Integrity Versus the Preservation of Life." *Rutgers Law Review* 26 (Winter 1972): 228-264.

Catholic Hospital Association. *Christian Affirmation of Life.* St. Louis: Catholic Hospital Association, 1974.

Dinello, Daniel. "On Killing and Letting Die." *Analysis* 31 (January 1971): 83-86.

Downing, A. B. *Euthanasia and the Right To Die.* New York: Humanities Press, 1970. (Appendix contains Voluntary Euthanasia Bill proposed in British Parliament.)

Fletcher, George. "Prolonging Life." *Washington Law Review* 42 (1967): 999-1016.

Geddes, Leonard. "On the Intrinsic Wrongness of Killing Innocent People." *Analysis* 33 (January 1973): 93-97.

Gruman, Gerald J. "An Historical Introduction to Ideas about Voluntary Euthanasia: With a Bibliographic Survey and Guides for Interdisciplinary Studies." *Omega* 4 (Summer 1973): 87-138.

In the Matter of Karen Quinlan: The Complete Legal Briefs, Court Proceedings, and Decision in the Superior Court of New Jersey. Arlington, Va.: University Publications of America, 1975.

Kelly, Gerald. "The Duty of Using Artificial Means of Preserving Life." *Theological Studies* 11 (June 1950): 203-220.

———. "The Duty To Preserve Life." *Theological Studies* 12 (December 1951): 550-556.

Kluge, Eike-Henner W. *The Practice of Death*. New Haven: Yale University Press, 1975.

Kohl, Marvin, ed. *Beneficent Euthanasia*. Buffalo: Prometheus Books, 1975.

_____. *The Morality of Killing*. New York: Humanities Press, 1974.

Maguire, Daniel C. *Death by Choice*. Garden City, N.Y.: Doubleday, 1974.

Mansson, Helge H. "Justifying the Final Solution." *Omega* 3 (May 1972): 79-87.

McKegney, F. P., and Lange, P. "The Decision To No Longer Live on Chronic Hemodialysis." *American Journal of Psychiatry* 128 (September 1971): 267-274.

Pius XII. "The Pope Speaks: Prolongation of Life." *Osservatore Romano* 4 (1957): 393-398.

Potter, Ralph B. "The Paradoxical Preservation of a Principle." *Villanova Law Review* 13 (1968): 784-792.

Rachels, James. "Active and Passive Euthanasia." *New England Journal of Medicine* 292 (Jan. 9, 1975): 78-80.

Ramsey, Paul. *The Patient as Person*. New Haven: Yale University Press, 1970. (See esp. ch. 3.)

Silving, Helen. "Euthanasia: A Study in Comparative Criminal Law." *University of Pennsylvania Law Review* 103 (1954): 350-389.

Sullivan, Michael T. "The Dying Person—His Plight and His Right." *New England Law Review* 8 (1973): 197-216.

Veatch, Robert M. *Death, Dying, and the Biological Revolution: Our Last Quest for Responsibility*. New Haven: Yale University Press, 1976.

Wassmer, Thomas A. "Between Life and Death: Ethical and Moral Issues Involved in Recent Medical Advances." *Villanova Law Review* 13 (1968): 759-783.

Williams, Robert H. "Our Role in the Generation, Modification and Termination of Life." *Journal of the American Medical Association* 209 (Aug. 11, 1969): 914-917.

_____. *To Live and To Die*. New York: Springer-Verlag, 1974.

Euthanasia and Neonatal Care

Duff, Raymond S., and Campbell, A. G. M. "Moral and Ethical Dilemmas in the Special-Care Nursery." *New England Journal of Medicine* 289 (Oct. 25, 1973): 890-894.

Fletcher, John. "Abortion, Euthanasia, and Care of Defective Newborns." *New England Journal of Medicine* 292 (Jan. 9, 1975): 75-78.

_____. "Attitudes Towards Defective Newborns." *Hastings Center Studies* 2 (January 1974): 21-32.

Gustafson, James M. "Mongolism, Parental Desires, and the Right to Life." *Perspectives in Biology and Medicine* 16 (Summer 1973): 529-557.

Heymann, Philip B., and Holtz, Sara. "The Severely Defective Newborn: The Dilemma and the Decision Process." *Public Policy* 23 (Fall 1975): 381-418.

Jonsen, A. R.; Phibbs, R. H.; Tooley, W. H.; and Garland, M. J. "Critical Issues in Newborn Intensive Care: A Conference Report and Policy Proposal." *Pediatrics* 55 (June 1975): 756-768.

Lorber, John. "Selective Treatment of Myelomeningocele: To Treat or Not To

Treat." *Pediatrics* 53 (March 1974): 307-308.

McCormick, Richard A. "To Save or Let Die: The Dilemma of Modern Medicine." *Journal of the American Medical Association* 229 (July 8, 1974): 172-176.

Shaw, Anthony. "Dilemmas of 'Informed Consent' in Children." *New England Journal of Medicine* 289 (Oct. 25, 1973): 885-890.

Working Party of the Newcastle Regional Hospital Board. "Ethics of Selective Treatment of Spina Bifida." *Lancet* 1 (Jan. 11, 1975): 85-88.

Suicide

Choron, Jacques. *Suicide.* New York: Charles Scribner's Sons, 1972.

Durkheim, E. *Suicide.* Glencoe, Ill.: Free Press, 1951.

Perlin, Seymour. *A Handbook for the Study of Suicide.* New York: Oxford University Press, 1975.

Shneidman, Edwin S., ed. *Essays in Self-Destruction.* New York: Science House, 1967.

————, ed. *On the Nature of Suicide.* San Francisco: Jossey-Bass, 1969.

Defining Death

Alderete, J. F., et al. "Irreversible Coma: A Clinical, Electroencephalographic, and Neuropathological Study." *Transactions of the American Neurological Association* 93 (1968): 16-20.

Bleich, J. David. "Establishing Criteria of Death." *Tradition* 13 (Winter 1973).

Brierley, J. B., et al. "Neocortical Death after Cardiac Arrest." *Lancet,* Sept. 11, 1971, pp. 560-565.

Capron, Alexander M., and Kass, Leon R. "A Statutory Definition of the Standards for Determining Human Death: An Appraisal and a Proposal." *University of Pennsylvania Law Review* 121 (November 1972): 87-118.

Harvard Medical School, Ad Hoc Committee To Examine the Definition of Brain Death. "A Definition of Irreversible Coma." *Journal of the American Medical Association* 205 (1968): 337-340.

Institute of Society, Ethics and the Life Sciences, Task Force on Death and Dying. "Refinements in Criteria for the Determination of Death." *Journal of the American Medical Association* 221 (July 3, 1972): 48-53.

Jonas, Hans. "Against the Stream." *Philosophical Essays: From Ancient Creed to Technological Man.* Englewood Cliffs, N.J.: Prentice-Hall, 1974.

Kennedy, Ian McColl. "The Kansas Statute on Death—An Appraisal." *New England Journal of Medicine* 285 (1975): 946-950.

Korein, Julius, and Maccario, Micheline. "On the Diagnosis of Cerebral Death: A Prospective Study on 55 Patients To Define Irreversible Coma." *Clinical Electroencephalography* 2 (1971): 178-199.

Mills, Don Harper. "The Kansas Death Statute—Bold and Innovative." *New England Journal of Medicine* 285 (Oct. 21, 1971): 968-969.

Morison, Robert, and Kass, Leon. "Death—Process or Event?" *Science* 173 (Aug. 20, 1971): 694-702.

Parsons, Talcott; Fox, Renée C.; and Lidz, Victor M. "The 'Gift of Life' and Its Reciprocation." *Social Research* 39 (1972): 367-415.

Ramsey, Paul. *The Patient as Person.* New Haven: Yale University Press, 1970. (See esp. ch. 2.)

Silverman, D., et al. "Irreversible Coma Associated with Electrocerebral Silence." *Neurology* 20 (1970): 525-533.

Veatch, Robert M. "The Whole-Brain-Oriented Concept of Death: An Outmoded Philosophical Formulation." *Journal of Thanatology* 3, no. 1 (1975): 13-30.

Wasmuth, Carl E., Jr. "The Concept of Death." *Ohio State Law Journal* 30 (1969): 32-60.

Bibliographies

Clouser, K. Danner, and Zuker, Arthur. *Abortion and Euthanasia: An Annotated Bibliography.* Philadelphia: Society for Health and Human Values, 1974.

Euthanasia Educational Fund. "Euthanasia—An Annotated Bibliography." May 1970. (Available from Euthanasia Educational Fund, 250 W. 57th St., New York, N.Y. 10019.)

Kalish, Richard A. "Death and Dying: A Briefly Annotated Bibliography." In *The Dying Patient,* ed. Orville G. Brim, Jr., et al. New York: Russell Sage Foundation, 1970.

Kutscher, A. *A Bibliography of Books on Death, Bereavement, Loss and Grief: 1955-1968.* New York: Health Sciences, 1969.

INTRODUCTION. FIVE QUESTIONS OF ETHICS

1. For basic surveys of ethical theory, see William K. Frankena, *Ethics,* 2nd ed. (Englewood Cliffs, N.J.: Prentice-Hall, 1973); G. J. Warnock, *Contemporary Moral Philosophy* (New York: St. Martin's Press, 1967). For a more detailed introduction, see Richard B. Brandt, *Ethical Theory* (Englewood Cliffs, N.J.: Prentice-Hall, 1959). For readers containing classical sources, see Richard B. Brandt, ed., *Value and Obligation* (New York: Harcourt, Brace and World, 1961); A. I. Melden, ed., *Ethical Theories,* 2nd ed. (Englewood Cliffs, N.J.: Prentice-Hall, 1967); W. S. Sellars and John Hospers, ed., *Readings in Ethical Theory,* 2nd ed. (New York: Appleton-Century-Crofts, 1970). For a shorter survey, see Robert M. Veatch, "Does Ethics Have an Empirical Basis?" *Hastings Center Studies* 1, no. 1 (1973): 50-65.

2. Immanuel Kant, *Groundwork of the Metaphysic of Morals* (New York: Harper and Row, 1964).

3. For the situationalist position, see Joseph Fletcher, *Situation Ethics: The New Morality* (Philadelphia: Westminster Press, 1966). For criticism of this position, see Paul Ramsey, *Deeds and Rules in Christian Ethics* (New York: Charles Scribner's Sons, 1967). For the difference between treating rules as summaries of past experience and as statements of acceptable practice, see John Rawls, "Two Concepts of Rules," *Philosophical Review* 64 (1955): 3-32. For the philosophical literature, see Michael D. Bayles, ed., *Contemporary Utilitarianism* (Garden City, N.Y.: Doubleday, 1968).

1. VALUES IN HEALTH AND ILLNESS

1. See Florence R. Kluckhohn and D. L. Strodtbeck, *Variations in Value Orientations* (Evanston, Ill.: Row, Peterson, 1961).

2. Walter B. Cannon, *The Wisdom of the Body* (New York: Norton, 1963).

3. Philip Rieff, *The Triumph of the Therapeutic: Uses of Faith after Freud* (New York: Harper and Row, 1968).

4. See Robert M. Veatch, "Drugs and Competing Drug Ethics," *Hastings Center Studies* 2 (January 1974): 68-80.

5. Guy F. Robbins, "Partial Mastectomy: Is It Only a Partial Answer," *Medical Consultant,* April 1973, p. 110.

6. Bernard Fisher, "Cooperative Clinical Trials in Primary Breast Cancer: A Critical Appraisal," *Cancer* 31 (May 1973): 1271-1286.

7. "A Survey: 'Radical' vs. 'Simple'," *Medical Opinion,* August 1972, pp. 60-62.

8. Morris Ploscowe, "Some Basic Problems in Drug Addiction and Suggestions for Research," in *Drug Addiction: Crime or Disease?* Interim and Final Reports of the Joint Committee of the American Bar Association and the American Medical Association on Narcotic Drugs (Bloomington: Indiana University Press, 1959), pp. 33-34.

9. Comments by Lynn A. White, in *Comments on Narcotic Drugs,* Report of the Advisory Committee of the Federal Bureau of Narcotics (Washington, D.C.: Treasury Department Bureau of Narcotics, 1959), pp. 66-70.

10. *Drug Addiction,* Report of the [Great Britain] Interdepartmental Committee [on Drug Addiction] (London: Her Majesty's Stationery Office, 1961), p. 9.

11. Richard Kunnes, *The American Heroin Empire: Power, Profits, and Politics* (New York, N.Y.: Dodd, Mead, and Co., 1972).

2. RESPONSIBILITY FOR THE DECISION

1. Based on Petition of *Nemser,* 51 Misc. 2d 616, 273 N.Y.S. 2d 624 (Sup. Ct. 1966).

2. Based on *Jane Doe and Herbert F. Santmire, M.D.,* v. *Bellin Memorial Hospital et al.,* Court of Appeals, Seventh Circuit, No. 73-1396, June 1, 1973.

3. DUTY TO THE PATIENT AND SOCIETY

1. Ludwig Edelstein, *Ancient Medicine* (Baltimore: Johns Hopkins, 1967), pp. 344-345n45.

2. *Levy* v. *Parker,* 478 F 2d 772 (1973).

3. *Levy* v. *Parker,* Brief of Petitioner, pp. 164-166. A third argument by Capt. Levy, that the order was illegal because it was motivated primarily by a desire to increase punishment, was important in the trial but did not directly raise the ethical question of the duty of the physician to society and to patients.

4. Robert F. Murray, commentator, "Case Studies in Bioethics: Drug Treatment or Drug Addiction?" *Hastings Center Report* 4 (June 1974): 11-12.

5. Alan Soble, commentator, "Case Studies in Bioethics: Drug Treatment or Drug Addiction?" *Hastings Center Report* 4 (June 1974): 12.

6. Daniel Callahan, commentator, "Case Studies in Bioethics: The Psychiatrist as Double Agent," *Hastings Center Report* 4 (February 1974): 12-13.

7. Willard Gaylin, commentator, "Case Studies in Bioethics: The Psychiatrist as Double Agent," *Hastings Center Report* 4 (February 1974): 13-14.

4. HEALTH CARE DELIVERY

1. Aristotle, *Nichomachean Ethics,* bk. V, ch. 3 (Indianapolis: Bobbs-Merrill, 1962), pp. 118-119.

2. Victor W. Sidel and Ruth Sidel, *Serve the People: Observations on Medicine in the People's Republic of China* (New York: Josiah Macy Jr. Foundation, 1973).

3. Excerpted from *Wyatt* v. *Stickney,* 334 Fc Supp. 1341 (M.D. Ala. 1971).

4. From opinion *Wyatt* v. *Stickney,* 325 F. Supp. 781 (Alabama 1971).

5. "Wyatt v. Stickney—Stickney Looks Back," *Psychiatric News,* Oct. 17, 1973, p. 23.

6. *Donaldson* v. *O'Connor,* 493 F 2d 507 (1974).

7. See *The Concept of Health,* a series of articles addressing various aspects of the problem of marginally medical conditions, in *Hastings Center Studies* 1, no. 3 (1973).

8. For classical description of the sick role, see Talcott Parsons, *The Social System* (New York: Free Press, 1951), pp. 428-479.

5. CONFIDENTIALITY

1. *Hastings Center Report* 2, no. 2 (1972): 1-3.

2. "General Medical Council: Disciplinary Committee," *British Medical Journal Supplement,* no. 3452, Mar. 20, 1971, pp. 79-80.

6. TRUTH-TELLING

1. Based on a case provided by Keith Sedlacek, M.D.

2. Herman Feifel et al., "Physicians Consider Death," *Proceedings, American Psychological Association,* 1967, pp. 201-202.

3. For this classical ethical debate, see Richard B. Brandt, *Ethical Theory: The Problems of Normative and Critical Ethics* (Englewood Cliffs, N.J.: Prentice-Hall, 1959), pp. 380-432; William Frankena, *Ethics* (Englewood Cliffs, N.J.: Prentice-Hall, 1963), pp. 11-46. For utilitarian ethics, see David Lyons, *Forms and Limits of Utilitarianism* (Oxford: Oxford University Press, 1965); W. D. Ross, *The Right and the Good* (Oxford: Oxford University Press, 1939).

4. Immanuel Kant, "On the Supposed Right To Tell Lies from Benevolent Motives," in *Kant's Critique of Practical Reason and Other Works on the Theory of Ethics,* trans. Thomas Kingsmill Abbott (London: Longmans, 1909), pp. 361-365.

5. Donald Oken, "What To Tell Cancer Patients," *Journal of the American Medical Association* 175 (Apr. 1, 1961): 1120-1128.

6. W. D. Kelly and S. R. Friesen, "Do Cancer Patients Want To Be Told?" *Surgery* 27 (June 1950): 822-826.

7. Lewis Glickman, "Student Doctors," *New England Journal of Medicine* 284, no. 21 (May 27, 1971): 1216, reprinted by permission. See also Edward Coppola, "Taking Students Off the Hook," *New England Journal of Medicine* 284, no. 8 (Feb. 25, 1971): 450-451.

8. Paul S. Entmacher, "The Duty To Withhold," *Hastings Center Report* 3, no. 5 (November 1973): 9.

9. *Siemer v. Beebe,* 292 N.Y.S. 2d 806 (1968).

10. *Wallace v. University Hospitals of Cleveland,* 164 NE 2d 917 (Ohio, 1959).

11. Jeremiah S. Gutman, "The Right To Know," *Hastings Center Report* 3, no. 5 (November 1973): 10.

7. ABORTION, STERILIZATION, AND CONTRACEPTION

1. Suggested by Jerome Le Jeune as the last chance for a genetic change during the process of twinning in his lecture "On the Nature of Man," presented to the American Society of Human Genetics, October 1969.

2. Sissela Bok, commentator, "Case Studies in Bioethics: Options in Dealing with the Threat of Hemophilia," *Hastings Center Report* 4 (April 1974): 8-9.

3. Marc Lappé, commentator, "Case Studies in Bioethics: Options in Dealing with the Threat of Hemophilia," *Hastings Center Report* 4 (April 1974): 8-9.

4. Pius XI, cited in Charles J. McFadden, *Medical Ethics,* 6th ed. (Philadelphia: F. A. Davis, 1967), pp. 325-326.

5. Immanuel Jakobovits, *Jewish Medical Ethics* (New York: Philosophical Library, 1959), pp. 159-165.

6. See W. H. S. Jones, *The Doctor's Oath* (Cambridge: The University Press, 1924), p. 48. Cf. Ludwig Edelstein, "The Hippocratic Oath," in *Ancient Medicine* (Baltimore: Johns Hopkins University Press, 1967), pp. 3-63.

7. See also Robert M. Veatch, *Value-Freedom in Science and Technology* (Missoula, Mont.: Scholars Press, 1976), pp. 220-222.

8. Arthur T. Fort et al., "Counseling the Patient with Sickle Cell Disease about Reproduction: Pregnancy Outcome Does Not Justify the Maternal Risk!" *American Journal of Obstetrics and Gynecology* 3, no. 3 (Oct. 1, 1971): 324-327.

9. *Buck v. Bell,* 274 U.S. 200 (1927), cited in Patrick J. McKinley, "Compulsory Eugenic Sterilization: For Whom Does *Bell* Toll?" *Duquesne University Law Review* 6 (1967): 149.

10. Richard D. Lyons, "Doctors Scored on Sterilization," *The New York Times,* Oct. 31, 1973, p. 7.

11. William J. Curran, "Sterilization of the Poor: Judge Gesell's Roadblock," *New England Journal of Medicine* 291, no. 1 (July 4, 1974): 25-26.

12. Edward Pohlman, commentator, "Case Studies in Bioethics: Food Incentives for Sterilization: Can They Be Just?" *Hastings Center Report* 3 (February 1973): 10-11.

13. Daniel Callahan, commentator, "Case Studies in Bioethics: Food Incentives for Sterilization: Can They Be Just?" *Hastings Center Report* 3 (February 1973): 11-12.

14. Paul VI, *Humanae Vitae* "On Human Life," in Daniel Callahan, ed., *The Catholic Case for Contraception* (New York: Macmillan, 1969), p. 224. For Catholic positions on the rhythm method, see John T. Noonan, Jr., *Contraception: A History of Its Treatment by the Catholic Theologians and Canonists* (Cambridge: Harvard University Press, 1966), pp. 38-47.

15. Pius XI, "On Christian Marriage," *The Catholic Mind* 29 (Jan. 22, 1931): 38.

16. "Majority Papal Commission Report," in *The Catholic Case for Contraception,* p. 158.

17. Paul VI, *Humanae Vitae* "On Human Life," in Callahan, ed., *The Catholic Case for Contraception,* pp. 212-236.

18. Fred Rosner, "Contraception in Jewish Law," in *Modern Medicine and Jewish Law* (New York: Yeshiva University Press, 1972), ch. 3. See also David M. Feldman, *Marital Relations, Birth Control and Abortion in Jewish Law* (New York: Schocken Books, 1974).

8. GENETICS, BIRTH, AND THE BIOLOGICAL REVOLUTION

1. For ethical problems of human genetics and medical interventions in the process of procreation and birth, see Joseph Fletcher, *The Ethics of Genetic Control: Ending Reproductive Roulette* (Garden City, N.Y.: Doubleday, 1974); Bruce Hilton et al., eds., *Ethical Issues in Human Genetics* (New York: Plenum Press, 1973); Michael Hamilton, ed., *The New Genetics and the Future of Man* (Grand Rapids, Mich.: Eerdmans, 1972); Paul Ramsey, *Fabricated Man: The Ethics of Genetic Control* (New Haven: Yale University Press, 1970); Albert Rosenfeld, *The Second Genesis: The Coming Control of Life* (New York: Arena Books, 1972); Robert M. Veatch, "Ethical Issues in Genetics," in Arthur G. Steinberg and Alexander G. Bearn, eds., *Progress in Medical Genetics* (New York: Grune & Stratton, 1974), vol. 10.

2. Marc Lappé and Richard O. Roblin, "Newborn Genetic Screening as a Concept in Health Care Delivery: A Critique," in Daniel Bergsma et al., eds., *Ethical, Social and Legal Dimensions of Screening for Human Genetic Disease* (New York: Stratton Intercontinental, 1974).

3. Adapted from John Fletcher, "The Brink: The Parent-Child Bond in the Genetic Revolution," *Theological Studies* 33 (September 1972): 457-485.

4. Summary from Robert M. Veatch, "Ethical Issues in Genetics," in Steinberg and Bearn, eds., *Progress in Medical Genetics,* pp. 249-250. For full text of the report, see Marc Lappé, James M. Gustafson, and Richard Roblin, "Ethical and Social Issues in Screening for Genetic Disease," *New England Journal of Medicine* 286 (May 25, 1972): 1129-1132. For the work of the group, see Bergsma et al., eds., *Ethical, Social and Legal Dimensions of Screening.*

5. David C. Duncombe et al., "Ethical Issues in Genetic Screening," *New England Journal of Medicine* 287 (1972): 204.

6. James E. Bowman, "Ethical Issues in Genetic Screening," *New England Journal of Medicine* 287 (1972): 204-205.

7. Based on *John E. Del Zio and Doris Del Zio* v. *The Presbyterian Hospital in the City of New York and Raymond L. Vande Wiele,* Complaint 74 Civ. 3588.

8. Supplied by Dr. Richard Roblin of the Basic Research Program, Frederick Cancer Research Center, Frederick, Md., whose cooperation is gratefully acknowledged.

9. Robert S. Morison, commentator, "Case Studies in Bioethics: The Human Fetus as Useful Research Material," *Hastings Center Report* 3 (April 1973): 8-9.

10. Sumner B. Twiss, Jr., commentator, "Case Studies in Bioethics: The Human Fetus as Useful Research Material," *Hastings Center Report* 3 (April 1973): 10-11.

11. Lewis Mumford, *The Myth of the Machine: The Pentagon of Power* (New York: Harcourt, Brace, Jovanovich, 1970).

12. Robert L. Sinsheimer, "The Prospect of Designed Genetic Change," *Engineering and Science* 32 (1969): 8-13.

13. Joseph Fletcher, "Indicators of Humanhood: A Tentative Profile of Man," *Hastings Center Report* 2 (November 1972): 2. See also Joseph Fletcher, *The Ethics of Genetic Control* (Garden City, N.Y.: Doubleday Anchor, 1974).

14. Joseph Fletcher, "Indicators of Humanhood," p. 3.

15. Lynn White, "The Historical Roots of Our Ecological Crisis," *Science* 155 (1967): 1203-1207.

16. Leon R. Kass, "Making Babies—The New Biology and the 'Old' Morality," *Public Interest* 26 (Winter 1972): 48.

17. Johan Huizinga, *Homo Ludens: A Study of the Play Element in Culture* (Boston: Beacon Press, 1955).

18. Harvey Cox, *The Feast of Fools* (Cambridge: Harvard University Press, 1969).

19. See e.g. Paul Ramsey, "Genetic Therapy: A Theologian's Response," in Michael P. Hamilton, ed., *The New Genetics and the Future of Man* (Grand Rapids, Mich.: Eerdmans, 1972), pp. 157-175.

20. See e.g. Marc Lappé, "Risk-taking for the Unborn," *Hastings Center Report* 2 (February 1972): 1-3.

9. TRANSPLANTATION, HEMODIALYSIS, AND THE ALLOCATION OF SCARCE RESOURCES

1. For the ethics of transplantation, see Paul Ramsey, *The Patient as Person* (New Haven: Yale University Press, 1970), esp. chs. 2, 4-6; James B. Nelson, *Human Medicine* (Minneapolis: Augsburg, 1973), ch. 7; William May, "Attitudes Toward the Newly Dead," *Hastings Center Studies* 1, no. 1 (1973): 3-13; Robert M. Veatch, *Death, Dying and the Biological Revolution* (New Haven: Yale University Press, 1976), pp. 249-270.

2. *Strunk* v. *Strunk,* 445 SW 2d 145, 35 ALR3d 683 (Ky, 1969).

3. See Kenneth Vaux, *Biomedical Ethics: Morality for the New Medicine* (New York: Harper and Row, 1974), p. 74.

4. See Renée C. Fox, "A Sociological Perspective on Organ Transplantation and Hemodialysis," *Annals, New York Academy of Sciences* 169 (January 1970): 406-428.

5. Another exotic reproductive intervention on the horizon is in vitro fertilization using donated eggs which are then fertilized and implanted in the recipient woman's uterus. At the time that the events in this case took place, in vitro fertilization and reimplantation were creating public excitement. While the procedure had been attempted, it had not yet been successful. The ovary transplant was considered an alternative with a possibility of clinical success. The moral problems raised by in vitro fertilization with donated eggs would be similar to those raised in the transplant case.

6. Paul Ramsey, "Screening: An Ethicist's View," in Bruce Hilton et al., eds., *Ethical Issues in Human Genetics* (New York: Plenum Press, 1973), pp. 147-161.

7. Originally appeared in John E. Schowalter, Julian B. Ferholt, and Nancy M. Mann, "The Adolescent Patient's Decision To Die." *Pediatrics* 51 (January 1973): 97-102. It was also discussed in "Case Studies in Bioethics: Saying 'No' to Hemodialysis," *Hastings Center Report* 4 (September 1974): 8-10.

8. Pius XII, "The Prolongation of Life," *The Pope Speaks* 3-4 (1956-1958): 395-396.

9. H. S. Abram, "The Psychiatrist, the Treatment of Chronic Renal Failure, and the Prolongation of Life," *American Journal of Psychiatry* 126 (1969): 157-167; R. G. Wright; P. Sand; and G. Livingston, "Psychological Stress During Hemodialysis for Chronic Renal Failure," *Annals of Internal Medicine* 64 (1966): 611-624; A. DeNour; J. Shaltiel; and J. W. Czaczkles, "Emotional Reactions of Patients on Chronic Hemodialysis," *Psychosomatic Medicine* 30 (1968): 521-533: Fox, "A Sociological Perspective on Organ Transplantation and Hemodialysis."

10. F. Patrick McKegney and Paul Lange, "The Decision To No Longer Live on Chronic Hemodialysis," *American Journal of Psychiatry* 128 (1971): 270.

11. See "The Totally Implantable Artificial Heart," Report of the Artificial Heart Assessment Panel, National Heart and Lung Institute, June 1973; Albert R. Jonsen, "The Totally Implantable Artificial Heart: Assessing the Impact of a Dramatic Development in Bio-engineering," *Hastings Center Report* 3 (November 1973): 1-4.

12. Edmond Cahn, *The Moral Decision* (Bloomington: Indiana University Press, 1955), p. 71.

10. PSYCHIATRY AND THE CONTROL OF HUMAN BEHAVIOR

1. Supplied by Dr. Gerald C. Davison, Department of Psychiatry, State University of New York, Stony Brook, whose cooperation is gratefully acknowledged.

2. Reprinted from *PACAF Surgeon's Newsletter* 7 (December 1966): 5.

3. Robert G. Newman, commentator, "Case Studies in Bioethics: Fear of Flying: The Psychiatrist's Role in War," *Hastings Center Report* 6 (February 1976): 22.

4. H. Tristram Engelhardt, Jr., commentator, "Case Studies in Bioethics: Fear of Flying: The Psychiatrist's Role in War," *Hastings Center Report* 6 (February 1976): 21.

5. Perry London, commentator, "Case Studies in Bioethics: Fear of Flying: The Psychiatrist's Role in War," *Hastings Center Report* 6 (February 1976): 20-21.

6. For the procedures and arguments in favor of psychosurgery, see Vernon H. Mark and Frank R. Ervin, *Violence and the Brain* (New York: Harper and Row, 1970). See also José Delgado, *Physical Control of the Mind* (New York: Harper and Row, 1969); Arthur Winter, *Surgical Control of the Brain* (Springfield, Ill.: Charles C. Thomas, 1971). For the ethical issues, see Vernon Mark and Robert Neville, "Brain Surgery in Aggressive Epileptics," *Journal of the American Medical Association* 266 (Nov. 12, 1973): 765-772.

7. Peter R. Breggin, "The Return of Lobotomy and Psychosurgery," *Congressional Record* 118 (Feb. 24, 1972): E1608. See also John D. Hodson, "Reflections Concerning Violence and the Brain," *Criminal Law Bulletin* 9 (October 1973): 684-702.

8. James M. Gustafson, commentator, "Case Studies in Bioethics: 'Ain't Nobody Gonna Cut on My Head!' " *Hastings Center Report* 5 (February 1975): 49-50.

9. Francis C. Pizzuli, commentator, "Case Studies in Bioethics: 'Ain't Nobody Gonna Cut on My Head!' " *Hastings Center Report* 5 (February 1975): 49-50.

10. P. H. Wender, *Minimal Brain Dysfunction in Children* (New York: Wiley-Interscience, 1971). See also Leon Eisenberg, "The Clinical Use of Stimulant Drugs in Children," *Pediatrics* 49 (May 1972): 709-715.

11. James H. Satterfield, Dennis P. Cantwell, Leonard I. Lesser, and Robert L. Podosin, "Physiological Studies of the Hyperkinetic Child," pt. I, *American Journal of Psychiatry* 128 (May 1972): 1418-1424. See also Charles Bradley, "The Behavior of Children Receiving Benzedrine," *American Journal of Psychiatry* 94 (1937): 577.

12. Barbara Fish, "The 'One Child, One Drug' Myth of Stimulants in Hyperkinesis," *Archives of General Psychiatry* 25 (September 1971): 193-203; Lester Grinspoon and Susan Singer, "Amphetamines in the Treatment of Hyperkinetic Children," *Harvard Educational Review* 43 (November 1973): 515-555.

13. Usually these are cases in which relatively minor medical treatments would be lifesaving, as in the case of a blood transfusion refused by Jehovah's Witnesses on behalf of their child. See William P. Cannon, "The Right To Die," *Houston Law Review* 7 (1970): 654-670; John C. Ford, "Refusal of Blood Transfusions by Jehovah's Witnesses," *Catholic Lawyer* 10 (Summer 1964): 212-226; Gary L. Milhollin, "The Refused Blood Transfusion: An Ultimate Challenge for Law and Morals," *Natural Law Forum* 10 (1965): 202-214. Occasionally, however, courts have ordered treatments on the same grounds in cases where the treatment is not lifesaving. In *Mitchell* v. *Davis,* 205 S.W. 2d 812

(Tex. Civ. App. 1947), for example, the court ordered standard medical treatment of a 12-year-old boy afflicted with pain and impaired movement from arthritis on the ground that the mother's home remedies and faith healing constituted neglect. In *Rotkowitz,* 175 Misc. 948, 25 N.Y.S. 2d 624 (Dom. Rel. Ct. 1941), the court ordered a corrective operation for a 10-year-old whose leg was infected with polio against objections of the father, asserting that the state has a right to interfere not only in emergency cases but also in instances where "the health, the limb, the person or the future of the child is at stake." In *Vascko,* 238 App. Div. 128, 263 N.Y. Supp. 552 (1933), the court ordered the removal of the eye of a two-year-old who had been permanently blinded in that eye by a growth which was probably malignant, would probably spread, and was likely to cause death in the future.

14. Based on Lloyd H. Cotter, "Operant Conditioning in a Vietnamese Mental Hospital," *American Journal of Psychiatry* 124 (July 1967): 23-28. Copyright 1967, the American Psychiatric Association. Reprinted by permission.

11. EXPERIMENTATION ON HUMAN BEINGS

1. *Kaimowitz* v. *Department of Mental Health,* Michigan Circuit Court for Wayne County, Civil Action No. 73-19434-AW (July 10, 1973). There is some dispute in the record as to whether John Doe's parents gave consent for the innovative surgical procedures. They testified that they had given consent only to the insertion of depth electrodes.

2. Based on William McGlothlin, Sidney Cohen, and Marcella S. McGlothlin, "Long Lasting Effects of LSD on Normals," *Archives of General Psychiatry* 17 (November 1967): 521-532.

3. Saul Krugman, "Experiments at the Willowbrook State School," *The Lancet,* May 8, 1971, p. 967. This account is based on a real case. See also Robert Ward, Saul Krugman, Joan P. Giles, A. Milton Jacobs, and Oscar Bodansky, "Infectious Hepatitis," *New England Journal of Medicine* 258 (1958): 407-416; Saul Krugman, Joan P. Giles, and Jack Hammond, "Infectious Hepatitis," *Journal of the American Medical Association* 200 (1967): 365-373; Saul Krugman, Joan P. Giles, and Jack Hammond, "Viral Hepatitis Type B (MS-2-Strain)," *Journal of the American Medical Association* 218 (1971): 1665-1670; Saul Krugman and Joan P. Giles, "Viral Hepatitis, Type B (MS-2-Strain)," *New England Journal of Medicine* 288 (1973): 755-760; "Proceedings of the Symposium on Ethical Issues in Human Experimentation," The Case of Willowbrook State Hospital Research, May 4, 1972, Sponsored by Student Council of New York University School of Medicine.

4. Based on Philip S. Hench, "Effects of Cortisone Acetate and Pituitary ACTH on Rheumatoid Arthritis, Rheumatic Fever, and Certain Other Conditions," *Archives of Internal Medicine* 85 (April 1950): 545-666. Copyright 1950, American Medical Association.

5. See Max Weber, *The Methodology of the Social Sciences* (New York: Free Press, 1949).

6. F. J. Ingelfinger, "Ethics of Experiments on Children," *New England*

Journal of Medicine 288 (1973): 791.

    7. Robert J. Levine, "Ethical Considerations in the Publication of the Results of Research Involving Human Subjects," *Clinical Research* 21 (1973): 763.

12. CONSENT AND THE RIGHT TO REFUSE TREATMENT

    1. Chauncey D. Leake, *Percival's Medical Ethics* (Baltimore: Williams & Wilkins, 1927), p. 76.

    2. *Jackson* v. *Burnham,* 20 Colo. 532, 39 Pac. 577 (1895), reversing 28 Pac. 250 (1891), cited in Jay Katz, Alexander Morgan Capron, and Elinor Swift Glass, *Experimentation with Human Beings* (New York: Russell Sage Foundation, 1972), p. 528.

    3. *Schloendorff* v. *New York Hospital,* 211 N.Y. 127, 129, 105 N.E. 92, 93 (1914).

    4. Based on *Halushka* v. *University of Saskatchewan,* 52 W.W.R. 608 (Sask. 1965).

    5. U.S. Department of Health, Education, and Welfare, "The Institutional Guide to DHEW Policy on Protection of Human Subjects," Dec. 1, 1971.

    6. William J. Curran and Henry K. Beecher, "Experimentation in Children," *Journal of the American Medical Association* 210 (Oct. 6, 1969): 80, 81.

    7. "Institutional Guide to DHEW Policy on Protection of Human Subjects," p. 7.

    8. *Federal Register* 38, no. 221 (Nov. 16, 1973): 31738-31749.

    9. S. E. Asch, "Effects of Group Pressure upon the Modification and Distortion of Judgments," in H. Proshansky and B. Seidenberg, eds., *Basic Studies in Social Psychology* (New York: Holst, 1965), pp. 393-401.

    10. Based on *Berkey* v. *Anderson,* 1 Cal. App. 3d 790, 82 Cal. Rptr. 67 (1969).

    11. See e.g. *Dow* v. *Permanente Medical Group* (90 Cal. Rptr. 747, Cal. 1970): *Cooper* v. *Roberts* (286 A 2d 647, Pa. 1971); *Hunter* v. *Brown* (484 P 2d 1162, Wash. 1971); *Cobbs* v. *Grant* (502 P 2d I, Cal. 1972); *Wilkinson* v. *Vesey* (295 A 2d 676, R.I., 1972). See also David S. Rubsamen, "Changes in 'Informed Consent,' " *Medical World News,* Feb. 9, 1973, pp. 66-67; Joseph E. Simonaitis, "Recent Decisions on Informed Consent," *Journal of the American Medical Association* 221, no. 4 (July 24, 1972): 441-442; Joseph E. Simonaitis, "More about Informed Consent," pt. 1, *Journal of the American Medical Association* 224 (June 25, 1973): 1831-1832.

    12. *Natanson* v. *Kline,* 186 Kan. 393 P. 2d 1093 (1960).

    13. Jack Himmelstein, commentator, "Case Studies in Bioethics: The Right To Refuse Psychoactive Drugs," *Hastings Center Report* 3 (June 1973): 9-10.

    14. Robert Michels, commentator, "Case Studies in Bioethics: The Right To Refuse Psychoactive Drugs," *Hastings Center Report* 3 (June 1973): 10-11.

    15. State of New York, Mental Hygiene Law, 1973, Article 15.03.4.

    16. *New York City Health and Hospitals Corporation* v. *Paula Stein,* 335 N.Y.S. 2nd. 461, 1972.

17. In the Court of Common Pleas of Northampton County, Orphans' Court Division, In re the Appointment of a Guardian of the Person of *Maida Yetter,* an alleged incompetent, No. 1973-533.

13. DEATH AND DYING

1. From Robert M. Veatch, *Death, Dying, and the Biological Revolution: Our Last Quest for Responsibility* (New Haven: Yale University Press, 1976), pp. 1-2, reprinted by permission of the publisher.

2. Based on *Tucker* v. *Lower,* No. 2831 (Richmond, Va., L + Eq. Ct., May 23, 1972). An earlier version of this case appeared in the *Hastings Center Report* (Nov. 1972), pp. 10-13.

3. "Virginia Jury Rules That Death Occurs When Brain Dies," *New York Times,* May 27, 1972, p. 15.

4. Harvard Medical School, Ad Hoc Committee of the Harvard Medical School To Examine the Definition of Brain Death, "A Definition of Irreversible Coma," *Journal of the American Medical Association* 205 (Aug. 5, 1968): 337-340.

5. "Virginia Jury Rules That Death Occurs When Brain Dies," p. 15.

6. Based on an account by Elisabeth K. Ross, M.D.

7. See Lev. 3:17, 7:26-27, 17:10-14, 19:26; Acts 15:29. See also John C. Ford, "Refusal of Blood Transfusions by Jehovah's Witnesses," *Catholic Lawyer* 10 (1964): 212-226.

8. Paraphrased from In re *Osborne,* 294 A.2d 373 (D.C. Ct. of Appl, July 12, 1972).

9. Leo Alexander, "Medical Science under Dictatorship," *New England Journal of Medicine* 241 (July 14, 1949): 44.

10. See Paul Ramsey, *The Patient as Person* (New Haven: Yale University Press, 1970), pp. 151-152.

11. Department of Health Affairs, United States Catholic Conference, "Ethical and Religious Directives for Actholic Health Facilities" (Washington, D.C., 1971), p. 8.

12. In the Interest of *Kenneth Clark,* a Minor, 21 Ohio Opinions 2d Series (Juvenile Docket No. 59723, 1962), pp. 86-90.

13. *People ex rel. Wallace et al.* v. *Labrenz et al.* 104 NE 2 769, Mar. 20, 1952, Supreme Court of Illinois.

14. *State* v. *Perricone,* 37 N.J. 463, 181A. 2d 751, cert. denied 371 U.S. 890 (1962).

15. "The Living Will," from the Euthanasia Educational Council, 250 West 57th Street, New York, N.Y. 10019. Reprinted with permission.

16. A. B. Downing, ed., *Euthanasia and the Right To Die: The Case for Voluntary Euthanasia* (New York: Humanities Press, 1970); Veatch, *Death, Dying, and the Biological Revolution,* pp. 164-203.

APPENDIXES

1. Reprinted with permission from Owsei Temkin and C. Lilian Temkin,

eds., *Ancient Medicine: Selected Papers of Ludwig Edelstein* (Baltimore: The Johns Hopkins University Press, 1967), p. 6.

2. Reprinted with the permission of the American Hospital Association.

3. Reprinted with permission from American Medical Association, *Judicial Council Opinions and Reports* (Chicago: American Medical Association, 1971), pp. VI-VII.

4. Reprinted with permission from the World Medical Association.

5. Reprinted with permission from the World Medical Association.

6. *Trials of War Criminals Before the Nuremburg Military Tribunals* (Washington, D.C.: U.S. Government Printing Office, 1948). Text from Jay Katz, *Experimentation with Human Beings* (New York: Russell Sage Foundation, 1972), pp. 305-306.

7. Reprinted with permission from the World Medical Association.

8. *Opinions and Reports of the Judicial Council* (Chicago: American Medical Association, 1971), pp. 10-12, reprinted with the permission of the American Medical Association.

9. Department of Health, Education, and Welfare, "Protection of Human Subjects," *Federal Register* 39 (May 30, 1974): 18914-18920.

Aas' hypnotic susceptibility tests, 272
Abortion, (case 4) 31; hospital abortion
  panel, (case 9) 48-49; hospital's right to
  refuse, (case 10) 49-51; *Roe* v. *Wade*
  Supreme Court decision, 168; conflict
  between spouses, (case 53) 173-174; for
  psychiatric reasons, (case 54) 174-175;
  for teenage pregnancy, (case 55) 175; for
  possible hemophiliac son, (case 56) 175-
  176; attempted abortion resulting in live
  birth, (case 57) 179-180; research on
  women scheduled for abortion, (case 92)
  285-289
Abram, H. S., 408
Absolutism. *See* Ethics
Achromycin, 32
Addiction, (case 1) 17-19, (case 3) 25-30,
  (case 18) 72-76, 84-85
Alcoholism, 251-254
Alexander, Leo, 330, 412
Alexander, M. R., 133-134
Allen, Francis A., 268
Allergy, development of, 295
Allocation of resources, 236-239; moral
  foundations of, 240-265.
American Bar Association and American
  Medical Association, Joint Committee
  on Narcotic Drugs, 25-26, 30
American Hospital Association: Patient's
  Bill of Rights, 352-354

American Law Institute Model Penal Code,
  172
American Medical Association, 25, 35,
  122-125, 307; Principles of Medical Eth-
  ics, 117, 118, 125, 131, 135, 354, 355;
  Ethical Guidelines for Clinical Investiga-
  tion, 297, 361-363
American Orthopsychiatric Society, 269
Amniocentesis, 137, 175, (case 61) 197-198;
  mandatory, 205
Amobarbitol, 310
Amphetamines, (case 12) 53-54, 259, (case
  81) 259-262, 272, 409
Amputation, (case 8) 44-48
Anderson, Frank A., 303
Anglicans on contraception, 190
Antigone, 127
Aquinas, Thomas, 6-7
Archives of Dermatology, 123
Archives of Internal Medicine, 124
Arginase, 208
Aristotle on justice in distribution, 8, 91,
  404
Armed Forces Epidemiological Board, 275
Artificial Heart Assessment Panel, 235, 237
Artificial insemination, (case 68) 207-208,
  (case 69) 214-216, 218
Asbestosis, (case 20) 82-83
Asch, Solomon, 301, 411
Asthma, 295

414

pulsory public service, (case 17) 69-72; as
drug reformer, (case 18) 72-76; company
physicians, (case 20) 82. *See also* Hip-
pocratic oath; Confidentiality
Pius XI, 181-182; on sterilization and con-
traception, 189-190; on dialysis, 405, 406,
408
Pizzulli, Francis C., 257-259, 409
Placebo, ethics of giving, (case 46) 151-153,
299, 300, 301
Plasmapheresis, 112
Plato, 193
Ploscowe, Morris, 26, 403
Podosin, Robert L., 409
Pohlman, Edward, 186-188, 406
Prescription writing, (case 5) 32-34
Primum non nocere, 8
Prisoners, (case 84) 267-271
Prochlorperazine, 337
Promise-keeping, 101, 145, 346
Propoxyphene, (case 1) 17-19, 336
Proshansky, H., 411
Protection of Human Subjects Committee,
295, 297
Protestant, 20, 21; on sterilization, 181; on
contraception, 190
Psychiatrist: as double agent, (case 19)
76-77; role of, (case 77) 241-245; in war,
(case 78) 245; political uses of, 247-249
Psychiatry and behavior control, 240-265
Psychosurgery, (cases 79-80) 251-259; for
sexual psychopath, (case 84) 267-271; for
violent alcoholic, (case 79) 251-253. *See
also* Behavior control techniques
Psychotherapy. *See* Behavior control techniques
Public responsibility, (cases 28-30) 104-108
Public service, compulsory, 69-72

Quinlan, Karen, 4

Ramsey, Paul, 402, 406, 407, 408, 412
Rawls, John, 402
Reasonable person standard, (case 96) 303-
304
Renal transplants. *See* Transplants
Research Group on Ethical, Social and
Legal Issues in Genetic Counseling and
Genetic Engineering at the Institute of
Society, Ethics and the Life Sciences,
179; principles of design and operation of
screening programs, 203
Retardation, (case 6) 36-42; mentally re-
tarded as kidney donors, (case 70) 222-

223, 225; mentally retarded as subjects of
experimentation, (case 87) 274-277. *See
also* Mongolism
Retinoblastoma, 194, 199-200
Rickenberg, Dr., 303
Rieff, Philip, 20, 403
Rights: 12, 168-169; to health care, 100-
104; of committed patients to care, 101-
104, 278-279; of patients to their own
medical records, (cases 50-52) 158-163;
to refuse hemodialysis, (case 74) 230-231;
to refuse psychoactive drugs and to refuse treatment, (cases 99-100) 309-315
Robbins, Guy F., 23, 403
Roblin, Richard, 406, 407
Rodin, Ernst, 267
Rolleston, Humphrey, 28-29
Roman Catholics: ethics of, 6-7; on brith
control (sterilization), 31, 187, 189-190,
406; care of dying, (case 6) 36, 42; on
abortion, (case 9) 49; on dialysis, 231-
232; on experimentation, 274; on eutha-
nasia, 332. *See also* "Ethical and Reli-
gious Directives for Catholic Hospitals"
Rosenfeld, Albert, 406
Rosner, Fred, 406
Ross, Elizabeth K., 412
Ross, W. D., 8, 404
Rotkowitz, 410
Rousseau, J. J., 346
Rubsamen, David S., 411
Rules-situation debate, 10-13

Sand, P., 408
Satterfield, James H., 409
Sawher, Clifford, 268
Schizophrenia, (case 19) 76-82, (case 35)
118-119, (case 100) 310-311
Schloendorff v. *New York Hospital,* 411
Schowalter, John E., 408
Scientific Review Committee, 268
Secobarbital, 151
Sedlacek, Keith, 404
Seidenberg, B., 411
Sellars, W. S., 402
Sex, premarital, (case 40), 131-134
Shaltiel, J., 408
Shettles, Landrum, 207-208
Shope papilloma virus, (case 67) 208
Sickle cell anemia (S-S hemoglobinopathy),
(case 18) 72-76; genetic counseling in cases
of, (case 42) 139-141, (case 58) 182-185;
screening for carriers, (case 64) 202-205
Sidel, Ruth, 404